D0150276

pocket posh® complete calorie counter

your guide to thousands of foods
from grocery stores and restaurants

D. Milton Stokes, MPH, RD

**Andrews McMeel
Publishing, LLC**

Kansas City • Sydney • London

Produced by
DOWNTOWN
BOOKWORKS INC.

President   Julie Merberg
Senior Vice President   Patty Brown
Layout by   Jennifer Richman/Richman Creative Group
Special Thanks   Sarah Parvis, LeeAnn Pemberton,
Pam Abrams, Felicia Stoler, Jenna Bell,
Maggie Moon, Kristen Carlucci, Dina Aronson

POCKET POSH® COMPLETE CALORIE COUNTER

Copyright © 2010 by Downtown Bookworks, Inc. All rights
reserved. Printed in China. No part of this book may be used or
reproduced in any manner whatsoever without written permission
except in the case of reprints in the context of reviews.

Andrews McMeel Publishing, LLC
an Andrews McMeel Universal company
1130 Walnut Street, Kansas City, Missouri 64106

www.andrewsmcmeel.com

12 13 14 15 16 LEO 10 9 8 7 6 5 4 3

ISBN: 978-1-4494-0150-4

Library of Congress Control Number: 2010934819

ATTENTION: SCHOOLS AND BUSINESSES
Andrews McMeel books are available at quantity discounts with bulk
purchase for educational, business, or sales promotional use. For information,
please email the Andrews McMeel Publishing Special Sales Department:
specialsales@amuniversal.com

This book does not serve as a replacement for professional or nutritional
advice or treatment. The publisher, packager, and authors are not responsible
for your specific medical, health or allergy needs that may require medical
or other professional supervision, or for any adverse consequences
based upon your use of the information contained in this book.

Nutritional information for all brand-name products was provided based
upon nutritional information provided by such companies or nutritional analysis
software databases and that information is subject to change from time to time.
Further, nutrition analysis of food products is not an exact science. Various
factors, including but not limited to the variations in testing conditions and food
preparation, as well as regular recipe modifications, guarantee variability
in actual counts. Accordingly, the publisher, packager, and authors are not
responsible for any inaccuracies caused by those variations or factors.

FOOD COUNTS

DINING OUT

preface

Knowing what's in your food is essential to making better choices to reach and maintain a healthy weight. The challenge is that with so many choices in grocery stores and restaurants today, it's impossible to instinctively know just how nutritious (or not) many foods are. In a lot of cases, a handful of very similar products can have wildly different amounts of calories or sodium, for example. That's what makes this book an invaluable companion.

Notable exceptions are fresh fruits and vegetables, which are always healthy choices. The simple goal to include a fruit or vegetable every time you eat, whether it's a meal or snack, is a smart way to get into the habit of eating a nutrient-rich diet. There's also a good chance that you'll naturally be taking in fewer calories, saturated fats, and sodium and a whole lot more fiber,vitamins, and minerals.

A well-balanced diet will also include whole grains, lean proteins, and good fats. For all of these foods and everything in between, knowing what you put in your body is going to help you balance your calories in with your calories out.

I hope you make the most of this pocket guide to help you keep track of what you eat and that you'll feel empowered to make better choices for your waistline and your overall health and well-being.

Eating right really works, and I am honored that you've picked up this book as an important part of getting there. Here's to a healthier you.

D. Milton Stokes, MPH, RD

introduction

Healthy Weight Fundamentals

Reaching and maintaining a healthy weight is about balancing calories in with calories out. Calories are a way to think about the amount of energy you get out of food and the amount of energy your body burns during exercise.

- Protein and carbohydrates provide 4 calories per gram.
- Fat provides 9 calories per gram.
- Walking for 5 minutes burns about 15 calories; sleeping burns about 1 calorie per minute.

To lose weight, you have to burn more calories than you take in. This is not groundbreaking news, but it certainly can be challenging to put into action. In addition to keeping track of calories by using this pocket guide, here are seven tips to living healthfully:

1. **More produce.** Eat lots of vegetables and fruits in a variety of colors, without added sugars, fats, or salt. Fresh, roasted, and sautéed are healthier ways to enjoy these foods.

2. **Good carbs.** Choose better carbohydrates from high-fiber foods such as whole grains, beans, and vegetables over refined grains and fried potatoes. Better carbohydrates can also be found in fruits and low-fat dairy products.

3. **Proteins to prefer.** Pick healthy proteins from plant sources such as beans, nuts, and soy products. Seafood also offers good protein choices. If including poultry and meat, choose lean types and roast, bake, broil, poach, or sauté.

4. **Healthy fats.** Don't be afraid of healthy fats from unsaturated sources such as liquid oils (e.g., canola oil, vegetable oil, olive oil) and foods such as avocado, salmon and other fatty fish, nuts, and whole grains. Do limit saturated fats and avoid trans fats.

5. **Stay hydrated.** Drink water and tea to stay hydrated. Enjoying fruits and vegetables with high water content also contributes to hydration. Some examples are cucumbers, watermelon, grapefruit, celery, peppers, and tomatoes.

6. **Get moving.** Move more, every day. Look for opportunities to work physical activity into your day. If it's hard to find time to get to the gym, join a sports team or take a dance class. Look for other ways to move more: Take the stairs, take a walk, lift weights during commercial breaks — where there's a will, there's a way.

7. **Track and assess.** Keep track of how you're doing in a diet and exercise journal. See how you're doing compared to your goals, making adjustments where there's room for improvement. Simply being more aware of what you're eating every day is doing something right for your health.

Carbohydrates to Love

Our bodies love carbohydrates. What's not to love? They're the preferred fuel source for the brain; we can use them for energy now or store them for energy later; some provide dietary fiber; and we can get them from a variety of whole grains, fruits, and vegetables.

Fruits and Vegetables

• Aim for 2.5 to 4.5 cups of fruits and vegetables every day, and go a little heavier on the vegetables.

• Give them a center-of-plate role in your meals and snacks.

• Mix it up and choose from green, yellow, orange, red, purple, and white fruits and veggies to get the most out of the different vitamins, minerals, antioxidants, and other phytonutrients they have to offer. Deeper in color often means richer in nutrients.

• Fresh fruits and veggies are delicious and will be most affordable when they're in season for your local area.

• Frozen fruits and veggies are often flash-frozen to retain flavor, quality, and nutrients. They're a great choice. Just be sure to flip the package around to the Nutrition Facts Panel to make sure there's no added salt or sugar.

• Canned fruits and veggies are good to have in the pantry (canned and jarred tomato products come to mind). However, because they often come with added sugar, salt, and preservatives, seek out fresh and frozen before canned.

Whole Grains

• At least half of your daily grains should be whole grains, but why not aim for more? Whole grains offer important B vitamins, trace minerals, healthy fats, and good carbs.

• Many whole-grain ingredients will contain the word "whole" in their name, e.g., whole wheat.

• Some whole-grain foods don't include the word "whole," e.g., brown rice, oats, oatmeal, and wheatberries.

• Ingredients that are never whole grain are enriched flour, degerminated corn meal, bran, and wheat germ.

• Sometimes descriptors such as "durum," "semolina," "organic," or "multigrain" appear on packaging, but these terms don't necessarily mean the ingredient contains whole grain.

• When the first ingredient is a refined grain and the second ingredient is a whole grain, there's a chance that the food in question could contain anywhere from 1% to 49% whole grain.

• Fiber is important, but it's not everything when it comes to whole grain. Fiber contents in whole grain vary; plus, some high-fiber products contain bran or other added fiber without providing much whole grain.

To be fair, not all carbs are created equal, and carbohydrates deserve their bad reputation when thinking about sugar-sweetened beverages (e.g., sodas), fried potatoes, and snack foods, breads, and pastas made with refined grains. Most of these foods are not just poor-quality carbohydrates, they are overall poor-nutrition foods.

Make the most of your carbohydrate choices from a variety of vegetables, fruits, and whole grains; enjoy them without too much added sugar, fat, or salt, and you'll be on the right track.

Healthy Fats

Say yes to good fats! They're good for you, and they make food taste great. Including the right kinds of fats in your diet helps your body stay fuller longer than fat-free meals, and they also help the body absorb essential vitamins and minerals.

The U.S. Dietary Guidelines, the American Dietetic Association, and other experts agree that 20% to 35% of calories should be coming from fats every day. At 9 calories per gram, that means about 44 to 78 grams of fat per day for a 2000-calorie diet. Though there are different types of fats, it's important to remember that all fats have 9 calories per gram.

Most of your daily fat intake should come from unsaturated sources, that is, polyunsaturated fats (PUFA) and monounsaturated fats (MUFA). Keeping PUFAs and MUFAs straight can get confusing, so it may be helpful to remember that both types are good for you and that they will be liquid at room temperature (sorry, that rules out butter).

Both types of unsaturated fats are important in a healthy diet, and many foods will have a combination of fats in them, though some foods are known for higher PUFAs or higher MUFAs (see below for examples).

You may have heard about omega-3 and omega-6 fats. They are types of good-for-you PUFAs that can be found in seafood, walnuts, pecans, flaxseeds and flaxseed oil, and vegetable oils (soybean, corn, and safflower).

For MUFAs, one of the most popular sources is olive oil. You can also find plenty of MUFAs in avocados; nuts such as almonds, cashews, and peanuts; olives; peanut butter and peanut oil; canola oil; sunflower oil; or sesame seeds and sesame oil.

Healthy fats are important to weight loss and weight maintenance when they are included in a varied diet that balances calories from food (energy in) with calories burned through exercise (energy out). They do even more good when they are replacing saturated or trans fats.

Saturated fat is easy to spot because it will be solid at room temperature (e.g., butter, hard cheeses, shortening, lard, cream, bacon). You can still enjoy these foods, but in moderation. Experts agree that we should keep saturated fat below 10% of the day's calories (about 22 grams per day for a 2000-calorie diet). They also agree that trans fats should be limited as much as possible; they're most often found in commercially produced packaged food and will show up on the Nutrition Facts Panel.

Enjoy a variety of foods and reach for good fats more often than not, and you'll be on your way to a healthier way of eating for life.

Protein Power from Plants and Animals

The body needs protein for just about everything from healthy hair, skin, and nails; to transporting nutrients in the bloodstream to provide energy; to building, maintaining, and repairing muscle. We need to get protein just about every day since the body doesn't have a way to store amino acids, the building blocks of proteins.

Most adults need 50 to 65 grams of protein per day. Most Americans get much more than that, mostly from animal sources. There's room in a healthy diet for both plant and animal proteins.

The benefit of plant proteins is that they are cholesterol-free and will be low in saturated fats and high in fiber. They are also typically more affordable than meat. Examples are beans, nuts, tofu, and whole grains. Experts used to think that plant foods had to be carefully combined to provide complete proteins comparable to animal protein, but recent studies suggest that eating a variety of plant-based protein throughout the day does the job.

When choosing animal sources, look for lower-fat dairy products and the leanest cuts of meat. An exception may be fatty fish such as salmon, herring, and mackerel, which provide heart-healthy omega-3 fats, which are polyunsaturated fats. Recall that unsaturated fats are the better fats to choose; saturated fats should be limited (and trans fats should simply be avoided).

Tools for Success

Change can be hard, and that includes changing eating and exercising habits. Having useful resources on hand can make the process easier. To set yourself up for success, check out the suggestions on the next page for helpful kitchen tools, information about common portion sizes, tips on how to keep a food journal, and the ABCs of how to read a food label.

Handy Things to Have Around the Kitchen

If you're new to counting calories and tracking your intake, it can be helpful to have the tools listed on the next page so that you get a good sense of portion sizes. It may also be helpful to use the same cups, bowls, and plates at home during this process. This can be especially useful when measuring out cereals, grains, pastas, and drinks.

- Basic calculator

- Food scale that measures grams

- Set of measuring spoons (1 Tbsp, 1/2 Tbsp, 1 tsp, 1/2 tsp, 1/4 tsp)

- Set of dry measuring cups (1 cup, 1/2 cup, 1/3 cup, 1/4 cup, 1/8 cup)

- Measuring cup for liquids (with markings for both cups and ounces)

Common Portion Sizes and Conversions

Use the table below to convert measurements from food packages into more understandable terms. For example, maybe visualizing 237 milliliters doesn't come into focus right away, so you consult the chart and see that it's the same as 8 fluid ounces or 1 cup, which are measurements that you are more familiar with. Another way to use this table is to convert a portion size from this book to the portion size you plan on eating.

Liquid or Volume Measures

1 teaspoon		1/3 tablespoon	5 ml
1 tablespoon	1/2 fluid ounce	3 teaspoons	15 ml
2 tablespoons	1 fluid ounce	1/8 cup	30 ml
1/4 cup	2 fluid ounces	4 tablespoons	59 ml
1/3 cup	2 2/3 fluid ounces	5 tablespoons & 1 teaspoon	79 ml
1/2 cup	4 fluid ounces	8 tablespoons	118 ml
2/3 cup	5 1/3 fluid ounces	10 tablespoons & 2 teaspoons	158 ml
3/4 cup	6 fluid ounces	12 tablespoons	177 ml
7/8 cup	7 fluid ounces	14 tablespoons	207 ml
1 cup	8 fluid ounces / 1/2 pint	16 tablespoons	237 ml
2 cups	16 fluid ounces / 1 pint	32 tablespoons	473 ml
4 cups	32 fluid ounces	1 quart	946 ml
1 pint	16 fluid ounces / 1 pint	32 tablespoons	473 ml
2 pints	32 fluid ounces	1 quart	946 ml
8 pints	1 gallon / 128 fluid ounces	4 quarts	3.78 liters
4 quarts	1 gallon / 128 fluid ounces	1 gallon	3.78 liters
1 liter	1.057 quarts		1 liter
128 fluid ounces	1 gallon	4 quarts	3.78 liters

Dry or Weight Measurements

1 ounce		30 grams when rounded, 28.35 grams to be exact
2 ounces		55 grams
3 ounces		85 grams
4 ounces	1/4 pound	115 grams
8 ounces	1/2 pound	230 grams
12 ounces	3/4 pound	340 grams
16 ounces	1 pound	454 grams
32 ounces	2 pounds	907 grams

Expert Tips for Keeping a Food and Exercise Journal

The purpose of keeping a food journal is so that you know how you're doing compared to your goals. The more you know, the easier it is to see where you need to focus your efforts for improvement. You can keep your journal in a physical notebook, on your smart phone, on your computer, or some combination of those. Find what works best for your lifestyle. The important thing is to keep an accurate record. Here are some helpful tips and strategies:

• Write down the day, date, and that day's goals for intake and exercise.

• Food or beverage, if it passes your lips, write it down.

• Enter calories for all foods, plus any other nutrients you'd like to track.

• Note the eating occasion (meals and snacks) and the time of day, if possible.

• Note the cooking method if it applies (e.g., baked, fried, steamed).

• Note the brand name of a product if it applies.

• Don't forget foods like the bread rolls that come out before a main dish, beverages, condiments, and things that may have been added during preparation such as added fats, sugars, and salt — everything counts!

• Keep track of daily physical activity by noting the number of minutes, the intensity (e.g., light, medium, hard), and a brief description of the activity.

• Feel great when you meet your goals, and don't get discouraged about the ones you haven't reached yet. Keep working on them, and your hard work will pay off. Better yet, once eating right and exercising becomes a habit, it won't even be hard work; it'll be habit.

sample food and exercise journal

Day, Date: Saturday, 1/01
Today's Goals:
1500 calories
Fewer than 16.6 grams of saturated fat
At least 25 grams of fiber; less than 1500 milligrams of sodium
At least 30 minutes of any physical activity

Eating Occasion & Time	Food	Calories	Saturated Fat	Fiber	Sodium
Breakfast, 8 a.m.					
Morning snack, 10:30 a.m.					
Lunch, 1 p.m.					
Afternoon snack, 4 p.m.					
Dinner, 7 p.m.					
	Total IN				
	Goals	1500	<16.6g	>25g	<1500mg
	Differences (+/–)				

How to Read Food Labels

The Nutrition Facts Panel is based on a 2000-calorie diet and applies to people 4 years of age and older. It includes serving size, servings per container, calories, total fat, saturated fat, cholesterol, sodium, total carbohydrate, dietary fiber, sugars, protein, vitamins A and C, calcium, and iron. Most labels will also list trans fat, and some will voluntarily list additional vitamins and minerals.

• Serving size. Take a close look at the serving size, because that is what all the nutrition information is based on. If you eat more than the serving size, you're getting more calories than the label lists, and if you eat less than the serving size, you're getting fewer calories and other nutrients.

• Daily value. The percentage Daily Value (DV) shows how a food contributes to a 2000-calorie diet, which may or may not apply to your individual goals, but it does give a ballpark idea of how a food fits into an overall day's diet.

If a single snack food supplies 50% of the day's sodium, even if that number is for a 2000-calorie diet, it tells you that if you choose to eat that food, you'll need to keep the sodium down in the rest of the foods you eat that day.

For fiber, protein, vitamins, and minerals, if a food has 10% to 19% DV, it may qualify to say it's a "good" source of that nutrient; for 20% DV or higher, it may qualify to say it's a "great," "excellent," or "rich" source.

• Ingredient statement. Ingredients are in order by weight from high to low. If the first ingredient is whole wheat, it's a good sign. On the other hand, if it's sugar, you may want to think twice about that food. The eight major allergens will also be listed here (wheat, eggs, fish, shellfish, milk, tree nuts, peanuts, and soy).

Nutrition Facts

Serving Size 1 package
Servings Per Container 1

Amount Per Serving

Calories 230   Calories from Fat 130

	% Daily Value*
Total Fat 15g	**23%**
Saturated Fat 4g	**22%**
Cholesterol 0mg	**0%**
Sodium 270mg	**11%**
Total Carbohydrate 23g	**8%**
Dietary Fiber 1g	**6%**
Sugars 0g	
Protein 3g	

Vitamin A 0%	•	Vitamin C 15%
Calcium 0%	•	Iron 2%

*Percent Daily Values are based on a 2,000 calorie diet. Your daily values may be higher or lower depending on your calorie needs:

	Calories: 2,000	2,500
Total Fat	Less then 65 g	80 g
Sat Fat	Less than 20 g	25 g
Cholesterol	Less than 300 mg	300 mg
Sodium	Less than 2,400 mg	2,400 mg
Total Carbohydrate	300 g	375 g
Dietary Fiber	25 g	30 g

Calories per gram:
Fat 9 • Carbohydrate 4 • Protein 4

INGREDIENTS: POTATOES, VEGETABLE OIL (CONTAINS ONE OR MORE OF THE FOLLOWING: CORN, COTTONSEED, OR SUNFLOWER OIL), AND SALT.

food counts

BEANS AND LEGUMES

Item	Serving Size	Calories	Protein	Carb	Fiber	Sugar	Total Fat	Sat Fat	Sodium
Adzuki beans, Arrowhead Mills	1/4 cup	183	11	37	5	1	0.0	0.0	0
Adzuki beans, Eden, canned, unsalted, fat free	1/2 cup	124	8	21	6	0	0.0	0.0	11
Adzuki beans, canned, with salt	1/2 cup	147	9	28	8	0	0.1	0.0	280
Bean soup mix, 13 varieties, dry, Bob's Red Mill	1/2 cup	322	20	56	6	2	2.0	0.0	19
Bean sprouts, canned	1/2 cup	9	1	2	1	0	0.0	0.0	15
Black beans, canned	1/2 cup	127	8	24	6	5	0.0	0.0	178
Black beans, canned, 50% less salt, Del Monte	1/2 cup	70	5	17	6	1	0.0	0.0	260
Black beans, canned, unsalted, fat-free, Eden	1/2 cup	100	7	18	6	0	0.0	0.0	15
Black-eyed peas, cooked	1/2 cup	99	7	18	6	3	0.5	0.1	3
Black-eyed peas, cooked with salt	1/2 cup	99	7	18	6	3	0.5	0.1	204
Black-eyed peas, cooked without salt	1/2 cup	82	3	17	4	3	0.3	0.1	3
Broad beans, cooked with salt	1/2 cup	94	6	17	5	2	0.3	0.1	205
Broad beans, cooked without salt	1/2 cup	94	6	17	5	2	0.3	0.1	4
Broad beans, young, cooked with salt and drained	1/2 cup	53	4	9	3	2	0.4	0.1	235
Butter beans, canned, Del Monte	1/2 cup	70	6	18	5	1	0.0	0.0	440
Butter beans, frozen, Birds Eye	1/2 cup	100	5	18	4	2	0.0	0.0	220
Cannellini beans, canned	1/2 cup	110	8	20	6	2	0.0	0.0	340
Cannellini beans, canned, unsalted, Eden	1/2 cup	100	6	17	5	1	1.0	0.0	40

BEANS AND LEGUMES continued

Item	Serving Size	Calories	Protein	Carb	Fiber	Sugar	Total Fat	Sat Fat	Sodium
Chickpea or garbanzo beans, canned, unsalted, Eden	1/2 cup	130	7	23	5	1	1.0	0.0	30
Chili bean mix, canned, with kidney, pinto, & black beans	1/2 cup	100	7	19	5	2	0.0	0.0	150
Chili-style beans, canned, medium spicy, Bush Brothers	1/2 cup	120	6	20	6	0	1.0	0.5	480
Chili-style beans, canned, mild, Bush Brothers	1/2 cup	120	6	20	6	0	1.0	0.5	480
Chili-style beans, canned, spicy, Bush Brothers	1/2 cup	120	6	20	6	0	1.0	0.5	480
Fava beans, canned	1/2 cup	100	6	17	5	0	0.5	0.0	250
Fava beans, cooked with salt	1/2 cup	94	6	17	5	2	0.3	0.1	205
Fava beans, cooked without salt	1/2 cup	94	6	17	5	2	0.3	0.1	205
Garbanzo beans	1/4 cup	155	8	26	7	5	2.6	0.3	10
Garbanzo beans, cooked	1/2 cup	134	7	22	6	4	2.1	0.2	6
Garbanzo beans, cooked with salt	1/2 cup	139	8	23	6	4	2.2	0.2	207
Golden gram beans, cooked with salt	1/2 cup	89	6	16	6	2	0.3	0.1	202
Golden gram beans, cooked without salt	1/2 cup	89	6	16	6	2	0.3	0.1	2
Golden gram beans, dry	1/4 cup	147	10	27	7	3	0.5	0.1	6
Great northern beans	1/4 cup	144	9	27	9	1	0.5	0.2	6
Great northern beans, canned, Westbrae	1/2 cup	100	7	19	6	2	0.0	0.0	140
Green & yellow Italian beans, cut and frozen, Birds Eye	1/2 cup	35	1	5	2	2	0.0	0.0	0
Green beans, canned, drained	1/2 cup	15	1	3	1	1	0.1	0.0	170
Green beans, cooked from frozen with salt and drained	1/2 cup	17	1	4	2	1	0.1	0.0	159

BEANS AND LEGUMES continued

Item	Serving Size	Calories	Protein	Carb	Fiber	Sugar	Total Fat	Sat Fat	Sodium
Green beans, cooked from frozen without salt and drained	1/2 cup	18	1	4	2	1	0.1	0.0	1
Green beans, cooked with salt and drained	1/2 cup	23	1	5	2	1	0.2	0.0	155
Green beans, cooked without salt and drained	1/2 cup	23	1	5	2	1	0.2	0.0	1
Green beans, frozen	1/2 cup	25	1	5	2	1	0.1	0.0	2
Green gram beans, cooked with salt	1/2 cup	68	5	12	5	1	0.2	0.1	155
Green gram beans, cooked without salt	1/2 cup	68	5	12	5	1	0.2	0.1	1
Green gram beans, dry	1/4 cup	147	10	27	7	3	0.5	0.1	6
Green peas, canned with liquid	1/2 cup	42	3	8	3	3	0.2	0.0	200
Green peas, canned without salt	1/2 cup	42	3	8	3	3	0.2	0.0	7
Green peas, fresh	1/2 cup	59	4	11	4	4	0.3	0.1	4
Green peas, frozen	1/2 cup	62	4	11	4	4	0.3	0.1	86
Green split peas, cooked with salt	1/2 cup	93	7	16	7	2	0.3	0.0	190
Green split peas, cooked without salt	1/2 cup	94	7	17	7	2	0.3	0.0	2
Gungo peas, young, fresh	1/2 cup	99	5	17	4	2	1.2	0.3	4
Horse beans, young	1/2 cup	58	4	9	3	5	0.5	0.1	40
Jackson wonder beans, canned, heirloom, Westbrae	1/2 cup	100	5	19	5	0	0.0	0.0	135
Kidney beans	1/4 cup	142	10	26	11	1	0.4	0.1	10
Kidney beans, canned	1/2 cup	71	4	12	5	2	0.5	0.1	252
Kidney beans, canned, dark red, Bush Brothers	1/2 cup	111	7	18	6	2	0.9	0.0	221
Kidney beans, cooked with salt	1/2 cup	108	7	19	5	0	0.4	0.1	202
Kidney beans, cooked without salt	1/2 cup	108	7	19	5	0	0.4	0.1	1
Lentils	1/4 cup	169	12	29	15	1	0.5	0.1	3
Lentils, cooked with salt	1/2 cup	109	9	19	8	2	0.4	0.0	228

BEANS AND LEGUMES continued

Item	Serving Size	Calories	Protein	Carb	Fiber	Sugar	Total Fat	Sat Fat	Sodium
Lentils, cooked without salt	1/2 cup	109	9	19	8	2	0.4	0.0	2
Lentils, red, Bob's Red Mill	1/2 cup	320	24	54	5	5	0.0	0.0	9
Lima beans, baby, young, cooked from frozen with salt and drained	1/2 cup	89	6	17	5	1	0.3	0.1	225
Lima beans, baby, young, cooked from frozen without salt and drained	1/2 cup	89	6	17	5	1	0.3	0.1	25
Lima beans, large, cooked with salt	1/2 cup	98	7	18	6	2	0.3	0.1	202
Lima beans, large, cooked without salt	1/2 cup	98	7	18	6	2	0.3	0.1	2
Lima beans, large, young, cooked from frozen and drained	1/2 cup	88	5	16	5	1	0.3	0.1	59
Lupin beans, cooked with salt	1/2 cup	99	13	8	2	2	2.5	0.3	204
Mung bean sprouts, canned and drained	1/2 cup	7	1	1	0	1	0.0	0.0	87
Mung bean sprouts, cooked with salt and drained	1/2 cup	12	1	2	0	2	0.1	0.0	153
Mung bean sprouts, cooked without salt and drained	1/2 cup	13	1	3	0	2	0.1	0.0	6
Mung bean sprouts, fresh	1/2 cup	11	1	2	1	1	0.1	0.0	2
Mung beans, cooked with salt	1/2 cup	89	6	16	6	2	0.3	0.1	202
Mung beans, dry	1/4 cup	147	10	27	7	3	0.5	0.1	6
Mung beans, cooked without salt	1/2 cup	89	6	16	6	2	0.3	0.1	2
Mungo beans, cooked with salt	1/2 cup	89	6	16	5	2	0.5	0.0	207
Mungo beans, cooked without salt	1/2 cup	89	6	16	5	2	0.5	0.0	6
Natto, fermented soybeans	1/2 cup	180	15	12	5	4	9.4	1.4	6
Navy beans	1/4 cup	143	9	26	10	2	0.6	0.1	2

BEANS AND LEGUMES continued

Item	Serving Size	Calories	Protein	Carb	Fiber	Sugar	Total Fat	Sat Fat	Sodium
Navy beans, canned	1/2 cup	96	6	17	4	0	0.4	0.1	381
Navy beans, cooked with salt	1/2 cup	119	7	22	9	0	0.5	0.1	201
Navy beans, cooked without salt	1/2 cup	119	7	22	9	0	0.5	0.1	0
No-eyed peas, young, fresh	1/2 cup	116	6	20	4	3	1.4	0.3	4
Pigeon peas, cooked with salt	1/2 cup	103	6	20	6	1	0.3	0.1	205
Pigeon peas, young, cooked with salt and drained	1/2 cup	94	5	17	5	2	1.2	0.1	204
Pigeon peas, young, cooked without salt and drained	1/2 cup	111	6	19	6	2	1.4	0.1	4
Pigeon peas, young, fresh	1/2 cup	111	6	19	6	2	1.4	0.1	4
Pink beans, cooked with salt	1/2 cup	127	8	24	5	0	0.4	0.1	202
Pink beans, cooked without salt	1/2 cup	127	8	24	5	0	0.4	0.1	2
Pinto beans, canned	1/2 cup	73	4	13	4	0	0.7	0.1	250
Pinto beans, cooked and mashed	1/2 cup	73	4	13	4	0	0.7	0.1	250
Pinto beans, cooked with salt	1/2 cup	122	8	22	8	0	0.6	0.1	202
Pinto beans, cooked without salt	1/2 cup	122	8	22	8	0	0.6	0.1	1
Red beans, small, Bob's Red Mill	1/2 cup	306	22	55	6	0	1.0	0.0	22
Red gram peas, cooked with salt	1/2 cup	103	6	20	6	1	0.3	0.1	205
Red gram peas, young, cooked with salt and drained	1/2 cup	94	5	17	5	2	1.2	0.1	204
Red gram peas, young, cooked without salt and drained	1/2 cup	94	5	17	5	2	1.2	0.1	4
Red gram peas, young, fresh	1/2 cup	116	6	20	4	3	1.4	0.3	4
Red pinto beans, cooked	1/2 cup	96	6	18	7	1	0.3	0.1	4

BEANS AND LEGUMES continued

Item	Serving Size	Calories	Protein	Carb	Fiber	Sugar	Total Fat	Sat Fat	Sodium
Refried beans, canned, fat-free	1/2 cup	67	5	11	4	1	0.4	0.1	372
Refried beans, canned, vegetarian	1/2 cup	71	4	11	4	1	0.7	0.1	366
Runner beans, canned, scarlet heirloom, Westbrae	1/2 cup	100	6	20	7	1	0.0	0.0	140
Shellie beans, canned with liquid	1/2 cup	26	1	5	3	1	0.2	0.0	284
Soldier beans, canned, European heirloom, Westbrae	1/2 cup	90	6	16	5	0	0.0	0.0	140
Soybean sprouts, steamed with salt	1/2 cup	50	5	7	0	0	2.8	0.4	153
Soybean sprouts, steamed without salt	1/2 cup	50	5	7	0	0	2.8	0.4	6
Soybean sprouts, stir-fried with salt	1/2 cup	78	8	6	1	0	4.4	0.0	155
Soybeans, edamame, prepared from frozen without salt	1/2 cup	95	8	8	4	2	4.0	0.5	5
Trout beans, canned, heirloom, Westbrae	1/2 cup	100	7	18	6	0	0.0	0.0	140
White beans, canned	1/2 cup	97	6	18	4	0	0.2	0.1	4
White beans, cooked with salt	1/2 cup	118	8	21	5	0	0.3	0.1	206
White beans, cooked without salt	1/2 cup	118	8	21	5	0	0.3	0.1	5
Yam bean, fresh	1/2 cup	25	0	6	3	1	0.1	0.0	3

BEVERAGES, Alcohol

Item	Serving Size	Calories	Protein	Carb	Fiber	Sugar	Total Fat	Sat Fat	Sodium
Aquavit, 80 proof	1.5 fl oz	96	0	0	0	0	0	0	1
Aquavit, 86 proof	1.5 fl oz	104	0	0	0	0	0	0	1
Aquavit, 90 proof	1.5 fl oz	110	0	0	0	0	0	0	1
Aquavit, 94 proof	1.5 fl oz	115	0	0	0	0	0	0	1
Aquavit, 100 proof	1.5 fl oz	123	0	0	0	0	0	0	1
Beer, ale	12 fl oz	147	1	13	0	0	0	0	34

BEVERAGES, Alcohol continued

Item	Serving Size	Calories	Protein	Carb	Fiber	Sugar	Total Fat	Sat Fat	Sodium
Beer, amber	12 fl oz	169	2	14	0	0	0	0	44
Beer, amber bock	12 fl oz	166	1	15	0	0	0	0	9
Beer, black and tan	12 fl oz	174	2	18	0	0	0	0	9
Beer, dark	12 fl oz	150	1	13	0	0	0	0	34
Beer, dark, classic	12 fl oz	159	1	15	0	0	0	0	9
Beer, draft, genuine	12 fl oz	143	1	13	0	0	0	0	7
Beer, draft, genuine light	12 fl oz	110	1	7	0	0	0	0	6
Beer, draft, golden	12 fl oz	151	2	13	0	0	0	0	9
Beer, draft, golden light	12 fl oz	110	1	7	0	0	0	0	9
Beer, extra gold	12 fl oz	150	1	11	0	11	0	0	11
Beer, lager	12 fl oz	102	1	6	1	0	0	0	14
Beer, light	12 fl oz	104	0	2	0	0	0	0	4
Beer, nonalcoholic	12 fl oz	74	1	14	0	11	0	0	10
Beer, original	12 fl oz	151	1	11	0	11	0	0	11
Beer, pale ale	12 fl oz	179	2	17	0	0	0	0	9
Bourbon, 80 proof	1.5 fl oz	104	0	0	0	0	0	0	1
Bourbon, 86 proof	1.5 fl oz	113	0	0	0	0	0	0	1
Bourbon, 90 proof	1.5 fl oz	118	0	0	0	0	0	0	1
Bourbon, 94 proof	1.5 fl oz	124	0	0	0	0	0	0	1
Bourbon, 100 proof	1.5 fl oz	133	0	0	0	0	0	0	1
Brandy, 80 proof	1.5 fl oz	104	0	0	0	0	0	0	1
Brandy, 86 proof	1.5 fl oz	113	0	0	0	0	0	0	1
Brandy, 90 proof	1.5 fl oz	118	0	0	0	0	0	0	1
Brandy, 94 proof	1.5 fl oz	124	0	0	0	0	0	0	1
Brandy, 100 proof	1.5 fl oz	133	0	0	0	0	0	0	1
Daiquiri, frozen cocktail	8 fl oz	446	0	7	0	7	0	0	5
Gin, 80 proof	1.5 fl oz	104	0	0	0	0	0	0	1
Gin, 86 proof	1.5 fl oz	113	0	0	0	0	0	0	1
Gin, 90 proof	1.5 fl oz	118	0	0	0	0	0	0	2
Gin, 94 proof	1.5 fl oz	124	0	0	0	0	0	0	1
Gin, 100 proof	1.5 fl oz	133	0	0	0	0	0	0	1
Gin and tonic cocktail	6 fl oz	117	0	6	0	6	0	0	5
Highball cocktail	6 fl oz	118	0	0	0	0	0	0	16
Long Island iced tea	6 fl oz	142	0	11	0	0	0	0	7
Malt beverage, Zima	8 fl oz	126	0	21	0	11	0	0	20
Manhattan cocktail	6 fl oz	213	0	6	0	6	0	0	5

BEVERAGES, Alcohol continued

Item	Serving Size	Calories	Protein	Carb	Fiber	Sugar	Total Fat	Sat Fat	Sodium
Margarita	1.5 fl oz	94	0	6	0	6	0	0	2
Martini	1.5 fl oz	103	0	1	0	0	0	0	1
Mint julep cocktail	1.5 fl oz	108	0	6	0	6	0	0	1
Piña colada	1.5 fl oz	82	0	11	0	0	1	1	3
Rum, 80 proof	1.5 fl oz	104	0	0	0	0	0	0	1
Rum, 86 proof	1.5 fl oz	113	0	0	0	0	0	0	1
Rum, 90 proof	1.5 fl oz	118	0	0	0	0	0	0	1
Rum, 94 proof	1.5 fl oz	124	0	0	0	0	0	0	1
Rum, 100 proof	1.5 fl oz	133	0	0	0	0	0	0	1
Sangria	5 fl oz	98	0	13	0	0	0	0	10
Tequila, 80 proof	1.5 fl oz	104	0	0	0	0	0	0	1
Tequila, 86 proof	1.5 fl oz	113	0	0	0	0	0	0	1
Tequila, 90 proof	1.5 fl oz	118	0	0	0	0	0	0	1
Tequila, 94 proof	1.5 fl oz	124	0	0	0	0	0	0	1
Tequila, 100 proof	1.5 fl oz	133	0	0	0	0	0	0	1
Vodka, 86 proof	1.5 fl oz	113	0	0	0	0	0	0	1
Vodka, 90 proof	1.5 fl oz	118	0	0	0	0	0	0	1
Vodka, 94 proof	1.5 fl oz	124	0	0	0	0	0	0	1
Vodka, 100 proof	1.5 fl oz	133	0	0	0	0	0	0	1
Whiskey, 80 proof	1.5 fl oz	96	0	0	0	0	0	0	0
Whiskey, 86 proof	1.5 fl oz	104	0	0	0	0	0	0	0
Whiskey, 90 proof	1.5 fl oz	110	0	0	0	0	0	0	0
Whiskey, 94 proof	1.5 fl oz	115	0	0	0	0	0	0	0
Wine cooler	5 fl oz	71	0	8	0	0	0	0	12
Wine, port	5 fl oz	236	0	20	0	11	0	0	13
Wine, red	5 fl oz	125	0	4	0	1	0	0	6
Wine, white	5 fl oz	123	0	3	0	1	0	0	5

BEVERAGES, Coffee and Tea

Item	Serving Size	Calories	Protein	Carb	Fiber	Sugar	Total Fat	Sat Fat	Sodium
Cappuccino, with fat-free milk	8 fl oz	53	5	7	0	7	0	0	73
Cappuccino, with low fat milk	8 fl oz	73	5	7	0	7	0	0	73
Coffee, brewed	8 fl oz	2	0	0	0	0	0.02	0	0

BEVERAGES, Coffee and Tea continued

Item	Serving Size	Calories	Protein	Carb	Fiber	Sugar	Total Fat	Sat Fat	Sodium
Coffee, brewed, decaf	8 fl oz	0	0	0	0	0	0	0	0
Coffee, iced, sweetened	6 fl oz	52	1	17	0	16	0.5	0.5	20
Coffee, instant, powdered	1 tbsp	7	0	1	0	0	0	0.2	1
Coffee, instant, powdered, decaf	1 tbsp	12	1	2	0	0	0.2	0.09	1
Espresso, restaurant prepared	6 fl oz	4	0	0	0	0	0.18	0.09	14
Espresso, restaurant prepared, decaf	6 fl oz	0	0	0	0	0	0.18	0.09	14
Frappuccino, caramel, Starbucks on the Go	6 fl oz	116	5	30	0	26	2.5	1.5	85
Frappuccino, coffee, Starbucks on the Go	6 fl oz	116	5	31	0	27	2.5	1.5	85
Frappuccino, mocha, lite, Starbucks on the Go	6 fl oz	58	5	10	0	9	2.5	1.5	80
Frappuccino, mocha, Starbucks on the Go	6 fl oz	103	6	28	0	26	3	2	80
Frappuccino, vanilla, Starbucks on the Go	6 fl oz	116	5	31	0	26	2.5	1.5	85
Tea, black	8 fl oz	0	0	0	0	0	0	0	0
Tea, black, English breakfast	8 fl oz	0	0	0	0	0	0	0	0
Tea, chai, original	8 fl oz	0	0	0	0	0	0	0	0
Tea, chai, original, decaf	8 fl oz	0	0	0	0	0	0	0	0
Tea, green	8 fl oz	0	0	0	0	0	0	0	0
Tea, herbal, Bengal Spice	8 fl oz	0	0	0	0	0	0	0	0
Tea, herbal, caffeine free	8 fl oz	0	0	0	0	0	0	0	0
Tea, herbal, chamomile	8 fl oz	2	0	0	0	0	0	0	2
Tea, iced, black, sweetened	8 fl oz	85	0	22	0	22	0	0	15
Tea, iced, black, unsweetened	8 fl oz	0	0	0	0	0	0	0	0
Tea, mint	8 fl oz	0	0	0	0	0	0.01	0	0
Tea, sweet	8 fl oz	114	0	31	0	31	0	0	10
Tea, unsweetened	8 fl oz	2	0	0	0	0	0	0	3

BEVERAGES, Juice

Item	Serving Size	Calories	Protein	Carb	Fiber	Sugar	Total Fat	Sat Fat	Sodium
Apple cider drink	8 fl oz	127	0	30	0	26	0	0	25
Apple juice	8 fl oz	106	0	29	0	27	0	0	0
Apple juice, unsweetened	8 fl oz	110	0	11	0	10	0.13	0.02	4
Apricot juice	8 fl oz	124	0	32	0	29	0	0	15
Blueberry juice	8 fl oz	130	0	31	1	28	0	0	15
Cherry juice	8 fl oz	136	0	34	0	32	0	0	15
Cherry soft drink, Kool-Aid Bursts	8 fl oz	103	0	23	0	23	0	0	40
Clam and tomato juice	6 fl oz	115	1	11	0	3	0.2	0	362
Cranberry juice	8 fl oz	104	0	26	0	26	0	0	15
Diet cranberry grapefruit juice, SoBe Lean	8 fl oz	5	0	1	0	0	0	0	15
Diet cranberry raspberry juice	8 fl oz	10	0	2	0	2	0	0	10
Diet white grape juice	8 fl oz	10	0	2	0	2	0	0	10
Energy drink, Amp Energy	8 fl oz	110	0	12	0	12	0	0	27
Energy drink, sugar free, Amp Energy	8 fl oz	5	0	1	0	0	0	0	31
Energy drink, with caffeine & vitamin B complex	8 fl oz	108	0	11	0	10	0.08	0	84
Flavored water, Blackberry Rush, Clear Fruit	8 fl oz	91	0	23	0	23	0	0	0
Flavored water, Cherry Blast, Clear Fruit	8 fl oz	91	0	23	0	23	0	0	0
Fruit punch	8 fl oz	133	0	50	0	50	0	0	45
Fruit punch, Tropicana	8 fl oz	165	1	40	0	40	0	0	30
Grape juice	8 fl oz	152	0	38	0	38	0	0	10
Grape juice, Capri Sun	8 fl oz	95	0	25	0	25	0	0	15
Grape juice, Kool-Aid Bursts	8 fl oz	114	0	24	0	24	0	0	35
Grapefruit juice	8 fl oz	122	0	29	0	28	0	0	0
Grapefruit, ruby red cocktail, 20% juice	8 fl oz	132	0	32	0	32	0	0	0
Guava nectar	8 fl oz	143	0	15	1	14	0.09	0.03	3
Kiwi strawberry drink, 10% juice	8 fl oz	122	0	30	0	30	0	0	0
Lemonade, Country Time	8 fl oz	87	0	23	0	23	0	0	90
Lemonade, pink	8 fl oz	106	0	29	0	28	0	0	5

BEVERAGES, Juice continued

Item	Serving Size	Calories	Protein	Carb	Fiber	Sugar	Total Fat	Sat Fat	Sodium
Lemonade, sugar-free, Crystal Light	8 fl oz	5	0	0	0	0	0	0	10
Lemonade, Tropicana	8 fl oz	122	0	29	0	28	0	0	20
Mandarin orange mango drink, 10% juice	8 fl oz	122	0	29	0	29	0	0	0
Mango juice	8 fl oz	133	1	34	0	28	0	0	70
O2 Perform, Fierce Grape, Gatorade	8 fl oz	62	0	6	0	5	0	0	39
O2 Perform, Fruit Punch, Gatorade	8 fl oz	62	0	6	0	5	0	0	39
O2 Perform, Glacier Freeze, Gatorade	8 fl oz	62	0	6	0	5	0	0	39
O2 Perform, Lemon-Lime, Gatorade	8 fl oz	62	0	6	0	5	0	0	39
O2 Perform, Lemonade, Gatorade	8 fl oz	62	0	6	0	5	0	0	39
O2 Perform, Rain Lime, Gatorade	8 fl oz	62	0	6	0	5	0	0	39
Papaya drink, premium, 20% juice	8 fl oz	142	0	35	0	35	0	0	0
Peach mango juice	8 fl oz	10	0	2	0	2	0	0	65
Peach mango juice, V8 Splash	8 fl oz	89	1	8	0	7	0	0	29
Peach mango juice, V8 V-Fusion	8 fl oz	118	0	11	0	11	0	0	28
Pineapple orange juice, Tropicana Tropics	8 fl oz	126	1	32	0	32	0	0	25
Prune juice	8 fl oz	173	1	42	3	16	0	0	35
Sparkling clementine juice, IZZE	8 fl oz	87	0	33	0	31	0	0	15
Sparkling grapefruit juice, IZZE	8 fl oz	96	1	37	0	37	0	0	15
Strawberry banana juice, V8 V-Fusion	8 fl oz	118	0	12	0	10	0	0	28
Strawberry banana smoothie	8 fl oz	124	1	29	1	27	0	0	10
Strawberry juice	8 fl oz	72	1	7	0	7	0.4	0.02	1
Sunrise, classic orange, Crystal Light	8 fl oz	5	0	0	0	0	0	0	20
Tangerine juice	8 fl oz	143	1	37	0	31	0	0	75

BEVERAGES, Juice continued

Item	Serving Size	Calories	Protein	Carb	Fiber	Sugar	Total Fat	Sat Fat	Sodium
Tomato juice	8 fl oz	48	1	4	1	3	0	0	280
Tropical Colada Smoothie, V8 Splash	8 fl oz	98	1	9	0	7	0	0	20
Vegetable juice, V8	8 fl oz	50	1	4	1	3	0	0	198
Vita-Boom cranberry grapefruit, SoBe	8 fl oz	98	0	28	0	27	0	0	10
Vita-Boom orange carrot, SoBe	8 fl oz	88	0	24	0	23	0	0	10

BEVERAGES, Milk and Nondairy

Item	Serving Size	Calories	Protein	Carb	Fiber	Sugar	Total Fat	Sat Fat	Sodium
Almond milk, Almond Breeze	8 fl oz	63	1	8	1	7	3	0	153
Almond milk, chocolate, Almond Breeze	8 fl oz	120	1	21	1	20	3	0	160
Breakfast drink, orange	8 fl oz	103	0	11	0	7	0	0	2
Breakfast drink, orange, prepared from powdered	8 fl oz	118	0	13	0	12	0	0	5
Breakfast drink, orange, reduced sugar	8 fl oz	10	0	1	0	0	0	0	5
Breakfast drink, orange, with add nutrients	8 fl oz	127	0	13	0	8	0	0	54
Breakfast drink, orange, with pulp, prepared from frozen conc with water	8 fl oz	118	0	12	0	12	0.14	0.02	10
Diet shake, cappuccino delight, Slim-Fast	8 fl oz	123	10	25	5	18	6	2	200
Diet shake, creamy chocolate, Slim-Fast	8 fl oz	130	20	6	4	1	9	1.5	260
Diet shake, French vanilla, Slim-Fast	8 fl oz	123	10	24	5	17	6	2.5	200
Diet shake, high protein, chocolate, extra creamy, Slim-Fast	8 fl oz	130	15	24	5	13	5	2	220
Diet shake, lower carb, vanilla cream, Slim-Fast	8 fl oz	123	20	4	2	1	9	1.5	220
Diet shake, rich chocolate royale, Slim-Fast	8 fl oz	151	10	40	5	35	3	1	220

BEVERAGES, Milk and Nondairy continued

Item	Serving Size	Calories	Protein	Carb	Fiber	Sugar	Total Fat	Sat Fat	Sodium
Hot cocoa, prepared from dry mix with water	8 fl oz	132	1	12	1	9	0.55	0.33	73
Hot cocoa, prepared from recipe with milk	8 fl oz	185	4	11	1	10	2.34	1.43	44
Milk, fat-free	8 fl oz	90	9	13	0	12	0	0	130
Milk, low fat 1%	8 fl oz	118	10	14	0	11	3	2	143
Milk, reduced fat 2%	8 fl oz	122	8	11	0	11	5	3	100
Milk, whole	8 fl oz	146	8	11	0	11	8	5	98
Rice milk	8 fl oz	144	3	28	2	0	2	0	86
Rice milk, Rice Dream Heartwise	8 fl oz	130	1	27	3	9	2	0	80
Soy milk	8 fl oz	127	11	12	3	1	5	1	135
Soy milk, all flavors, enhanced	8 fl oz	102	7	8	1	6	4.5	0.5	50
Soy milk, assorted flavors, light, with calcium, vitamins A & D	8 fl oz	107	5	19	2	16	1.5	0.1	46
Soy milk, assorted flavors, lowfat, with calcium, vitamins A & D	8 fl oz	98	4	16	2	8	1.4	0.0	37
Soy milk, chocolate	8 fl oz	143	5	23	1	18	3.5	0.5	53
Soy milk, chocolate, light, with calcium, vitamins A & D	8 fl oz	107	5	19	2	16	1.5	0.1	46
Soy milk, chocolate, nonfat, with calcium, vitamins A & D	8 fl oz	100	6	19	0	8	0.1	0.0	57
Soy milk, chocolate, with calcium, vitamins A & D	8 fl oz	143	5	23	1	18	3.5	0.5	53
Soy milk, unsweetened, Silk	8 fl oz	80	7	4	1	1	4	0.5	85
Soy milk, vanilla & original, with calcium and vitamins A & D, unsweetened	8 fl oz	77	6	9	1	1	1.9	0.2	63
Soy milk, vanilla, light, Silk	8 fl oz	80	6	10	1	7	2	0	95
Soy milk, vanilla, Silk	8 fl oz	100	6	10	1	7	3.5	0.5	95
Soy milk, with calcium, vitamins A & D	8 fl oz	98	6	11	0	8	3.3	0.5	47

BEVERAGES, Soda and Water

Item	Serving Size	Calories	Protein	Carb	Fiber	Sugar	Total Fat	Sat Fat	Sodium
7Up	8 fl oz	100	0	26	0	26	0	0	50
7Up, cherry	8 fl oz	98	0	26	0	26	0	0	50
A&W cream soda	8 fl oz	117	0	31	0	31	0	0	30
Black cherry soda	8 fl oz	113	0	41	0	41	0	0	45
Cherry-citrus soda	8 fl oz	110	0	31	0	31	0	0	70
Cherry Coke	8 fl oz	100	0	28	0	28	0	0	4
Cherry cola	8 fl oz	107	0	39	0	39	0	0	45
Cherry lemon-lime soda	8 fl oz	103	0	39	0	39	0	0	10
Chocolate flavored soda	8 fl oz	101	0	11	0	11	0	0	88
Club soda	8 fl oz	0	0	0	0	0	0	0	45
Coke Classic	8 fl oz	94	0	27	0	27	0	0	9
Coke Classic, caffeine-free	8 fl oz	94	0	27	0	27	0	0	9
Cola	8 fl oz	89	0	10	0	9	0.02	0	4
Cola, caffeine-free	8 fl oz	98	0	11	0	11	0	0	4
Cranberry ginger ale	8 fl oz	89	0	25	0	25	0	0	15
Diet 7Up	8 fl oz	0	0	0	0	0	0	0	35
Diet 7Up, cherry	8 fl oz	0	0	0	0	0	0	0	35
Diet black cherry soda	8 fl oz	0	0	0	0	0	0	0	45
Diet cherry-citrus soda	8 fl oz	0	0	0	0	0	0	0	25
Diet Cherry Coke	8 fl oz	1	0	0	0	0	0	0	4
Diet cherry cola	8 fl oz	0	0	0	0	0	0	0	45
Diet Coke	8 fl oz	1	0	0	0	0	0	0	4
Diet cranberry ginger ale	8 fl oz	0	0	0	0	0	0	0	50
Diet cream soda	8 fl oz	0	0	0	0	0	0	0	35
Diet Doc Shasta	8 fl oz	0	0	0	0	0	0	0	45
Diet Dr Pepper	8 fl oz	0	0	0	0	0	0	0	35
Diet Dr Pepper, caffeine-free	8 fl oz	0	0	0	0	0	0	0	35
Diet French vanilla cream soda	8 fl oz	1	0	0	0	0	0	0	20
Diet ginger ale	8 fl oz	0	0	0	0	0	0	0	60
Diet grape soda	8 fl oz	0	0	0	0	0	0	0	45
Diet orange soda	8 fl oz	0	0	0	0	0	0	0	45
Diet orange soda, with saccharin & aspartame	8 fl oz	0	0	0	0	0	0	0	55
Diet Pepsi, caffeine-free	8 fl oz	0	0	0	0	0	0	0	25

BEVERAGES, Soda and Water continued

Item	Serving Size	Calories	Protein	Carb	Fiber	Sugar	Total Fat	Sat Fat	Sodium
Diet Pepsi Jazz	8 fl oz	0	0	0	0	0	0	0	25
Diet Pepsi lime	8 fl oz	0	0	0	0	0	0	0	25
Diet Pibb Xtra	8 fl oz	1	0	0	0	0	0	0	2
Diet root beer	8 fl oz	0	0	0	0	0	0	0	45
Diet Sierra Mist, lemon-lime	8 fl oz	0	0	0	0	0	0	0	25
Diet Sprite	8 fl oz	3	0	0	0	0	0	0	0
Dr Pepper	8 fl oz	98	0	27	0	27	0	0	35
Dr Pepper, caffeine-free	8 fl oz	98	0	27	0	27	0	0	35
Dr. Shasta	8 fl oz	107	0	39	0	39	0	0	45
French vanilla cream soda	8 fl oz	107	0	30	0	30	0	0	20
Fresca	8 fl oz	3	0	0	0	0	0	0	1
Ginger ale	8 fl oz	79	0	22	0	22	0	0	25
Grape Fanta	8 fl oz	112	0	31	0	31	0	0	9
Grape soda	8 fl oz	127	0	48	0	48	0	0	45
Mello Yello soda	8 fl oz	114	0	32	0	32	0	0	9
Mountain Dew	8 fl oz	105	0	31	0	31	0	0	40
Mountain Dew, caffeine-free	8 fl oz	105	0	31	0	31	0	0	40
Orange cream soda	8 fl oz	116	0	44	0	44	0	0	10
Orange soda	8 fl oz	133	0	49	0	49	0	0	45
Orange soda, Crush	8 fl oz	116	0	34	0	34	0	0	30
Orange soda, Sunkist	8 fl oz	126	0	35	0	35	0	0	30
Peach soda	8 fl oz	113	0	43	0	43	0	0	45
Pepsi lime	8 fl oz	96	0	27	0	27	0	0	20
Pibb Xtra	8 fl oz	94	0	26	0	26	0	0	7
Root beer	8 fl oz	106	0	30	0	30	0	0	24
Sierra Mist, lemon-lime	8 fl oz	100	0	26	0	26	0	0	25
Sprite	8 fl oz	96	0	10	0	9	0.02	0	9
Tab soda	8 fl oz	1	0	0	0	0	0	0	4
Water, bottled, noncarbonated	8 fl oz	0	0	0	0	0	0	0	0
Water, seltzer	8 fl oz	0	0	0	0	0	0	0	0
Water, sparkling, Perrier	8 fl oz	0	0	0	0	0	0	0	2
Water, tonic	8 fl oz	89	0	24	0	24	0	0	15

BREADS AND CRACKERS

Item	Serving Size	Calories	Protein	Carb	Fiber	Sugar	Total Fat	Sat Fat	Sodium
Bagel, cinnamon raisin, 3"	1	188	7	38	2	4	1.0	0.0	222
Bagel, cinnamon raisin, 3.5"–4"	1	273	10	55	2	6	1.7	0.3	322
Bagel, cinnamon raisin, 4.5"	1	358	13	72	3	8	2.0	0.4	422
Bagel, cinnamon raisin, mini, 2.5"	1	71	3	14	1	2	2.0	0.0	84
Bagel, cinnamon raisin, toasted, 3.5"	1	191	7	39	2	4	1.2	0.2	225
Bagel, cinnamon raisin, toasted, 4"	1	291	11	59	3	6	1.8	0.3	343
Bagel, cinnamon raisin, toasted, 4.5"	1	362	13	73	3	8	2.0	0.4	426
Bagel, cinnamon raisin, toasted, mini, 2.5"	1	71	3	14	1	2	0.4	0.0	83
Bagel, oat bran, 3"	1	176	7	37	3	1	0.8	0.1	350
Bagel, oat bran, 3.5"–4"	1	268	11	56	4	2	1.3	0.2	532
Bagel, oat bran, 4.5"	1	334	14	70	5	2	1.6	0.3	664
Bagel, oat bran, mini, 2.5"	1	66	3	14	1	0	0.3	0.0	132
Bagel, onion, enriched, with calcium propionate, 3'	1	171	7	35	2	4	1.0	0.3	309
Bagel, onion, enriched, with calcium propionate, 3", toasted	1	187	7	37	2	4	1.1	0.2	312
Bagel, onion, enriched, with calcium propionate, 3.5"	1	270	11	53	2	5	1.7	0.4	470
Bagel, onion, enriched, with calcium propionate, 3.5", toasted	1	285	11	57	3	6	1.7	0.3	475
Bagel, onion, enriched, with calcium propionate, 4"	1	270	11	53	2	5	1.7	0.4	470
Bagel, onion, enriched, with calcium propionate, 4", toasted	1	285	11	57	3	6	1.7	0.3	475
Bagel, onion, enriched, with calcium propionate, 4.5"	1	337	13	66	3	7	2.1	0.5	587
Bagel, onion, enriched, with calcium propionate, 4.5", toasted	1	354	14	70	3	7	2.1	0.4	590
Bagel, onion, mini, enriched, with calcium propionate, 2.5"	1	67	3	13	1	1	0.4	0.3	116

BREADS AND CRACKERS continued

Item	Serving Size	Calories	Protein	Carb	Fiber	Sugar	Total Fat	Sat Fat	Sodium
Bagel, onion, mini, enriched, with calcium propionate, 2.5", toasted	1	69	3	14	1	1	0.4	0.1	115
Bagel, plain, enriched, with calcium propionate, 3"	1	171	7	35	2	4	1.0	0.3	309
Bagel, plain, enriched, with calcium propionate, 3", toasted	1	187	7	37	2	4	1.1	0.2	312
Bagel, plain, enriched, with calcium propionate, 3.5"	1	270	11	53	2	5	1.7	0.4	470
Bagel, plain, enriched, with calcium propionate, 3.5", toasted	1	285	11	57	3	6	1.7	0.3	475
Bagel, plain, enriched, with calcium propionate, 4"	1	270	11	53	2	5	1.7	0.4	470
Bagel, plain, enriched, with calcium propionate, 4", toasted	1	285	11	57	3	6	1.7	0.3	475
Bagel, plain, enriched, with calcium propionate, 4.5"	1	337	13	66	3	7	2.1	0.5	587
Bagel, plain, enriched, with calcium propionate, 4.5", toasted	1	354	14	70	3	7	2.1	0.4	590
Bagel, plain, mini, enriched, with calcium propionate, 2.5"	1	67	3	13	1	1	0.4	0.3	116
Bagel, plain, mini, enriched, with calcium propionate, 2.5", toasted	1	69	3	14	1	1	0.4	0.1	115
Bagel, poppy seed, enriched, with calcium propionate, 3"	1	171	7	35	2	4	1.0	0.3	309
Bagel, poppy seed, enriched, with calcium propionate, 3", toasted	1	187	7	37	2	4	1.1	0.2	312
Bagel, poppy seed, enriched, with calcium propionate, 3.5"	1	270	11	53	2	5	1.7	0.4	470
Bagel, poppy seed, enriched, with calcium propionate, 3.5', toasted	1	285	11	57	3	6	1.7	0.3	475
Bagel, poppy seed, enriched, with calcium propionate, 4"	1	270	11	53	2	5	1.7	0.4	470

BREADS AND CRACKERS continued

Item	Serving Size	Calories	Protein	Carb	Fiber	Sugar	Total Fat	Sat Fat	Sodium
Bagel, poppy seed, enriched, with calcium propionate, 4", toasted	1	285	11	57	3	6	1.7	0.3	475
Bagel, poppy seed, enriched, with calcium propionate, 4.5"	1	337	13	66	3	7	2.1	0.5	587
Bagel, poppy seed, enriched, with calcium propionate, 4.5", toasted	1	354	14	70	3	7	2.1	0.4	590
Bagel, poppy seed, mini, enriched, with calcium propionate, 2.5"	1	67	3	13	1	1	0.4	0.3	116
Bagel, poppy seed, mini, enriched, with calcium propionate, 2.5", toasted	1	69	3	14	1	1	0.4	0.1	115
Bagel, sesame seed, enriched, with calcium propionate, 3.5"	1	270	11	53	2	5	1.7	0.4	470
Bagel, sesame seed, enriched, with calcium propionate, 3.5", toasted	1	285	11	57	3	6	1.7	0.3	475
Bagel, sesame, enriched, with calcium propionate, 3"	1	171	7	35	2	4	1.0	0.3	309
Bagel, sesame, enriched, with calcium propionate, 3", toasted	1	187	7	37	2	4	1.1	0.2	312
Bagel, sesame, enriched, with calcium propionate, 4"	1	270	11	53	2	5	1.7	0.4	470
Bagel, sesame, enriched, with calcium propionate, 4", toasted	1	285	11	57	3	6	1.7	0.3	475
Bagel, sesame, enriched, with calcium propionate, 4.5"	1	337	13	66	3	7	2.1	0.5	587
Bagel, sesame, enriched, with calcium propionate, 4.5', toasted	1	354	14	70	3	7	2.1	0.4	590
Bagel, sesame, mini, enriched, with calcium propionate, 2.5"	1	67	3	13	1	1	0.4	0.3	116
Bagel, sesame, mini, enriched, with calcium propionate, 2.5", toasted	1	69	3	14	1	1	0.4	0.1	115
Biscuit, buttermilk, lower fat, refrigerated dough, 2"	1	59	2	11	0	2	1.0	0.3	287

BREADS AND CRACKERS continued

Item	Serving Size	Calories	Protein	Carb	Fiber	Sugar	Total Fat	Sat Fat	Sodium
Biscuit, buttermilk, prepared from recipe, 1.5"	1	49	1	6	0	0	2.3	0.6	81
Biscuit, buttermilk, prepared from recipe, 2.5"	1	212	4	27	1	1	9.8	2.6	348
Biscuit, buttermilk, prepared from recipe, 4"	1	357	7	45	2	2	16.5	4.4	586
Biscuit, buttermilk, small, 2.5"	1	128	2	17	1	1	5.8	0.9	368
Biscuit, cheese	1	112	3	13	0	1	5.7	1.7	222
Biscuit, plain, dry mix, prepared	1	95	2	14	1	0	3.4	0.8	271
Biscuit, plain, higher fat, refrigerated dough	1	138	3	19	0	3	5.9	1.5	430
Biscuit, plain, higher fat, refrigerated dough, baked, 2.5"	1	95	2	13	0	2	4.0	1.0	292
Biscuit, plain, lower fat, refrigerated dough, 2.25"	1	186	3	25	1	2	8.4	1.3	537
Biscuit, plain, lower fat, refrigerated dough, 2"	1	59	2	11	0	2	1.0	0.3	287
Biscuit, plain, prepared from recipe, 1.5"	1	49	1	6	0	0	2.3	0.6	81
Biscuit, plain, prepared from recipe, 2.5"	1	212	4	27	1	1	9.8	2.6	348
Biscuit, plain, small, 2.5"	1	128	2	17	1	1	5.8	0.9	368
Biscuit, whole wheat	1	116	3	21	4	0	2.5	0.6	295
Bread, barley	1 slice	73	2	14	2	1	0.9	0.2	5
Bread, bran, whole grain, Bran For Life	1 slice	80	4	17	5	1	1.0	0.0	140
Bread, buckwheat	1 slice	70	2	13	1	1	1.0	0.2	4
Bread, buckwheat, toasted	1 slice	72	2	13	1	1	1.1	0.2	4
Bread, cheese	1 slice	71	2	12	1	1	1.3	0.5	141
Bread, cheese, toasted	1 slice	72	2	13	1	1	1.3	0.5	142
Bread, cheese-onion	1 slice	71	2	12	1	1	1.3	0.5	141
Bread, cheese-onion, toasted	1 slice	72	2	13	1	1	1.3	0.5	142
Bread, coffee, Spanish	1 slice	89	2	15	1	3	2.3	0.4	4
Bread, corn & molasses	1 slice	71	2	13	1	2	1.4	0.4	7
Bread, corn & molasses, toasted	1 slice	73	2	13	1	2	1.4	0.4	7

BREADS AND CRACKERS continued

Item	Serving Size	Calories	Protein	Carb	Fiber	Sugar	Total Fat	Sat Fat	Sodium
Bread, Cuban/Spanish/Portuguese	1 slice	71	2	14	1	0	0.8	0.2	158
Bread, Cuban/Spanish/Portuguese, toasted	1 slice	72	2	13	1	0	0.8	0.2	159
Bread, egg	1 slice	113	4	19	1	1	2.4	0.6	197
Bread, egg, toasted	1 slice	117	4	20	1	1	2.4	0.6	200
Bread, French, large slice	1 slice	277	11	54	2	3	1.8	0.5	624
Bread, French, medium slice	1 slice	185	8	36	2	2	1.2	0.3	416
Bread, French, small slice	1 slice	92	4	18	1	1	0.6	0.2	208
Bread, French, toasted, large slice	1 slice	281	11	55	3	3	1.9	0.4	634
Bread, French, toasted, medium slice	1 slice	188	8	37	2	2	1.3	0.3	425
Bread, French, toasted, small slice	1 slice	93	4	18	1	1	0.6	0.2	209
Bread, Indian fry, with lard, Apache	1 slice	87	2	13	1	1	2.8	1.0	188
Bread, Italian, large slice	1 slice	81	3	15	1	0	1.1	0.3	175
Bread, Italian, medium slice	1 slice	54	2	10	1	0	0.7	0.2	117
Bread, Italian, small slice	1 slice	27	1	5	0	0	0.4	0.1	58
Bread, millet, whole grain, wheat, gluten-free	1 slice	100	2	21	1	3	0.5	0.0	170
Bread, multigrain	1 slice	69	4	11	2	2	1.1	0.2	109
Bread, multigrain, large slice	1 slice	109	6	18	3	3	1.7	0.4	172
Bread, multigrain, toasted	1 slice	69	4	11	2	2	1.1	0.2	110
Bread, multigrain, toasted, large slice	1 slice	109	6	18	3	3	1.8	0.4	174
Bread, oat bran	1 slice	71	3	12	1	2	1.3	0.2	122
Bread, oat bran, reduced calorie	1 slice	46	2	10	3	1	0.7	0.1	81
Bread, oat bran, reduced calorie, toasted	1 slice	45	2	9	3	1	0.7	0.1	79
Bread, oat bran, toasted	1 slice	70	3	12	1	2	1.3	0.2	121
Bread, oatmeal	1 slice	73	2	13	1	2	1.2	0.2	162
Bread, oatmeal, toasted	1 slice	73	2	13	1	2	1.2	0.2	163

BREADS AND CRACKERS continued

Item	Serving Size	Calories	Protein	Carb	Fiber	Sugar	Total Fat	Sat Fat	Sodium
Bread, Pan De Torta Salvadoran	1 slice	214	4	28	1	10	9.6	1.7	214
Bread, Pan Dulce	1 slice	231	6	36	1	8	7.3	1.4	144
Bread, piki, with blue cornmeal, Hopi	1 slice	117	3	22	3	1	2.2	0.2	18
Bread, pita, Bible, original	1 slice	160	7	31	2	1	1.5	0.0	115
Bread, pita, Bible, very low salt	1 slice	160	7	30	1	1	2.0	0.0	30
Bread, pita, white, enriched, large, 6 1/2"	1 slice	165	5	33	1	1	0.7	0.1	322
Bread, pita, white, enriched, small, 4"	1 slice	77	3	16	1	0	0.3	0.1	150
Bread, pita, whole wheat, large, 6 1/2"	1 slice	170	6	35	5	1	1.7	0.3	340
Bread, pita, whole wheat, 4"	1 slice	74	3	15	2	0	0.7	0.1	149
Bread, pound cake type	1 slice	214	4	28	1	10	9.6	1.7	214
Bread, protein	1 slice	47	2	8	1	0	0.4	0.1	104
Bread, protein, toasted	1 slice	46	2	8	1	0	0.4	0.1	102
Bread, pumpernickel	1 slice	65	2	12	2	0	0.8	0.1	174
Bread, pumpernickel, toasted	1 slice	80	3	15	2	0	1.0	0.1	214
Bread, Quesadilla Salvadoran	1 slice	206	4	26	0	14	9.4	2.5	280
Bread, raisin pecan, wheat, gluten-free	1 slice	130	2	25	2	6	3.0	0.0	5
Bread, raisin, enriched	1 slice	71	2	14	1	2	1.1	0.3	101
Bread, raisin, enriched, toasted	1 slice	71	2	14	1	2	1.2	0.3	102
Bread, rice almond, wheat, gluten-free	1 slice	120	2	22	2	3	2.5	0.0	5
Bread, rice bran	1 slice	66	2	12	1	1	1.2	0.2	119
Bread, rice bran, toasted	1 slice	66	2	12	1	1	1.3	0.2	120
Bread, rice pecan, wheat, gluten-free	1 slice	130	2	24	2	3	3.0	0.0	5
Bread, rice, Bhutanese red, whole grain, wheat, gluten-free	1 slice	90	1	19	1	2	1.5	0.0	105

BREADS AND CRACKERS continued

Item	Serving Size	Calories	Protein	Carb	Fiber	Sugar	Total Fat	Sat Fat	Sodium
Bread, rice, brown, whole grain, wheat, gluten-free	1 slice	110	2	21	2	3	2.0	0.0	120
Bread, rice, China black, whole grain, wheat, gluten-free	1 slice	90	2	18	1	2	2.0	0.0	105
Bread, rice, white, wheat, gluten-free	1 slice	110	1	22	1	3	2.0	0.0	230
Bread, rye	1 slice	83	3	16	2	1	1.1	0.2	211
Bread, rye, reduced calorie	1 slice	47	2	9	3	1	0.7	0.1	93
Bread, rye, toasted, large slice	1 slice	82	3	15	2	1	1.0	0.2	210
Bread, rye, toasted, regular slice	1 slice	68	2	13	2	1	0.9	0.2	174
Bread, rye, toasted, thin slice	1 slice	51	2	10	1	1	0.7	0.1	130
Bread, Salvadoran sweet cheese	1 slice	206	4	26	0	14	9.4	2.5	280
Bread, sourdough, large slice	1 slice	277	11	54	2	3	1.8	0.5	624
Bread, sourdough, medium slice	1 slice	185	8	36	2	2	1.2	0.3	416
Bread, sourdough, small slice	1 slice	92	4	18	1	1	0.6	0.2	208
Bread, sourdough, toasted, large slice	1 slice	281	11	55	3	3	1.9	0.4	634
Bread, sourdough, toasted, medium slice	1 slice	188	8	37	2	2	1.3	0.3	425
Bread, sourdough, toasted, small slice	1 slice	92	4	18	1	1	0.6	0.2	208
Bread, soy	1 slice	69	3	12	1	2	1.0	0.3	6
Bread, soy, toasted	1 slice	71	3	12	1	2	1.0	0.3	7
Bread, spelt, whole grain	1 slice	110	4	20	3	1	2.0	0.0	160
Bread, sprouted, 7 whole grain, flourless	1 slice	80	4	15	3	1	0.5	0.0	80
Bread, sprouted, carrot raisin	1 slice	130	5	27	5	10	0.0	0.0	6
Bread, sprouted, cinnamon raisin, 7 grain, flourless	1 slice	80	3	19	2	6	0.5	0.0	65

BREADS AND CRACKERS continued

Item	Serving Size	Calories	Protein	Carb	Fiber	Sugar	Total Fat	Sat Fat	Sodium
Bread, sprouted, cinnamon raisin, whole grain, flourless	1 slice	80	3	18	2	5	0.0	0.0	65
Bread, sprouted, millet rice	1 slice	130	5	28	5	9	0.0	0.0	3
Bread, sprouted, sesame, whole grain, flourless	1 slice	80	4	14	3	0	0.5	0.0	80
Bread, sprouted, SunSeed	1 slice	160	6	29	7	11	2.0	0.0	3
Bread, sprouted, whole grain, flourless	1 slice	80	4	15	3	0	0.5	0.0	75
Bread, sprouted, whole grain, low sodium, flourless	1 slice	80	4	15	3	0	0.5	0.0	0
Bread, sprouted, whole grain & seed, flourless	1 slice	80	4	14	3	0	2.0	0.0	65
Bread, sweet, pannetone, Italian style	1 slice	84	2	14	1	5	2.2	1.1	27
Bread, sweet potato	1 slice	77	2	13	1	3	1.6	0.4	21
Bread, sweet yeast	1 slice	231	6	36	1	8	7.3	1.4	144
Bread, tennis, plain, Apache	1 slice	77	3	16	1	1	0.3	0.1	243
Bread, triticale	1 slice	66	2	12	2	1	1.0	0.2	154
Bread, triticale, toasted	1 slice	67	2	13	2	1	1.0	0.2	158
Bread, Vienna, large slice	1 slice	277	11	54	2	3	1.8	0.5	624
Bread, Vienna, medium slice	1 slice	185	8	36	2	2	1.2	0.3	416
Bread, Vienna, small slice	1 slice	92	4	18	1	1	0.6	0.2	208
Bread, Vienna, toasted, large slice	1 slice	281	11	55	3	3	1.9	0.4	634
Bread, Vienna, toasted, medium slice	1 slice	188	8	37	2	2	1.3	0.3	425
Bread, Vienna, toasted, small slice	1 slice	92	4	18	1	1	0.6	0.2	208
Bread, wheat	1 slice	66	3	12	1	1	0.9	0.2	130
Bread, wheat, reduced calorie	1 slice	46	2	10	3	1	0.5	0.1	118
Bread, wheat, toasted	1 slice	75	3	13	1	2	1.0	0.2	147
Bread, wheat bran	1 slice	89	3	17	1	4	1.2	0.3	75
Bread, wheat germ	1 slice	73	3	14	1	1	1.0	0.2	155

BREADS AND CRACKERS continued

Item	Serving Size	Calories	Protein	Carb	Fiber	Sugar	Total Fat	Sat Fat	Sodium
Bread, wheat germ, toasted	1 slice	73	3	14	1	1	0.8	0.2	155
Bread, white, reduced calorie	1 slice	48	2	10	2	1	0.6	0.1	104
Bread, white, soft	1 slice	66	2	13	1	1	0.8	0.2	170
Bread, white, soft, cubes	1 slice	93	3	18	1	2	1.2	0.3	238
Bread, white, soft, large slice	1 slice	80	2	15	1	1	1.0	0.2	204
Bread, white, soft, thin slice	1 slice	53	2	10	1	1	0.7	0.1	136
Bread, white, soft, toasted	1 slice	64	2	12	1	1	0.9	0.1	130
Bread, white, soft, very thin slice	1 slice	40	1	8	0	1	0.5	0.1	102
Bread, white, soft, without crust	1 slice	32	1	6	0	1	0.4	0.1	82
Bread, white, soft, without crust, toasted	1 slice	32	1	6	0	1	0.4	0.1	65
Bread, white, very low sodium	1 slice	67	2	12	1	1	0.9	0.2	7
Bread, whole grain	1 slice	69	4	11	2	2	1.1	0.2	109
Bread, whole grain, toasted, large slice	1 slice	109	6	18	3	3	1.8	0.4	174
Bread, white, soft	1 slice	66	2	13	1	1	0.8	0.2	170
Bread, whole wheat, prepared from recipe	1 slice	70	2	13	2	1	1.4	0.2	87
Bread, whole wheat, toasted	1 slice	73	4	12	2	1	1.0	0.2	140
Breadsticks, plain, 7.5"	1	41	1	7	0	0	1.0	0.1	66
Breadsticks, plain, 9"	1	25	1	4	0	0	0.6	0.1	39
Breadsticks, plain, small, 4"	1	21	1	3	0	0	0.5	0.1	33
Bun, hamburger	1	120	4	21	1	3	1.9	0.5	206
Bun, hamburger, mixed grain	1	113	4	19	2	3	2.6	0.6	197
Bun, hamburger, reduced calorie	1	84	4	18	3	2	0.9	0.1	190
Bun, hamburger, whole wheat	1	114	4	22	3	4	2.0	0.4	206
Bun, hot dog / frankfurter	1	120	4	21	1	3	1.9	0.5	206
Bun, hot dog / frankfurter, mixed grain	1	113	4	19	2	3	2.6	0.6	197

BREADS AND CRACKERS continued

Item	Serving Size	Calories	Protein	Carb	Fiber	Sugar	Total Fat	Sat Fat	Sodium
Bun, hot dog / frankfurter, reduced calorie	1	84	4	18	3	2	0.9	0.1	190
Bun, hot dog / frankfurter, whole wheat	1	114	4	22	3	4	2.0	0.4	206
Cornbread, hush puppies, prepared from recipe	1	74	2	10	1	1	3.0	0.5	147
Crackers, Ak Mak,	5	115	5	20	4	5	2.0	0.0	220
Crackers, animal	2 oz	254	4	42	1	8	7.9	2.0	224
Crackers, cheese, bite size	1 cup	312	6	36	2	0	15.7	5.8	617
Crackers, cheese, cheddar, thin crisps, 100 Calorie pack Kraft Cheese Nips	1 oz	100	2	15	1	0	3.0	1.0	250
Crackers, cheese, goldfish	1 oz	141.75	0	0	0	0	9.45	4.725	283.5
Crackers, cheese, low sodium	1 oz	141.75	0	28.35	0	0	8.505	2.835	141.75
Crackers, cheese, small square	1 oz	141.75	0	28.35	0	0	8.505	2.835	283.5
Crackers, Cuban	1 oz	567	0	113.4	0	28.35	8.505	2.835	368.55
Crackers, garden veggie	1 oz	110	3	18	1	1	3.5	1.5	370
Crackers, graham, chocolate coated, 2 1/2" square	3	203	2	28	1	18	9.7	5.6	122
Crackers, graham, plain, squares	3	89	2	16	1	7	2.1	0.3	127
Crackers, matzo, plain	3/4 oz	84	2	18	1	0	0.3	0.1	0
Crackers, saltine	6	76	2	13	1	0	1.6	0.4	201
Crackers, saltines, low sodium, fat-free	6	76	2	13	1	0	1.6	0.4	114
Crackers, sandwich, cheese, with cheese filling	3	96	2	12	0	2	4.8	0.0	171
Crackers, sandwich, cheese, with peanut butter filling	3	97	2	11	1	1	4.9	0.9	138
Crackers, sandwich, with cheese filling	3	100	2	13	0	1	4.4	1.3	294
Crackers, sandwich, with peanut butter filling	3	104	2	12	1	2	5.2	1.0	151
Crackers, whole wheat, low sodium	7	124	3	19	3	0	4.8	1.0	69
Croissant, butter, large	1	272	6	31	2	8	14.1	7.8	498

BREADS AND CRACKERS continued

Item	Serving Size	Calories	Protein	Carb	Fiber	Sugar	Total Fat	Sat Fat	Sodium
Croissant, butter, medium	1	231	5	26	2	7	12.0	6.7	424
Croissant, butter, mini	1	114	2	13	1	3	5.9	3.3	208
Croissant, butter, small	1	171	3	19	1	5	8.8	4.9	312
Matzo balls	1	48	2	6	0	0	1.7	0.4	12
Roll, cheese	1	238	5	29	1	0	12.0	4.0	236
Roll, dinner, brown & serve	1	87	3	15	1	2	1.8	0.4	150
Roll, dinner, egg, 2 1/2"	1	107	3	18	1	2	2.2	0.6	191
Roll, dinner, large	1	133	5	22	1	2	2.8	0.6	230
Roll, dinner, oat bran	1	78	3	13	1	2	1.5	0.2	136
Roll, dinner, rye, large, 3 1/2"–4"	1	123	4	23	2	1	1.5	0.3	384
Roll, dinner, rye, medium	1	103	4	19	2	0	1.2	0.2	321
Roll, dinner, rye, small, 2 3/8"	1	80	3	15	1	0	1.0	0.2	250
Roll, dinner, small, 2" x 2"	1	78	3	13	1	2	1.6	0.4	134
Roll, dinner, wheat	1	76	2	13	1	1	1.8	0.4	95
Roll, dinner, whole wheat	1	74	2	14	2	2	1.3	0.2	134
Roll, dinner, whole wheat, medium, 2 1/2"	1	96	3	18	3	3	1.7	0.3	172
Roll, French	1	105	3	19	1	0	1.6	0.4	231
Roll, garlic	1	84	2	14	1	1	2.0	0.5	145
Roll, hard, 3 1/2"	1	167	6	30	1	1	2.5	0.4	310
Roll, hoagie, whole wheat, large	1	359	12	69	10	11	6.3	1.1	645
Roll, kaiser, 3 1/2"	1	167	6	30	1	1	2.5	0.4	310
Roll, Mexican, bolillo	1	198	7	39	1	0	1.2	0.3	233
Roll, onion, large	1	133	5	22	1	2	2.8	0.6	230
Roll, pan, small	1	87	3	15	1	2	1.8	0.4	150
Roll, pumpernickel, medium, 2 1/2"	1	100	4	19	2	0	1.0	0.2	205
Roll, pumpernickel, small, 2" cubic square	1	78	3	15	2	0	0.8	0.1	159
Roll, submarine, whole wheat, large	1	359	12	69	10	11	6.3	1.1	645
Roll, submarine, whole wheat, medium	1	250	8	48	7	8	4.4	0.8	449
Rolls, submarine, whole wheat, small	1	173	6	33	5	6	3.1	0.5	311

CEREALS

Item	Serving Size	Calories	Protein	Carb	Fiber	Sugar	Total Fat	Sat Fat	Sodium
Arrowhead Mills, hot cereal, 4 Grain Plus Flax	1 packet	140	6	28	9	0	1.5	0.0	0
Arrowhead Mills, hot cereal, 7 Grain	1 packet	220	12	41	5	8	2.5	0.0	210
Arrowhead Mills, amaranth flakes	3/4 cup	100	3	24	4	5	0.0	0.0	90
Arrowhead Mills spelt flakes	1 cup	120	4	24	3	3	1.0	0.0	100
Barbara's Bakery Puffins, cinnamon	3/4 cup	100	2	26	6	6	1.0	0.0	150
Barbara's Bakery Puffins, honey rice	3/4 cup	120	2	25	2	6	1.5	0.0	125
Barbara's Bakery Puffins, original	3/4 cup	90	2	23	5	5	1.0	0.0	190
Barbara's Bakery Puffins, peanut butter	3/4 cup	110	3	23	2	6	2.0	0.5	230
Barbara's Bakery Weetabix	1 biscuit	67	2	14	2	2	0.5	0.1	70
Bob's Red Mill hot cereal, 5 grain rolled	1 packet	120	5	24	5	0	1.5	0.0	0
Bob's Red Mill hot cereal, 7 grain	1 packet	140	6	28	5	1	1.5	0.0	0
Bob's Red Mill hot cereal, 8 grain, wheatless	1 packet	110	4	20	3	0	2.0	1.0	5
Bob's Red Mill hot cereal, kamut, organic whole grain	1/4 cup	120	5	26	4	0	1.0	0.0	0
Bob's Red Mill hot cereal, Mighty Tasty, dry	1/4 cup	150	4	31	4	0	1.5	0.0	5
Bob's Red Mill hot cereal, Right Stuff, 6 grain with flaxseed	1 packet	140	6	27	4	2	2.0	2.0	2
Bob's Red Mill hot cereal, Scottish oatmeal	1 packet	140	6	27	4	0	2.5	0.5	0

CEREALS continued

Item	Serving Size	Calories	Protein	Carb	Fiber	Sugar	Total Fat	Sat Fat	Sodium
Bob's Red Mill muesli, old country style	1/4 cup	110	4	21	4	5	3.0	0.0	0
Bran flakes	3/4 cup	96	3	24	5	6	0.7	0.1	220
Cap'N Crunch	3/4 cup	108	1	23	1	12	1.6	0.4	202
Cap'N Crunch, crunch berries	3/4 cup	104	1	22	1	12	1.5	0.4	182
Cap'N Crunch, peanut butter crunch	3/4 cup	112	2	21	1	9	2.5	0.5	200
Corn, puffed, frosted, chocolate-flavored	1 cup	122	1	26	1	14	1.1	0.3	201
Corn and Rice	1 cup	110	2	25	0	3	0.3	0.1	231
Cornflakes, low sodium	1 cup	100	2	22	0	2	0.1	0.0	2
Frosted oat, with marshmallows	1 cup	109	2	24	1	12	1.0	0.2	158
General Mills, Basic 4	1 cup	210	4	44	3	14	3.0	0.5	320
General Mills, Cheerios	1 cup	111	3	22	3	1	1.8	0.4	273
General Mills, Cheerios, apple cinnamon	3/4 cup	118	2	25	1	13	1.5	0.3	120
General Mills, Cheerios, berry burst, triple berry	1 cup	110	3	24	2	11	1.5	0.5	180
General Mills, Cheerios, frosted	1 cup	115	2	26	1	13	0.9	0.2	210
General Mills, Cheerios, fruity	3/4 cup	100	1	23	2	9	1.0	0.0	135
General Mills, Cheerios, honey nut	1 cup	112	3	24	2	11	1.2	0.2	269
General Mills, Cheerios, multigrain	1 cup	108	2	24	3	6	1.2	0.3	201
General Mills, Cheerios, yogurt burst, strawberry	1 cup	120	2	24	2	9	1.5	0.5	180
General Mills Chex, chocolate	3/4 cup	130	2	26	1	8	2.5	0.5	230
General Mills, Chex, corn	1 cup	112	2	26	1	3	0.3	0.1	288

CEREALS continued

Item	Serving Size	Calories	Protein	Carb	Fiber	Sugar	Total Fat	Sat Fat	Sodium
General Mills, Chex, honey nut	3/4 cup	114	2	26	0	10	0.6	0.1	224
General Mills, Chex, multibran	1 cup	166	3	41	6	11	1.2	0.2	322
General Mills, Chex, rice	1 1/4 cup	117	2	27	0	3	0.3	0.1	292
General Mills, Chex, wheat	1 cup	104	3	24	3	3	0.6	0.1	267
General Mills, Cinnamon Toast Crunch	3/4 cup	127	2	24	1	10	3.3	0.5	206
General Mills, Cocoa Puffs	3/4 cup	108	1	23	1	13	1.4	0.0	144
General Mills, Cookie Crisp	1 cup	120	1	26	1	13	1.5	0.0	170
General Mills, Cookie Crisp, double chocolate	1 1/4 cup	130	1	26	1	15	2.5	0.0	140
General Mills, Fiber One	1/2 cup	60	2	25	14	0	1.0	0.1	105
General Mills, Fiber One, caramel delight	1 cup	180	3	41	9	10	3.0	0.0	260
General Mills, Fiber One, honey clusters	1 cup	160	5	42	13	6	1.5	0.0	280
General Mills, Fiber One, raisin bran clusters	1 cup	170	4	45	11	13	1.0	0.0	260
General Mills, Golden Grahams	3/4 cup	120	1	26	1	10	1.0	0.1	270
General Mills, Hearty Morning	1 cup	200	5	43	8	11	2.5	0.5	360
General Mills, Kix	1 1/4 cup	110	2	25	3	3	1.0	0.2	199
General Mills, Kix, berry berry	3/4 cup	104	1	23	1	8	1.3	0.0	139
General Mills, Lucky Charms	3/4 cup	110	2	22	1	11	1.0	0.2	183
General Mills Lucky Charms, chocolate	3/4 cup	110	1	25	1	12	1.0	0.2	149
General Mills, raisin bran	1 cup	164	3	41	5	18	1.0	0.0	231

CEREALS continued

Item	Serving Size	Calories	Protein	Carb	Fiber	Sugar	Total Fat	Sat Fat	Sodium
General Mills raisin nut bran	3/4 cup	178	4	38	5	13	3.1	0.5	223
General Mills, Reese's Puffs	3/4 cup	126	2	22	1	12	3.4	0.5	193
General Mills, Total, cinnamon crunch	1 cup	190	4	40	4	9	2.5	0.0	200
General Mills, Total, cornflakes	1 1/3 cup	112	2	26	1	3	0.5	0.1	209
General Mills, Total, cranberry crunch	1 1/4 cup	190	4	48	4	16	1.6	0.2	230
General Mills, Total, honey nut clusters	1 cup	218	4	48	3	18	2.6	0.0	290
General Mills, Total, raisin bran	1 cup	164	3	41	5	18	1.0	0.2	231
General Mills, Trix	1 cup	128	1	28	1	12	1.6	0.2	180
General Mills, Wheaties	3/4 cup	99	3	22	3	4	0.9	0.1	189
Granola, homemade	1 oz	139	4	15	3	6	6.8	1.2	7
Grits, corn, white, regular, enriched, cooked with water & salt	1 cup	182	4	38	2	0	1.2	0.2	573
Grits, corn, white, regular, enriched, cooked with water, without salt	1 cup	182	4	38	2	0	1.2	0.2	5
Grits, corn, white, regular, enriched, dry	1/3 cup	206	4	45	2	0	0.8	0.2	1
Grits, corn, white, regular, unenriched, cooked with water & salt	3/4 cup	107	3	23	1	0	0.4	0.0	406
Grits, corn, white, regular, unenriched, cooked with water, without salt	3/4 cup	107	3	23	1	0	0.4	0.0	4
Grits, corn, white, regular, unenriched, dry	1/3 cup	191	5	41	1	0	0.6	0.1	1
Grits, corn, white, quick, enriched, cooked with water & salt	1 cup	182	4	38	2	0	1.2	0.2	573
Grits, corn, white, quick, enriched, cooked with water without salt	1 cup	182	4	38	2	0	1.2	0.2	5

CEREALS continued

Item	Serving Size	Calories	Protein	Carb	Fiber	Sugar	Total Fat	Sat Fat	Sodium
Grits, corn, white, quick, enriched, dry	1/3 cup	206	4	45	2	0	0.8	0.2	1
Grits, corn, white, quick, unenriched, cooked with water & salt	3/4 cup	107	3	23	1	0	0.4	0.0	406
Grits, corn, white, quick, unenriched, ckd with water without salt	3/4 cup	107	3	23	1	0	0.4	0.0	4
Grits, corn, white, quick, unenriched, dry	1/3 cup	191	5	41	1	0	0.6	0.1	1
Grits, corn, yellow, regular, enriched, cooked with water & salt	1 cup	151	3	32	2	0	0.9	0.1	520
Grits, corn, yellow, regular, enriched, cooked with water without salt	1 cup	151	3	32	2	0	0.9	0.1	5
Grits, corn, yellow, regular, unenriched, cooked with water & salt	3/4 cup	107	3	23	1	0	0.4	0.1	406
Grits, corn, yellow, regular, unenriched, cooked with water, without salt	3/4 cup	107	3	23	1	0	0.4	0.0	4
Grits, corn, yellow, regular, unenriched, dry	1/3 cup	191	5	41	1	0	0.6	0.1	1
Grits, corn, yellow, quick, enriched, cooked with water & salt	1 cup	151	3	32	2	0	0.9	0.1	520
Grits, corn, yellow, quick, enriched, cooked with water, without salt	1 cup	151	3	32	2	0	0.9	0.1	5
Grits, corn, yellow, quick, unenriched, cooked with water & salt	3/4 cup	107	3	23	1	0	0.4	0.1	406
Grits, corn, yellow, quick, unenriched, cooked with water, without salt	3/4 cup	107	3	23	1	0	0.4	0.0	4
Grits, corn, yellow, quick, unenriched, dry	1/3 cup	191	5	41	1	0	0.6	0.1	1
Hain Celestial, Healthy Fiber, multigrain flakes	3/4 cup	100	3	23	4	3	0.0	0.0	15

CEREALS continued

Item	Serving Size	Calories	Protein	Carb	Fiber	Sugar	Total Fat	Sat Fat	Sodium
Health Valley Fiber 7	3/4 cup	100	3	24	4	5	0.0	0.0	90
Health Valley Fiber 7, multigrain flakes	3/4 cup	100	3	24	4	5	0.0	0.0	90
Hot cereal, farina, enriched, cooked with water & salt	1 cup	123	4	25	2	2	0.8	0.2	294
Hot cereal, farina, enriched, cooked with water, without salt	1 cup	127	4	26	2	2	0.8	0.2	43
Hot cereal, farina, unenriched, dry	1 cup	649	19	137	3	0	0.9	0.1	5
Hot cereal, oatmeal, cinnamon spice, fortified, instant	1 packet	170	4	35	3	16	2.2	0.4	246
Hot cereal, oatmeal, cinnamon spice, fortified, instant, prepared with water	1 packet	177	4	36	3	16	2.2	0.4	249
Hot cereal, oatmeal, plain, fortified, instant, prepared with water	1 packet	120	4	21	3	1	2.4	0.5	87
Hot cereal, oatmeal, plain, unenriched, cooked, with water & salt	3/4 cup	119	5	20	3	0	2.5	0.5	119
Hot cereal, oatmeal, plain, unenriched, cooked with water, without salt	3/4 cup	124	5	21	3	1	2.7	0.5	7
Hot cereal, oatmeal, plain, unenriched, dry	1/3 cup	102	4	18	3	0	1.8	0.3	2
Hot cereal, oatmeal, raisin spice, fortified, instant	1 packet	155	3	33	3	16	1.8	0.2	242
Hot cereal, oatmeal, raisin spice, fortified, instant, prepared with water	1 packet	162	3	33	3	16	1.9	0.3	245
Hot cereal, whole wheat, natural, cooked with water & salt	3/4 cup	113	4	25	3	0	0.7	0.1	424

CEREALS continued

Item	Serving Size	Calories	Protein	Carb	Fiber	Sugar	Total Fat	Sat Fat	Sodium
Hot cereal, whole wheat, natural, cooked with water, without salt	3/4 cup	113	4	25	3	0	0.7	0.1	0
Hot cereal, whole wheat, natural, dry	1/3 cup	106	4	23	3	0	0.6	0.1	1
Kellogg's 7 whole grain, flakes	3/4 cup	105	3	25	3	3	0.6	0.1	91
Kellogg's 7 whole grain, puffs	3/4 cup	29	1	7	1	0	0.1	0.0	0
Kellogg's Apple Jacks	1 cup	102	1	25	3	12	0.6	0.1	124
Kellogg's Cocoa Krispies	3/4 cup	118	2	27	1	11	0.9	0.6	197
Kellogg's Corn Pops	1 cup	110	1	26	0	14	0.2	0.1	112
Kellogg's Crispix	1 cup	109	2	25	0	3	0.4	0.1	222
Kellogg's Froot Loops	1 cup	118	1	27	0	13	0.6	0.4	141
Kellogg's Froot Loops, with marshmallow	1 cup	120	1	27	1	16	1.0	0.5	110
Kellogg's Frosted Flakes	3/4 cup	110	1	27	1	12	0.1	0.0	139
Kellogg's Frosted Flakes, reduced sugar	1 cup	117	2	28	0	8	0.1	0.0	178
Kellogg's Frosted Krispies	3/4 cup	115	2	27	0	12	0.3	0.1	193
Kellogg's Frosted Mini Wheats	5 biscuits	175	5	42	5	11	0.8	0.2	5
Kellogg's Frosted Mini Wheats, bite-size	27 biscuits	203	6	48	6	12	0.9	0.2	5
Kellogg's Frosted Mini Wheats, maple & brown sugar, bite-size	24 biscuits	185	4	43	5	13	0.8	0.2	1
Kellogg's Frosted Mini Wheats, strawberry delight	25 biscuits	180	4	43	5	12	0.9	0.2	0

CEREALS continued

Item	Serving Size	Calories	Protein	Carb	Fiber	Sugar	Total Fat	Sat Fat	Sodium
Kellogg's Frosted Mini Wheats, strawberry delight, bite-size	26 biscuits	180	4	43	5	12	0.9	0.2	0
Kellogg's Fruit Harvest, strawberry blueberry	3/4 cup	107	2	25	1	10	0.4	0.1	137
Kellogg's Go Lean	1 cup	148	14	30	10	6	1.0	0.2	86
Kellogg's Go Lean Crunch!	1 cup	200	9	36	8	13	3.1	0.3	204
Kellogg's Go Lean Crunch!, honey almond flax	1 cup	202	9	36	9	12	4.4	0.4	138
Kellogg's Good Friends	1 cup	167	5	43	12	9	1.9	0.2	129
Kellogg's Heart to Heart, honey toasted oat	3/4 cup	118	4	25	5	5	1.7	0.3	79
Kellogg's Heart to Heart, oat flakes & wild blueberry	1 cup	204	6	42	4	12	2.6	0.5	133
Kellogg's Honey Smacks	3/4 cup	104	2	24	1	15	0.5	0.1	50
Kellogg's Mueslix, with raisins, dates, & almonds	2/3 cup	196	5	40	4	17	3.0	0.4	170
Kellogg's Product 19	1 cup	100	2	25	1	4	0.4	0.1	207
Kellogg's Raisin Bran	1 cup	190	5	46	7	18	1.3	0.2	342
Kellogg's Raisin Bran Crunch	1 cup	188	3	45	4	20	1.0	0.2	209
Kellogg's Rice Krispies	1 1/4 cup	128	2	28	0	3	0.3	0.1	299
Kellogg's Rice Krispies Treats	3/4 cup	120	1	25	0	9	1.4	0.3	166
Kellogg's Smart Start, strong heart, antioxidants	1 cup	182	4	43	3	14	0.7	0.1	275

CEREALS continued

Item	Serving Size	Calories	Protein	Carb	Fiber	Sugar	Total Fat	Sat Fat	Sodium
Kellogg's Smart Start, strong heart, maple brown sugar	1 1/4 cup	220	6	48	5	17	2.2	0.4	140
Kellogg's Special K	1 cup	117	7	22	1	4	0.5	0.1	224
Kellogg's Special K, chocolatey delight	3/4 cup	120	2	26	1	9	1.8	1.5	180
Kellogg's Special K, fruit & yogurt	3/4 cup	122	2	28	2	11	0.9	0.5	137
Kellogg's Special K, red berries	1 cup	114	4	25	1	10	0.3	0.1	220
Kellogg's Special K, vanilla almond	3/4 cup	115	2	25	2	8	1.5	0.2	164
Malt-O-Meal frosted flakes	3/4 cup	116	2	27	1	11	0.1	0.0	172
Muesli, dried fruit & nut	1 cup	289	8	66	6	26	4.2	0.7	196
Nature's Path hot oatmeal, Optimum, cranberry ginger	1 packet	150	5	30	3	11	2.5	0.5	170
Nature's Path hot oatmeal, OptimumCinnamon, blueberry flaxseed	1 packet	150	5	29	4	9	3.0	0.5	120
Nature's Path Kamut Puffs	1 cup	50	2	11	2	0	0.0	0.0	0
Nature's Path Millet Puffs	1 cup	50	2	14	1	0	0.0	0.0	0
Nature's Path Millet Rice Flakes	3/4 cup	110	3	21	3	3	1.5	0.5	110
Nature's Path MesaSunrise Flakes, gluten-free	3/4 cup	120	3	24	3	4	1.5	0.0	130
Nature's Path Multigrain Oatbran Flakes	3/4 cup	110	4	24	5	4	1.0	0.0	115
Nature's Path Optimum Slim	1 cup	180	9	38	11	10	2.5	0.0	250

CEREALS continued

Item	Serving Size	Calories	Protein	Carb	Fiber	Sugar	Total Fat	Sat Fat	Sodium
Nature's Path Optimum Rebound	3/4 cup	190	10	35	6	9	6.0	1.0	140
Nature's Path spelt flakes	3/4 cup	80	3	20	3	3	0.5	0.0	150
Oat, corn, & wheat, maple flavor, squares, with added sugars	1 cup	129	2	24	1	11	2.9	0.4	130
Rice, puffed, fortified	1 cup	56	1	13	0	0	0.1	0.0	0
Rice crisps	1 1/4 cup	126	2	28	0	3	0.4	0.1	280
Shredded wheat, without sugar & salt, rectangle biscuits	2 biscuits	155	5	36	6	0	1.0	0.2	3
Shredded wheat, without sugar & salt, round biscuits	2 biscuits	128	4	30	5	0	0.8	0.2	2
Wheat, puffed, fortified	1 cup	44	2	10	1	0	0.1	0.0	0
Wheat & bran, fruit & nuts, with added sugars	1 cup	212	4	42	5	16	3.1	0.4	280
Wheat & malt barley flakes	3/4 cup	106	3	24	3	5	0.8	0.2	140
Wheat germ, toasted	1 oz	108	8	14	4	2	3.0	0.5	1
Whole wheat, rolled oats, & pecans, with added sugars	2/3 cup	216	5	38	4	8	6.3	0.7	214

CHEESE

Item	Serving Size	Calories	Protein	Carb	Fiber	Sugar	Total Fat	Sat Fat	Sodium
American, pasteurized	1.5 oz	159	9	1	0	0	13.3	8.4	276
American, pasteurized, fat-free	1.5 oz	63	10	6	0	4	0.3	0.2	650
American, pasteurized, low fat	1.5 oz	77	10	1	0	0	3.0	1.9	608
American, pasteurized, low sodium	1.5 oz	160	9	1	0	0	13.3	8.4	3
American, pasteurized, with disodium phosphate	1.5 oz	159	9	1	0	0	13.3	8.4	633
Blue	1.5 oz	150	9	1	0	0	12.2	7.9	593
Blue, crumbled	1.5 oz	150	9	1	0	0	12.2	7.9	593
Brick	1.5 oz	158	10	1	0	0	12.6	8.0	238
Brie	1.5 oz	142	9	0	0	0	11.8	7.4	267
Camembert	1.5 oz	128	8	0	0	0	10.3	6.5	358
Cheddar	1.5 oz	171	11	1	0	0	14.1	9.0	264
Cheddar, low fat	1.5 oz	74	10	1	0	0	3.0	1.8	260
Cheddar, low sodium	1.5 oz	169	10	1	0	0	13.9	8.8	9
Cheddar, pasteurized, fat-free	1.5 oz	63	10	6	0	4	0.3	0.2	650
Cheddar, pasteurized, low sodium	1.5 oz	160	9	1	0	0	13.3	8.4	3
Cheddar, reduced fat	1.5 oz	120	12	1	0	0	7.8	4.9	308
Cheese product, American, pasteurized	1.5 oz	140	8	3	0	3	10.7	6.3	538
Cheese product, American, pasteurized, reduced fat	1.5 oz	102	7	5	0	3	6.0	3.8	675
Cheese product, American, pasteurized, reduced fat, with vitamin D	1.5 oz	102	7	5	0	3	6.0	3.8	675
Cheese product, American, pasteurized, with disodium phosphate	1.5 oz	139	8	3	0	3	10.5	6.6	679
Cheese product, cheddar, pasteurized, reduced fat	1.5 oz	102	7	5	0	3	6.0	3.8	675
Cheese spread, American	1.5 oz	123	7	4	0	3	9.0	5.7	572

CHEESE continued

Item	Serving Size	Calories	Protein	Carb	Fiber	Sugar	Total Fat	Sat Fat	Sodium
Cheese spread, cream cheese base	1.5 oz	125	3	1	0	1	12.2	7.7	286
Cheese substitute, American, low cholesterol	1.5 oz	166	11	0	0	0	13.6	2.5	285
Cheese substitute, American cheddar	1.5 oz	102	7	5	0	3	6.0	3.7	572
Cheese substitute, cheddar, low cholesterol	1.5 oz	166	11	0	0	0	13.6	2.5	285
Cheese substitute, mozzarella	1.5 oz	105	5	10	0	10	5.2	1.6	291
Chevres, soft	1.5 oz	114	8	0	0	0	9.0	6.2	156
Colby	1.5 oz	168	10	1	0	0	13.7	8.6	257
Colby, low fat	1.5 oz	74	10	1	0	0	3.0	1.8	260
Colby, low sodium	1.5 oz	169	10	1	0	0	13.9	8.8	9
Cottage cheese, 1% fat	1.5 oz	31	5	1	0	1	0.4	0.3	173
Cottage cheese, 1% fat, reduced lactose	1.5 oz	31	5	1	0	1	0.4	0.3	94
Cottage cheese, 1% fat, unsalted	1.5 oz	31	5	1	0	1	0.4	0.3	6
Cottage cheese, 1% fat, with vegetables	1.5 oz	28	5	1	0	1	0.4	0.3	171
Cottage cheese, 2% fat	1.5 oz	37	5	2	0	2	1.0	0.4	140
Cottage cheese, creamed, large curd, not packed	1.5 oz	42	5	1	0	1	1.8	0.7	155
Cottage cheese, creamed, small curd, not packed	1.5 oz	42	5	1	0	1	1.8	0.7	155
Cottage cheese, creamed, with fruit	1.5 oz	41	5	2	0	1	1.6	1.0	146
Cottage cheese, low fat, low sodium	1.5 oz	31	5	1	0	1	0.4	0.3	6
Cottage cheese, nonfat, large curd, dry	1.5 oz	31	4	3	0	1	0.1	0.1	140
Cottage cheese, nonfat, small curd, dry	1.5 oz	31	4	3	0	1	1.8	1.1	171
Cottage cheese, with vegetables	1.5 oz	40	5	1	0	1	14.6	8.2	137
Cream cheese	1.5 oz	145	3	2	0	0	14.8	9.3	126
Cream cheese, fat-free	1.5 oz	45	7	3	0	2	6.5	3.9	200

CHEESE continued

Item	Serving Size	Calories	Protein	Carb	Fiber	Sugar	Total Fat	Sat Fat	Sodium
Cream cheese, low fat	1.5 oz	85	3	3	0	2	6.5	3.9	200
Cream cheese, low fat, whipped	1.5 oz	85	3	3	0	1	9.7	5.4	142
Cream cheese, Neufchâtel	1.5 oz	108	4	2	0	1	9.7	5.4	142
Cream cheese, whipped	1.5 oz	145	3	2	0	0	3.4	0.9	57
Edam	1.5 oz	152	11	1	0	1	11.8	7.5	410
Emmentaler	1.5 oz	162	11	2	0	1	11.8	7.6	82
Feta	1.5 oz	112	6	2	0	2	9.0	6.4	475
Fontina	1.5 oz	165	11	1	0	1	13.2	8.2	340
Goat, hard	1.5 oz	192	13	1	0	1	15.1	10.5	147
Goat, semi-soft	1.5 oz	155	9	1	0	1	12.7	8.8	219
Goat, soft	1.5 oz	114	8	0	0	0	9.0	6.2	156
Gouda	1.5 oz	151	11	1	0	1	11.7	7.5	348
Gruyère	1.5 oz	176	13	0	0	0	13.8	8.0	143
Limburger	1.5 oz	139	9	0	0	0	11.6	7.1	340
Mexican, queso añejo, crumbled	1.5 oz	159	9	2	0	2	12.7	8.1	481
Mexican, queso asadero	1.5 oz	151	10	1	0	1	12.0	7.6	279
Mexican, queso chihuahua	1.5 oz	159	9	2	0	2	12.6	8.0	262
Mexican blend, reduced fat	1.5 oz	120	10	1	0	0	8.2	4.9	330
Monterey Jack	1.5 oz	159	10	0	0	0	12.9	8.1	228
Monterey, low fat	1.5 oz	132	12	0	0	0	9.2	6.0	240
Mozzarella, low moisture, part skim	1.5 oz	128	11	2	0	0	8.5	4.6	225
Mozzarella, low moisture, whole milk	1.5 oz	135	9	1	0	0	10.5	6.6	176
Mozzarella, low sodium	1.5 oz	119	12	1	0	1	7.3	4.6	7
Mozzarella, nonfat, shred	1.5 oz	60	13	1	1	1	0.0	0.0	316
Mozzarella, part skim	1.5 oz	108	10	1	0	0	6.8	4.3	263
Mozzarella, whole milk	1.5 oz	128	9	1	0	0	9.5	5.6	267
Muenster	1.5 oz	156	10	0	0	0	12.8	8.1	267
Muenster, low fat	1.5 oz	115	11	1	0	1	7.5	4.7	255

CHEESE continued

Item	Serving Size	Calories	Protein	Carb	Fiber	Sugar	Total Fat	Sat Fat	Sodium
Parmesan	1.5 oz	176	16	1	0	0	11.6	7.4	721
Parmesan, dried, grated, reduced fat	1.5 oz	113	9	1	0	0	8.5	5.7	650
Parmesan, fat-free, topping	1.5 oz	157	17	17	0	1	2.1	1.3	489
Parmesan, grated	1.5 oz	183	16	2	0	0	12.2	7.4	650
Parmesan, hard	1.5 oz	167	15	1	0	0	11.0	7.0	681
Parmesan, low sodium	1.5 oz	192	18	2	0	0	12.8	8.1	27
Pimento, pasteurized	1.5 oz	159	9	1	0	0	13.3	8.4	607
Port du Salut	1.5 oz	150	10	0	0	0	12.0	7.1	227
Provolone	1.5 oz	149	11	1	0	0	11.3	7.3	373
Provolone, reduced fat	1.5 oz	117	11	1	0	0	7.5	4.8	373
Ricotta, part skim	1.5 oz	59	5	2	0	0	3.4	2.1	53
Ricotta, whole milk	1.5 oz	74	5	1	0	0	5.5	3.5	36
Romano	1.5 oz	165	14	2	0	0	11.5	7.3	510
Samsor	1.5 oz	162	11	2	0	1	11.8	7.6	82
Sweitzer	1.5 oz	162	11	2	0	1	11.8	7.6	82
Swiss	1.5 oz	162	11	2	0	1	11.8	7.6	82
Swiss, low fat	1.5 oz	74	12	1	0	1	2.2	1.4	111
Swiss, low sodium	1.5 oz	159	12	1	0	1	11.7	7.5	6
Swiss, pasteurized, low fat	1.5 oz	70	11	2	0	1	2.2	1.4	608
Swiss, pasteurized, with disodium phosphate	1.5 oz	142	11	1	0	1	10.6	6.8	583

CONDIMENTS, DRESSINGS, MARINADES, AND SPREADS

Item	Serving Size	Calories	Protein	Carb	Fiber	Sugar	Total Fat	Sat Fat	Sodium
Dip, sour cream, with onion soup mix, reduced calorie	2 oz	83	2	4	0	3	6.5	4.0	400
Dressing, mayonnaise, light	2 oz	184	0	5	0	2	18.8	3.0	382
Dressing, mayonnaise, low sodium, low calorie	2 oz	131	0	9	0	2	10.9	1.9	62
Dressing, mayonnaise, reduced calorie, cholesterol-free	2 oz	189	1	4	0	2	18.9	2.6	416
Dressing, mayonnaise, soybean & safflower oil	2 oz	407	1	2	0	0	45.0	4.9	322
Dressing, mayonnaise, soybean oil	2 oz	407	1	2	0	1	45.0	6.7	322
Dressing, mayonnaise-type	2 oz	221	1	14	0	4	18.9	2.8	403
Dressing, mayonnaise-type, fat-free	2 oz	48	0	9	1	6	1.5	0.3	447
Dressing, mayonnaise-type, low calorie	2 oz	149	1	14	0	2	10.8	1.7	392
Dressing, mayonnaise-type, no cholesterol	2 oz	390	0	0	0	0	44.1	6.1	276
Dressing, mayonnaise-type, no cholesterol, diet	2 oz	221	1	14	0	4	18.9	2.8	403
Dressing, mayonnaise-type, soybean	2 oz	132	0	9	0	3	10.9	1.9	282
Dressing, mayonnaise-type, soybean, no cholesterol	2 oz	273	0	9	0	3	27.0	4.3	200
Dressing, mayonnaise-type, tofu	2 oz	183	3	2	1	0	18.0	1.7	438
Dressing, sour, non-butterfat, cultured, filled cream-type	2 oz	101	2	3	0	3	9.4	7.5	27
Fruit butter, apple	2 oz	98	0	24	1	20	0.2	0.0	9
Gravy, beef, canned	2 oz	30	2	3	0	0	1.3	0.7	318
Gravy, chicken, canned	2 oz	45	1	3	0	0	3.2	0.8	327

CONDIMENTS, DRESSINGS, MARINADES, AND SPREADS continued

Item	Serving Size	Calories	Protein	Carb	Fiber	Sugar	Total Fat	Sat Fat	Sodium
Gravy, meat, low sodium, prepared	2 oz	30	2	3	0	0	1.4	0.6	10
Gravy, poultry, low sodium, prepared	2 oz	30	2	3	0	0	1.4	0.6	10
Gravy, sausage, country style, canned	2 oz	67	2	3	0	1	5.8	1.4	260
Gravy, turkey, canned	2 oz	29	1	3	0	0	1.2	0.4	327
Horseradish, prepared	2 oz	27	1	6	2	5	0.4	0.1	178
Jam	2 oz	158	0	39	1	27	0.0	0.0	18
Jam, any flavor, with sodium saccharin	2 oz	75	0	30	1	21	0.2	0.0	0
Jam, apricot	2 oz	137	0	37	0	25	0.1	0.0	23
Jelly	2 oz	151	0	40	1	29	0.0	0.0	17
Jelly, reduced sugar, prepared from recipe	2 oz	101	0	26	0	26	0.0	0.0	1
Ketchup	2 oz	55	1	14	0	13	0.2	0.0	632
Ketchup, low sodium	2 oz	55	1	14	0	13	0.2	0.0	11
Lunchmeat spread, chicken, canned	2 oz	90	10	2	0	0	10.0	1.8	409
Lunchmeat spread, ham salad	2 oz	122	5	6	0	0	8.8	2.9	517
Lunchmeat spread, liverwurst	2 oz	173	7	3	1	1	14.4	5.6	397
Lunchmeat spread, pork & beef	2 oz	133	4	7	0	0	9.8	3.4	574
Lunchmeat spread, poultry salad	2 oz	113	7	4	0	0	7.7	2.0	214
Lunchmeat spread, roast beef	2 oz	126	9	2	0	0	9.2	3.6	411
Marmalade, orange	2 oz	139	0	38	0	34	0.0	0.0	32
Miso	2 oz	113	7	15	3	4	3.4	0.6	2114
Mustard, yellow, prepared	2 oz	38	2	3	2	0	2.3	0.1	644
Preserves	2 oz	158	0	39	1	27	0.0	0.0	18
Preserves, any flavor, with sodium saccharin	2 oz	75	0	30	1	21	0.2	0.0	0
Preserves, apricot	2 oz	137	0	37	0	25	0.1	0.0	23
Relish, pickle, hamburger	2 oz	73	0	20	2	17	0.3	0.0	621
Relish, pickle, hot dog	2 oz	52	1	13	1	12	0.3	0.0	619
Relish, pickle, sweet	2 oz	74	0	20	1	17	0.3	0.0	460

CONDIMENTS, DRESSINGS, MARINADES, AND SPREADS continued

Item	Serving Size	Calories	Protein	Carb	Fiber	Sugar	Total Fat	Sat Fat	Sodium
Salad dressing, assorted flavors	2 oz	94	0	9	0	8	6.1	0.9	625
Salad dressing, bacon & tomato	2 oz	185	1	1	0	1	19.8	3.1	615
Salad dressing, blue cheese	2 oz	270	1	3	0	2	29.0	4.7	527
Salad dressing, blue cheese, fat-free	2 oz	65	1	15	1	4	0.6	0.3	462
Salad dressing, blue cheese, low calorie	2 oz	56	3	2	0	2	4.1	1.5	680
Salad dressing, blue cheese, reduced calorie	2 oz	49	1	7	0	2	1.5	0.4	913
Salad dressing, blue cheese, unsalted	2 oz	286	3	4	0	4	29.7	5.6	17
Salad dressing, buttermilk, light	2 oz	115	1	12	1	2	7.0	0.7	515
Salad dressing, Caesar	2 oz	307	1	2	0	2	32.8	5.0	611
Salad dressing, Caesar, low calorie	2 oz	62	0	11	0	9	2.5	0.4	611
Salad dressing, coleslaw	2 oz	221	1	13	0	11	18.9	2.8	403
Salad dressing, coleslaw, reduced fat	2 oz	187	0	23	0	22	11.3	1.7	907
Salad dressing, creamy, with buttermilk, reduced calorie, no cholesterol	2 oz	79	1	9	0	2	4.5	0.8	528
Salad dressing, creamy, with sour cream, reduced calorie, no cholesterol	2 oz	79	1	9	0	2	4.5	0.8	528
Salad dressing, creamy, with sour cream and buttermilk, reduced calorie	2 oz	61	1	11	0	3	1.5	0.3	567
Salad dressing, French	2 oz	259	0	9	0	9	25.4	3.2	474
Salad dressing, French, fat-free	2 oz	75	0	18	1	9	0.2	0.0	453
Salad dressing, French, reduced calorie	2 oz	113	0	15	0	15	7.4	1.1	567
Salad dressing, French, reduced fat	2 oz	126	0	18	1	10	6.5	0.5	447
Salad dressing, French, reduced fat, unsalted	2 oz	132	0	17	1	16	7.6	0.6	17

CONDIMENTS, DRESSINGS, MARINADES, AND SPREADS continued

Item	Serving Size	Calories	Protein	Carb	Fiber	Sugar	Total Fat	Sat Fat	Sodium
Salad dressing, French, unsalted	2 oz	260	0	9	0	9	25.4	3.2	0
Salad dressing, honey mustard, reduced calorie	2 oz	117	1	17	0	10	5.7	0.5	510
Salad dressing, Italian	2 oz	165	0	6	0	5	16.1	2.5	938
Salad dressing, Italian, fat-free	2 oz	27	1	5	0	5	0.5	0.2	640
Salad dressing, Italian, reduced calorie	2 oz	113	0	4	0	1	11.3	1.6	806
Salad dressing, Italian, reduced fat	2 oz	43	0	3	0	3	3.6	0.3	775
Salad dressing, Italian, reduced fat, unsalted	2 oz	43	0	3	0	3	3.6	0.3	17
Salad dressing, Italian, unsalted	2 oz	166	0	6	0	5	16.1	2.5	17
Salad dressing, peppercorn	2 oz	320	1	2	0	1	34.8	6.0	604
Salad dressing, prepared from recipe, cooked	2 oz	89	2	8	0	5	5.4	1.6	416
Salad dressing, ranch	2 oz	274	1	4	0	1	29.1	4.5	463
Salad dressing, ranch, reduced fat	2 oz	111	1	12	1	2	7.0	0.7	515
Salad dressing, Roquefort	2 oz	270	1	3	0	2	29.0	4.7	527
Salad dressing, Roquefort, fat-free	2 oz	65	1	15	1	4	0.6	0.3	462
Salad dressing, Roquefort, low calorie	2 oz	56	3	2	0	2	4.1	1.5	680
Salad dressing, Roquefort, reduced calorie	2 oz	49	1	7	0	2	1.5	0.4	913
Salad dressing, Roquefort, unsalted	2 oz	286	3	4	0	4	29.7	5.6	17
Salad dressing, Russian	2 oz	201	0	18	0	10	14.8	1.4	563
Salad dressing, Russian, low calorie	2 oz	80	0	16	0	12	2.3	0.3	492
Salad dressing, sesame seed	2 oz	251	2	5	1	4	25.6	3.5	567
Salad dressing, sweet and sour	2 oz	9	0	2	0	2	0.0	0.0	118
Salad dressing, Thousand Island	2 oz	210	1	8	0	8	19.9	2.9	489

CONDIMENTS, DRESSINGS, MARINADES, AND SPREADS continued

Item	Serving Size	Calories	Protein	Carb	Fiber	Sugar	Total Fat	Sat Fat	Sodium
Salad dressing, Thousand Island, fat-free	2 oz	75	0	17	2	10	0.8	0.1	413
Salad dressing, Thousand Island, reduced fat	2 oz	111	0	14	1	10	6.4	0.4	472
Salad dressing, vinegar & oil, prepared from recipe	2 oz	255	0	1	0	1	28.4	5.2	1
Spread, hummus, prepared from recipe	2 oz	100	3	11	2	0	4.9	0.6	137
Spread, sandwich, with pickles & unspecified oil	2 oz	221	1	13	0	9	19.3	2.9	567

DAIRY PRODUCTS

Item	Serving Size	Calories	Protein	Carb	Fiber	Sugar	Total Fat	Sat Fat	Sodium
Buttermilk, cultured, reduced fat	1 fl oz	16	1	2	0	2	0.6	0.4	24
Buttermilk, dried	1 fl oz	110	10	14	0	14	1.6	1.0	147
Buttermilk, low fat, cultured	1 fl oz	11	1	1	0	1	0.2	0.2	30
Cream, half & half	1 fl oz	37	1	1	0	0	3.3	2.0	12
Cream, half & half, fat-free	1 fl oz	17	1	3	0	1	0.4	0.2	41
Cream, light	1 fl oz	55	1	1	0	0	5.5	3.4	11
Cream, whipping, heavy	1 fl oz	98	1	1	0	0	10.5	6.5	11
Cream, whipping, light	1 fl oz	83	1	1	0	0	8.8	5.5	10
Cream substitute, flavored, liquid	1 fl oz	71	0	10	0	9	3.8	0.7	23
Cream substitute, flavored, powder	1 fl oz	141	0	21	0	16	6.1	5.5	56
Cream substitute, hydrogenated vegetable oil & soy protein, liquid	1 fl oz	39	0	3	0	3	2.8	0.5	22
Cream substitute, light	1 fl oz	20	0	3	0	3	1.0	0.3	17
Cream substitute, light, powder	1 fl oz	122	1	21	0	21	4.5	1.1	65
Cream substitute, powder	1 fl oz	155	1	16	0	16	10.1	9.2	51

DAIRY PRODUCTS continued

Item	Serving Size	Calories	Protein	Carb	Fiber	Sugar	Total Fat	Sat Fat	Sodium
Eggnog	8 fl oz	200	10	18	0	18	9.5	5.9	122
Eggnog, prepared from dry mix with whole milk	8 fl oz	215	7	32	0	29	6.8	3.9	125
Milk, 1%	8 fl oz	95	8	11	0	11	2.2	1.4	100
Milk, 1%, low lactose	8 fl oz	95	7	11	0	11	2.4	1.5	115
Milk, 1%, protein fortified, with vitamins A & D	8 fl oz	109	9	13	0	10	2.7	1.7	132
Milk, 1%, with nonfat milk solids, vitamins A & D	8 fl oz	98	8	11	0	10	2.2	1.4	118
Milk, 1%, with vitamins A & D	8 fl oz	95	8	11	0	11	2.2	1.4	100
Milk, 2%	8 fl oz	113	7	11	0	11	4.5	2.3	107
Milk, 2%, protein fortified, with vitamins A & D	8 fl oz	127	9	12	0	12	4.5	2.8	134
Milk, 2%, with nonfat milk solids, vitamins A & D	8 fl oz	116	8	11	0	10	4.4	2.7	118
Milk, 2%, with vitamins A & D	8 fl oz	113	7	11	0	11	4.5	2.3	107
Milk, chocolate, 2%, with vitamins A & D	8 fl oz	172	7	28	2	22	4.3	2.7	150
Milk, chocolate, nonfat, prepared with syrup	8 fl oz	134	7	27	1	25	0.6	0.4	130
Milk, chocolate, prepared with syrup & whole milk	8 fl oz	204	7	29	1	26	6.7	3.8	107
Milk, chocolate, reduced fat, with calcium	8 fl oz	177	7	28	2	22	4.3	2.7	150
Milk, chocolate, with vitamins A & D	8 fl oz	188	7	23	2	22	7.7	4.8	136
Milk, condensed, sweetened, canned	8 fl oz	728	18	123	0	123	19.7	12.5	288
Milk, evaporated, canned	8 fl oz	306	15	23	0	23	17.1	10.4	240
Milk, evaporated, nonfat, with vitamins A & D, canned	8 fl oz	177	17	26	0	26	0.5	0.3	261
Milk, evaporated, with vitamins A, canned	8 fl oz	304	15	23	0	23	17.1	10.4	240

DAIRY PRODUCTS continued

Item	Serving Size	Calories	Protein	Carb	Fiber	Sugar	Total Fat	Sat Fat	Sodium
Milk, filled, fluid, with lauric acid oil	8 fl oz	143	8	11	0	11	7.7	7.0	129
Milk, goat, with vitamin D	8 fl oz	156	8	10	0	10	9.4	6.1	113
Milk, human breast	8 fl oz	159	2	16	0	16	9.9	4.6	39
Milk, low fat, chocolate, with vitamins A & D	8 fl oz	143	7	24	1	23	2.3	1.4	138
Milk, low fat, prepared from dry with water	8 oz	77	7	11	0	11	0.4	0.2	122
Milk, low sodium	8 oz	138	7	10	0	10	7.8	4.9	7
Milk, nonfat, calcium fortified	8 oz	79	8	11	0	11	0.4	0.3	118
Milk, nonfat, prepared from dry with water	8 oz	75	7	11	0	11	0.2	0.1	122
Milk, nonfat, protein fortified, with vitamins A & D	8 oz	93	9	13	0	10	0.6	0.4	134
Milk, nonfat, with nonfat milk solids & vitamins A & D	8 oz	84	8	11	0	11	0.6	0.4	120
Milk, nonfat, with vitamins A & D	8 oz	77	8	11	0	11	0.2	0.1	95
Milk, nonfat, without added vitamins A & D	8 oz	77	8	11	0	11	0.2	0.1	95
Milk, whole, 3.25%	8 oz	138	7	11	0	11	7.4	4.2	98
Milk, whole, 3.25%, with vitamins D	8 oz	138	7	11	0	11	7.4	4.2	98
Milk, whole, prepared from dry with water	8 oz	146	8	11	0	11	7.9	4.9	115
Milk substitute, non-soy	8 fl oz	104	4	12	0	12	4.5	0.6	125
Parfait, fruit & yogurt, lowfat, with granola	8 oz	191	8	36	2	26	2.3	1.2	111
Sour cream, cultured	1 oz	58	1	1	0	1	5.9	3.5	24
Sour cream, fat-free	1 oz	22	1	5	0	0	0.0	0.0	42
Sour cream, imitation, cultured	1 oz	62	1	2	0	2	5.9	5.3	31
Sour cream, light	1 oz	41	1	2	0	0	3.2	2.0	21
Sour cream, reduced fat	1 oz	54	2	2	0	0	4.2	2.6	21
Sour cream, reduced fat, cultured	1 oz	41	1	1	0	0	3.6	2.2	12

DAIRY PRODUCTS continued

Item	Serving Size	Calories	Protein	Carb	Fiber	Sugar	Total Fat	Sat Fat	Sodium
Yogurt, chocolate, nonfat	8 oz	254	8	53	3	34	0.0	0.0	135
Yogurt, chocolate, nonfat, with vitamin D	8 oz	254	8	53	3	34	0.0	0.0	135
Yogurt, chocolate, whole milk	8 oz	229	11	31	0	27	7.2	4.5	65
Yogurt, fruit, low fat	8 oz	231	10	43	0	43	2.4	1.6	58
Yogurt, fruit, low fat, with vitamin D	8 oz	231	10	43	0	43	2.4	1.6	58
Yogurt, fruit, low fat,	8 oz	225	9	42	0	42	2.6	1.7	53
Yogurt, fruit, low fat, with vitamin D	8 oz	225	9	42	0	42	2.6	1.7	53
Yogurt, fruit, low fat, reduced sugar, with vitamin D	8 oz	238	11	42	0	7	3.2	2.1	58
Yogurt, fruit, low fat, with artificial sweetener	8 oz	238	11	42	0	7	3.2	2.1	58
Yogurt, fruit, nonfat, with vitamin D	8 oz	215	10	43	0	43	0.5	0.3	58
Yogurt, lemon, low fat	8 oz	193	11	31	0	31	2.8	1.8	66
Yogurt, lemon, nonfat, reduced sugar, with vitamin D	8 oz	98	9	17	0	17	0.4	0.3	59
Yogurt, lemon, nonfat, with low-calorie sweetener	8 oz	98	9	17	0	17	0.4	0.3	59
Yogurt, maple, low fat	8 oz	193	11	31	0	31	2.8	1.8	66
Yogurt, plain, low fat	8 oz	143	12	16	0	16	3.5	2.3	70
Yogurt, plain, skim	8 oz	127	13	17	0	17	0.4	0.3	77
Yogurt, plain, whole milk	8 oz	138	8	11	0	11	7.4	4.8	46
Yogurt, tofu	8 oz	213	8	36	0	3	4.1	0.6	35
Yogurt, vanilla, low fat	8 oz	193	11	31	0	31	2.8	1.8	66
Yogurt, vanilla, low fat, with vitamin D	8 oz	193	11	31	0	31	2.8	1.8	66
Yogurt, vanilla, nonfat, reduced sugar, with vitamin D	8 oz	98	9	17	0	17	0.4	0.3	59
Yogurt, vanilla, nonfat, with low-cal sweetener	8 oz	98	9	17	0	17	0.4	0.3	59

DESSERTS AND SWEET TREATS

Item	Serving Size	Calories	Protein	Carb	Fiber	Sugar	Total Fat	Sat Fat	Sodium
Baking chips, milk chocolate	1/2 oz	80	1	9	1	8	4.4	2.8	12
Bread, sweet, Mex-pan dulce with crumb topping	2 oz	209	3	35	1	16	6.4	1.3	54
Brownie	2 oz	230	3	36	1	21	9.2	2.4	177
Brownie, sugar- & sodium-free, prepared from dry mix	2 oz	218	2	40	2	0	6.3	2.9	53
Cake, angel food, prepared from dry mix	2 oz	141	3	32	0	17	0.2	0.0	280
Cake, applesauce, without icing	2 oz	204	2	34	1	24	7.5	1.5	92
Cake, apricot, without icing	2 oz	204	2	34	1	24	7.5	1.5	92
Cake, blackberry, without icing	2 oz	204	2	34	1	24	7.5	1.5	92
Cake, Boston cream pie	2 oz	143	1	24	1	20	4.8	1.4	82
Cake, cherry fudge, with chocolate frosting	2 oz	150	1	22	1	19	7.1	2.9	128
Cake, coffee, cinnamon, with crumb topping prepared from mix	2 oz	180	3	30	1	17	5.4	1.1	239
Cake, date pudding	2 oz	176	2	26	1	18	7.6	4.0	88
Cake, fruit	2 oz	184	2	35	2	17	5.2	0.6	153
Cake, graham cracker	2 oz	200	3	28	1	20	8.6	2.0	238
Cake, ice cream, chocolate roll	2 oz	169	2	23	1	15	8.3	3.4	75
Cake, oatmeal, with icing	2 oz	211	2	36	1	34	7.2	1.5	86
Cake, plum pudding	2 oz	176	2	26	1	18	7.6	4.0	88
Cake, poppy seed, without icing	2 oz	224	4	27	1	14	11.3	4.2	197
Cake, pound, fat-free	2 oz	160	3	35	1	19	0.7	0.1	193
Cake, rhubarb, without icing	2 oz	204	2	34	1	24	7.5	1.5	92
Cake, snack, sponge, with cream filling	2 oz	212	2	36	1	21	6.5	2.3	227
Cake, spice, with icing	2 oz	191	2	32	1	31	6.1	1.6	146
Cake, white, with coconut frosting, prepared from recipe	2 oz	202	2	36	1	33	5.8	2.2	161

DESSERTS AND SWEET TREATS continued

Item	Serving Size	Calories	Protein	Carb	Fiber	Sugar	Total Fat	Sat Fat	Sodium
Cake, white, without frosting, prepared from recipe	2 oz	202	3	32	0	20	7.0	1.9	185
Candy, almonds, sugar coated	1.5 oz	202	4	29	1	27	7.6	0.8	6
Candy, butterscotch	1.5 oz	166	0	38	0	34	1.4	0.9	166
Candy, candy corn, prepared from recipe	1.5 oz	159	0	40	0	38	0.0	0.0	5
Candy, caramel, chocolate flavor roll	1.5 oz	168	1	37	0	24	2.2	0.4	19
Candy, caramel, with nuts, chocolate-covered	1.5 oz	200	4	26	2	18	8.9	2.0	10
Candy, caramels	1.5 oz	162	2	33	0	28	3.4	1.1	104
Candy, chocolate, dark	1.5 oz	234	2	26	3	20	13.7	8.1	10
Candy, chocolate, dark, 45%–59% cacao solids	1.5 oz	232	2	26	3	20	13.3	7.9	10
Candy, chocolate, dark, 60%–69% cacao solids	1.5 oz	246	3	22	3	16	16.3	9.4	4
Candy, chocolate, dark, 70%–85% cacao solids	1.5 oz	254	3	20	5	10	18.1	10.4	9
Candy, chocolate-covered, low calorie	1.5 oz	252	5	16	2	6	18.4	9.3	48
Candy, coffee beans, dark chocolate–covered	1.5 oz	230	3	25	3	18	12.8	6.4	11
Candy, coffee beans, milk chocolate–covered	1.5 oz	233	3	23	2	21	14.1	7.7	30
Candy, divinity, prepared from recipe	1.5 oz	155	1	38	0	34	0.0	0.0	14
Candy, fondant, prepared from recipe	1.5 oz	159	0	40	0	38	0.0	0.0	5
Candy, fruit & nut, squares, soft	1.5 oz	166	1	31	1	20	4.0	0.4	56
Candy, fudge, chocolate, prepared from recipe	1.5 oz	175	1	33	1	31	4.4	2.7	19
Candy, fudge, chocolate, with nuts, prepared from recipe	1.5 oz	196	2	29	1	27	8.0	2.8	17
Candy, fudge, chocolate marshmallow, prepared from recipe	1.5 oz	193	1	30	1	27	7.4	4.5	36

DESSERTS AND SWEET TREATS continued

Item	Serving Size	Calories	Protein	Carb	Fiber	Sugar	Total Fat	Sat Fat	Sodium
Candy, fudge, peanut butter, prepared from recipe	1.5 oz	165	2	33	0	31	2.8	0.7	50
Candy, fudge, vanilla, prepared from recipe	1.5 oz	163	0	35	0	34	2.3	1.4	20
Candy, fudge, vanilla, with nuts, prepared from recipe	1.5 oz	185	1	32	0	30	5.8	1.6	18
Candy, gumdrops	1.5 oz	168	0	42	0	25	0.0	0.0	19
Candy, gumdrops, low calorie	1.5 oz	69	0	37	8	30	0.1	0.0	3
Candy, gummy bears	1.5 oz	168	0	42	0	25	0.0	0.0	19
Candy, gummy dinosaurs	1.5 oz	168	0	42	0	25	0.0	0.0	19
Candy, gummy fish	1.5 oz	168	0	42	0	25	0.0	0.0	19
Candy, gummy worms	1.5 oz	168	0	42	0	25	0.0	0.0	19
Candy, hard, all flavors	1.5 oz	168	0	42	0	27	0.1	0.0	16
Candy, hard, low calorie	1.5 oz	168	0	42	0	40	0.0	0.0	0
Candy, jelly ring	1.5 oz	168	0	42	0	25	0.0	0.0	19
Candy, jellybeans	1.5 oz	159	0	40	0	30	0.0	0.0	21
Candy, Jordan almonds	1.5 oz	202	4	29	1	27	7.6	0.8	6
Candy, milk chocolate, with almonds	1.5 oz	224	4	23	3	19	14.6	7.5	31
Candy, nougat, with almonds	1.5 oz	169	1	39	1	35	0.7	0.7	14
Candy, peanut brittle, prepared from recipe	1.5 oz	207	3	30	1	22	8.1	1.8	189
Candy, peanuts, milk chocolate covered	1.5 oz	221	6	21	2	16	14.2	6.2	17
Candy, praline, prepared from recipe	1.5 oz	206	1	25	1	24	11.0	0.9	20
Candy, raisins, milk chocolate covered	1.5 oz	166	2	29	1	26	6.3	4.4	15
Candy, sesame crunch	1.5 oz	219	5	21	3	13	14.2	2.0	71
Candy, spice drops	1.5 oz	168	0	42	0	25	0.0	0.0	19
Candy, spice stick	1.5 oz	168	0	42	0	25	0.0	0.0	19
Candy, taffy, prepared from recipe	1.5 oz	169	0	39	0	29	1.4	0.9	22
Candy, toffee, prepared from recipe	1.5 oz	238	0	28	0	27	13.9	8.7	57
Candy, truffle, prepared from recipe	1.5 oz	217	3	19	1	16	14.4	7.9	29

DESSERTS AND SWEET TREATS continued

Item	Serving Size	Calories	Protein	Carb	Fiber	Sugar	Total Fat	Sat Fat	Sodium
Candy, yogurt-covered, with vitamin C	1.5 oz	176	0	37	0	28	3.2	0.5	32
Candy bar, caramel, chocolate flavor roll	1.5 oz	168	1	37	0	24	2.2	0.4	19
Candy bar, carob, unsweetened	1.5 oz	230	3	24	2	15	13.3	12.3	46
Candy bar, crispy	1.5 oz	230	4	24	1	17	13.3	5.5	112
Candy bar, milk chocolate	1.5 oz	228	3	25	1	22	12.6	7.9	34
Candy bar, milk chocolate, with crisped rice	1.5 oz	217	3	25	1	22	12.5	6.8	37
Candy bar, peanut	1.5 oz	222	7	20	2	18	14.3	2.0	66
Candy bar, sweet chocolate	1.5 oz	216	2	26	2	22	14.5	8.5	7
Cheesecake	4.5 oz	410	7	33	1	28	28.7	12.7	264
Cheesecake, no bake, prepared from dry mix	4.5 oz	350	7	45	2	34	16.2	8.5	485
Chewing gum, block	3 g	11	0	3	0	2	0.0	0.0	0
Chewing gum, Chiclets	3 g	11	0	3	0	2	0.0	0.0	0
Chewing gum, stick	3 g	11	0	3	0	2	0.0	0.0	0
Chewing gum, sugarless	3 g	8	0	3	0	0	0.0	0.0	0
Cookie, anisette sponge, with lemon juice & rind	1 oz	103	3	17	0	7	2.6	0.9	42
Cookie, applesauce	1 oz	104	1	18	1	12	3.4	0.7	61
Cookie, butter, enriched	1 oz	132	2	20	0	6	5.3	3.1	100
Cookie, butterscotch brownie	1 oz	127	2	16	0	12	6.4	1.2	75
Cookie, chocolate chip, enriched	1 oz	134	1	18	1	10	6.6	2.8	84
Cookie, chocolate chip, soft	1 oz	129	1	18	1	11	5.8	2.8	77
Cookie, chocolate chip, sugar- & sodium-free	1 oz	128	1	21	1	11	4.8	1.2	3
Cookie, chocolate, extra cream filling	1 oz	141	1	19	1	13	7.0	1.5	100
Cookie, chocolate wafer	1 oz	123	2	21	1	8	4.0	1.2	164
Cookie, coconut macaroon, prepared from recipe	1 oz	115	1	20	1	20	3.6	3.2	70
Cookie, fig bar	1 oz	99	1	20	1	13	2.1	0.3	99
Cookie, fortune	1 oz	107	1	24	0	13	0.8	0.2	78
Cookie, gingersnap	1 oz	118	2	22	1	6	2.8	0.7	185

DESSERTS AND SWEET TREATS continued

Item	Serving Size	Calories	Protein	Carb	Fiber	Sugar	Total Fat	Sat Fat	Sodium
Cookie, ladyfinger, with lemon juice & rind	1 oz	103	3	17	0	7	2.6	0.9	42
Cookie, marshmallow pie, chocolate-coated	1 oz	119	1	19	1	13	4.8	1.3	48
Cookie, marshmallow, fudge	1 oz	119	1	19	1	13	4.8	1.3	48
Cookie, molasses	1 oz	122	2	21	0	5	3.6	0.9	130
Cookie, oatmeal	1 oz	128	2	19	1	7	5.1	1.3	109
Cookie, oatmeal, fat-free	1 oz	92	2	22	2	12	0.4	0.1	84
Cookie, oatmeal raisin, low calorie, sugar- & sodium-free	1 oz	127	1	20	1	9	5.1	0.8	3
Cookie, peanut butter	1 oz	135	3	17	1	9	6.7	1.3	118
Cookie, raisin, soft type	1 oz	114	1	19	0	13	3.9	1.0	96
Cookie, sandwich, chocolate, with cream	1 oz	133	2	20	1	12	5.6	1.8	143
Cookie, sandwich, chocolate, with cream, chocolate-coated	1 oz	136	1	19	1	17	7.5	2.1	92
Cookie, sandwich, chocolate, with cream, sugar- & sodium-free	1 oz	131	1	19	1	7	6.3	1.1	69
Cookie, sandwich, peanut butter	1 oz	136	2	19	1	10	6.0	1.4	104
Cookie, sandwich, vanilla, with cream	1 oz	137	1	20	0	11	5.7	0.8	99
Cookie, shortbread, plain	1 oz	142	2	18	1	4	6.8	1.7	129
Cookie, sugar	1 oz	136	1	19	0	11	6.0	1.5	101
Cookie, sugar, prepared from recipe with margarine	1 oz	134	2	17	0	7	6.6	1.3	139
Cookie, sugar, prepared from refrigerated dough	1 oz	137	1	19	0	7	6.5	1.7	133
Cookie, sugar wafer, cream-filled	1 oz	145	1	20	0	10	6.9	1.0	42
Cookie, vanilla	1 oz	136	1	19	0	11	6.0	1.5	101
Cookie, vanilla wafer, lower fat	1 oz	125	1	21	1	11	4.3	1.1	88
Croissant, cheese	2 oz	235	5	27	1	6	11.9	6.0	315
Cupcake, snack, chocolate, with frosting & cream filling	3 oz	339	3	51	3	32	13.5	4.2	331

DESSERTS AND SWEET TREATS continued

Item	Serving Size	Calories	Protein	Carb	Fiber	Sugar	Total Fat	Sat Fat	Sodium
Cupcake, yellow with fruit & cream filling	3 oz	285	4	48	1	45	8.7	2.0	411
Danish, almond	2 oz	244	4	26	1	15	14.3	3.3	206
Danish, apple cinnamon, enriched	2 oz	210	3	27	1	16	10.5	2.8	201
Danish, cheese	2 oz	212	5	21	1	4	12.4	3.8	255
Danish, cinnamon nut	2 oz	244	4	26	1	15	14.3	3.3	206
Danish, lemon, enriched	2 oz	210	3	27	1	16	10.5	2.8	201
Danish, raisin nut	2 oz	244	4	26	1	15	14.3	3.3	206
Danish, raspberry, enriched	2 oz	210	3	27	1	16	10.5	2.8	201
Danish, strawberry, enriched	2 oz	210	3	27	1	16	10.5	2.8	201
Dessert, apple crisp, prepared from recipe	4.5 oz	201	2	39	2	25	4.3	0.9	439
Dessert, lemon, bar	4.5 oz	542	6	78	1	54	23.3	4.8	329
Doughnut, cake, chocolate, glazed, sugared	2 oz	236	3	33	1	18	11.3	2.9	193
Doughnut, cake, holes	2 oz	237	3	26	1	9	13.4	4.0	316
Doughnut, cake, wheat, glazed, sugared	2 oz	204	4	24	1	12	10.9	1.7	201
Doughnut, cake, with chocolate icing	2 oz	256	3	29	1	15	14.3	7.6	234
Doughnut, cream-filled	2 oz	205	4	17	0	8	13.9	3.1	175
Doughnut, French crullers	2 oz	234	2	34	1	20	10.4	2.6	196
Doughnut, glazed, enriched	2 oz	226	4	29	1	11	10.8	3.1	219
Doughnut, jelly-filled	2 oz	193	3	22	1	12	10.6	2.7	166
Frosting, chocolate, creamy, prepared from dry mix with butter	1 oz	116	0	20	1	0	3.7	2.4	35
Frosting, chocolate, creamy, ready to eat	1 oz	113	0	18	0	16	5.0	1.6	52
Frosting, chocolate, glaze, prepared from recipe with butter	1 oz	102	0	20	0	18	2.0	1.3	37
Frosting, coconut nut, ready to eat	1 oz	123	0	15	1	11	6.8	2.4	55
Frosting, cream cheese, creamy, ready to eat	1 oz	118	0	19	0	18	4.9	1.3	54
Frosting, glaze, prepared from recipe	1 oz	97	0	24	0	23	0.2	0.1	2

DESSERTS AND SWEET TREATS continued

Item	Serving Size	Calories	Protein	Carb	Fiber	Sugar	Total Fat	Sat Fat	Sodium
Frosting, vanilla, creamy, ready to eat	1 oz	119	0	19	0	18	4.6	0.8	52
Frozen dessert, ice milk, chocolate	3 oz	123	4	22	0	21	2.7	1.7	53
Frozen dessert, ice novelty, lime	3 oz	109	0	28	0	28	0.0	0.0	19
Frozen dessert, parfait, with fruits, nuts, whipped topping	3 oz	218	3	25	0	20	13.0	7.5	72
Frozen dessert, soft serve, light, with cookie pieces	3 oz	144	3	22	0	18	4.8	2.3	64
Frozen dessert, soft serve, light, with milk chocolate candies	3 oz	155	3	23	0	21	5.5	3.1	46
Frozen dessert bar, fruit juice	3 oz	74	1	17	1	15	0.1	0.0	3
Frozen dessert bar, ice novelty, fruit, no sugar added	3 oz	20	0	5	0	0	0.1	0.0	4
Frozen dessert bar, skim milk	3 oz	93	2	20	0	19	1.0	0.2	46
Frozen dessert pop, with low-calorie sweetener	3 oz	20	0	5	0	1	0.0	0.0	9
Frozen yogurt, all flavors, not chocolate	3 oz	108	3	18	0	17	3.1	2.0	54
Frozen yogurt, chocolate	3 oz	108	3	18	2	16	3.1	1.9	54
Frozen yogurt, chocolate, nonfat, with artificial sweetener	3 oz	91	4	17	2	11	0.7	0.4	69
Frozen yogurt, soft serve, vanilla	3 oz	135	3	21	0	20	4.8	2.9	74
Frozen yogurt bar, chocolate-coated	3 oz	226	3	25	0	21	13.9	11.1	58
Frozen yogurt cone, chocolate, large	3 oz	183	4	27	1	17	8.0	4.6	91
Frozen yogurt cone, chocolate, small	3 oz	183	4	27	1	17	8.0	4.6	91
Frozen yogurt cone, vanilla, fruit, large	3 oz	160	4	27	0	18	4.6	2.6	98
Frozen yogurt cone, vanilla, fruit, small	3 oz	160	4	27	0	18	4.6	2.6	98

DESSERTS AND SWEET TREATS continued

Item	Serving Size	Calories	Protein	Carb	Fiber	Sugar	Total Fat	Sat Fat	Sodium
Frozen yogurt sandwich	3 oz	181	4	32	0	21	4.4	2.3	57
Ice cream, chocolate, light, no sugar added	3 oz	147	3	23	1	5	4.9	3.1	64
Ice cream, chocolate, low carbohydrate	3 oz	201	3	23	4	5	10.8	5.8	65
Ice cream, chocolate, rich	3 oz	217	4	18	1	15	14.4	8.8	48
Ice cream, soft serve, French vanilla	3 oz	189	3	19	1	18	11.1	6.4	52
Ice cream, soft serve, vanilla, light	3 oz	107	4	19	0	16	2.2	1.4	60
Ice cream, vanilla	3 oz	176	3	20	1	18	9.4	5.8	68
Ice cream, vanilla, fat-free	3 oz	117	4	26	1	5	0.0	0.0	82
Ice cream, vanilla, light	3 oz	153	4	25	0	19	4.1	2.5	63
Ice cream, vanilla, light, no sugar added	3 oz	144	3	18	0	5	6.3	3.4	82
Ice cream, vanilla, low carbohydrate	3 oz	184	3	19	4	5	10.8	5.8	41
Ice cream bar, vanilla, chocolate coated, light, no sugar added	3 oz	188	5	22	1	7	8.6	4.7	88
Ice cream cone, sundae, individually packaged	3 oz	157	4	25	0	18	5.1	2.6	81
Marshmallows	1 oz	90	1	23	0	16	0.1	0.0	23
Milk shake, chocolate	8 oz	270	7	48	1	47	6.1	3.8	252
Milk shake, vanilla	8 oz	254	9	40	0	40	6.9	4.3	215
Pastry, cream puff, chocolate, custard-filled, prepared from recipe	2 oz	147	4	14	0	4	8.8	2.3	189
Pastry, cream puff, custard-filled, prepared from recipe	2 oz	144	4	13	0	5	8.7	2.1	191
Pastry, eclair, chocolate, custard-filled, prepared from recipe	2 oz	147	4	14	0	4	8.8	2.3	189
Pastry, eclair, custard-filled, prepared from recipe	2 oz	144	4	13	0	5	8.7	2.1	191
Pastry, pastelito de guava	2 oz	212	3	27	1	10	10.4	3.1	129
Pastry, toaster, apple	2 oz	219	3	39	1	16	5.9	1.5	187
Pastry, toaster, apple, frosted	2 oz	219	2	40	0	20	5.6	1.5	175

DESSERTS AND SWEET TREATS continued

Item	Serving Size	Calories	Protein	Carb	Fiber	Sugar	Total Fat	Sat Fat	Sodium
Pastry, toaster, apple, toasted	2 oz	229	3	41	1	16	6.2	1.5	198
Pastry, toaster, blueberry	2 oz	219	3	39	1	16	5.9	1.5	187
Pastry, toaster, blueberry, frosted	2 oz	219	2	40	0	20	5.6	1.5	175
Pastry, toaster, blueberry, toasted	2 oz	229	3	41	1	16	6.2	1.5	198
Pastry, toaster, cherry	2 oz	219	3	39	1	16	5.9	1.5	187
Pastry, toaster, cherry, frosted	2 oz	219	2	40	0	20	5.6	1.5	175
Pastry, toaster, cherry, toasted	2 oz	229	3	41	1	16	6.2	1.5	198
Pastry, toaster, fruit	2 oz	219	3	39	1	16	5.9	1.5	187
Pastry, toaster, fruit, frosted	2 oz	219	2	40	0	20	5.6	1.5	175
Pastry, toaster, fruit, toasted	2 oz	229	3	41	1	16	6.2	1.5	198
Pastry, toaster, strawberry	2 oz	219	3	39	1	16	5.9	1.5	187
Pastry, toaster, strawberry, frosted	2 oz	219	2	40	0	20	5.6	1.5	175
Pastry, toaster, strawberry, toasted	2 oz	229	3	41	1	16	6.2	1.5	198
Pie, apple, with enriched flour	4.5 oz	296	2	43	2	20	13.8	4.8	333
Pie, banana cream, prepared from recipe	4.5 oz	336	6	41	1	15	17.0	4.7	300
Pie, blackberry, prepared from recipe	4.5 oz	335	3	47	4	19	15.7	3.1	22
Pie, blueberry	4.5 oz	290	2	44	1	12	12.5	2.1	406
Pie, cherry	4.5 oz	325	3	50	1	18	13.8	3.2	308
Pie, coconut cream	4.5 oz	373	3	47	2	45	20.8	8.7	319
Pie, Dutch apple, prepared from recipe	4.5 oz	363	3	56	2	28	14.4	2.9	250
Pie, egg custard	4.5 oz	263	7	26	2	14	14.5	2.9	300
Pie, lemon meringue	4.5 oz	335	2	59	2	30	10.9	2.2	183
Pie, peach	4.5 oz	279	2	41	1	8	12.5	1.9	338
Pie, pecan	4.5 oz	509	6	75	3	31	20.9	3.3	300
Pie, pumpkin	4.5 oz	304	5	44	2	24	12.2	2.5	291

DESSERTS AND SWEET TREATS continued

Item	Serving Size	Calories	Protein	Carb	Fiber	Sugar	Total Fat	Sat Fat	Sodium
Pie, vanilla cream, prepared from recipe	4.5 oz	348	6	41	1	16	18.0	5.0	325
Sweet roll, butterhorn	2 oz	208	3	29	1	12	9.2	2.4	214
Sweet roll, honey bun, enriched	2 oz	223	3	28	1	11	10.7	3.0	217
Topping, chocolate fudge	1 oz	99	1	18	1	10	2.5	1.1	98
Topping, marshmallow creme	1 oz	91	0	22	0	13	0.1	0.0	23
Topping, pineapple	1 oz	72	0	19	0	6	0.0	0.0	12
Topping, strawberry	1 oz	72	0	19	0	8	0.0	0.0	6
Topping, syrup, with nuts	1 oz	127	1	16	1	10	6.2	0.6	12
Topping, whipped, dietetic, prepared from powder	1 oz	28	0	3	0	3	1.7	0.9	30
Topping, whipped, low fat, frozen	1 oz	64	1	7	0	7	3.7	3.2	20
Topping, whipped, semi-solid, frozen	1 oz	90	0	7	0	7	7.2	6.2	7
Topping, whipped cream, pressurized	1 oz	73	1	4	0	2	6.3	3.9	37

EGGS

Item	Serving Size	Calories	Protein	Carb	Fiber	Sugar	Total Fat	Sat Fat	Sodium
Egg substitute, Better 'n Eggs	2 oz	20	5	0	0	0	0.0	0.0	90
Egg substitute, egg replacer, dry mix	7 g	30	3	2	1	1	1.0	0.0	20
Egg whites, raw	1 white	14	3	0	0	0	0.1	0.0	50
Egg yolks, raw	1 yolk	57	3	1	0	0	4.8	1.7	48
Egg yolks, raw, frozen	1 yolk	55	3	0	0	0	4.6	1.4	67
Egg yolks, raw, large	1 yolk	57	3	1	0	0	4.8	1.7	48
Eggs, duck, whole, raw	1 egg	150	10	1	0	1	11.2	3.0	118
Eggs, goose, whole, raw	1 egg	266	20	2	0	1	19.1	5.2	199
Eggs, hard-boiled, large	1 egg	71	6	1	0	1	4.9	1.5	124
Eggs, large, cage-free, raw	1 egg	32	3	0	0	0	2.1	0.7	30
Eggs, large, with omega 3, raw	1 egg	32	3	0	0	0	2.1	0.7	30

EGGS continued

Item	Serving Size	Calories	Protein	Carb	Fiber	Sugar	Total Fat	Sat Fat	Sodium
Eggs, poached, large	1 egg	65	6	0	0	0	4.6	1.4	135
Eggs, quail, whole, raw	1 egg	73	6	0	0	0	5.1	1.6	65
Eggs, whole, large, fried	1 egg	90	6	0	0	0	7.0	2.0	94
Eggs, whole, raw, extra large	1 egg	82	7	0	0	0	5.7	1.8	80
Eggs, whole, raw, jumbo	1 egg	102	9	1	0	1	7.1	2.2	99
Eggs, whole, raw, large	1 egg	66	6	0	0	0	4.6	1.4	64
Eggs, whole, raw, medium	1 egg	72	6	0	0	0	5.0	1.6	70
Eggs, whole, raw, small	1 egg	61	5	0	0	0	4.3	1.3	60

ENTRÉES AND SIDE DISHES

Item	Serving Size	Calories	Protein	Carb	Fiber	Sugar	Total Fat	Sat Fat	Sodium
Bean cakes, Japanese style	3 oz	347	5	42	2	18	18.2	2.7	1
Bouillon, beef, condensed, prepared with water	1 cup	17	3	0	0	0	0.5	0.1	624
Bouillon, beef, prepared from powder with water	1 cup	7	1	1	0	0	0.2	0.1	624
Bouillon, chicken, prepared from dehydrated with water	1 cup	10	1	1	0	1	0.6	8.2	2561
Bouillon or broth, beef, low sodium, canned	1 cup	38	5	1	0	0	1.4	0.4	72
Broth, beef, prepared from dry cube with water	1 cup	7	1	1	0	0	0.2	0.1	624
Broth, beef, ready to serve	1 cup	17	3	0	0	0	0.5	0.1	314
Broth, chicken, low sodium, canned	1 cup	38	5	3	0	0	1.4	0.4	763
Broth, chicken, prepared from canned with water	1 cup	38	5	1	0	1	1.4	0.4	763
Broth, chicken, prepared from dehydrated with water	1 cup	10	1	1	0	1	0.6	0.0	554
Broth, chicken, reduced sodium, canned	1 cup	17	3	1	0	1	0.0	4.6	1529
Burrito, bean & cheese, microwave	5 oz	364	12	57	15	2	10.0	5.7	923
Burrito, beef & bean, microwave	5 oz	417	12	55	10	2	16.7	3.7	477

ENTRÉES AND SIDE DISHES continued

Item	Serving Size	Calories	Protein	Carb	Fiber	Sugar	Total Fat	Sat Fat	Sodium
Casserole, chicken, with cheese sauce	5 oz	214	25	5	0	1	9.5	3.7	429
Chili, beef, condensed	1 cup	281	12	45	6	12	6.1	1.5	931
Chili, beef, prepared from canned with water	1 cup	137	6	22	3	6	3.0	4.2	1018
Chili, con carne, with beans, canned	1 cup	290	17	27	9	5	12.6	5.6	1253
Chili, with beans, canned	1 cup	269	14	29	11	3	13.2	5.4	934
Chili, without beans, canned	1 cup	283	18	15	3	3	17.0	4.2	718
Chowder, clam, Manhattan style, chunky, ready to serve	1 cup	134	7	19	3	4	3.4	2.1	1001
Chowder, clam, Manhattan style, condensed	1 cup	146	4	23	3	6	4.2	0.7	1097
Chowder, clam, Manhattan style, prepared from canned with water	1 cup	72	2	11	1	3	2.1	2.3	1678
Chowder, clam, New England, condensed	1 cup	173	8	25	2	1	4.9	2.3	1678
Chowder, clam, New England, prepared from canned with milk	1 cup	146	8	18	1	7	4.8	1.1	826
Chowder, clam, New England, prepared from canned with water	1 cup	84	4	12	1	0	2.4	3.9	874
Dish, arroz con habichuelas coloradas	5 oz	199	6	33	4	0	4.8	4.9	487
Dish, beef, with cream or white sauce	5 oz	201	14	8	0	4	12.2	7.6	467
Dish, beef Bourguignon	5 oz	115	12	5	1	3	4.8	1.9	66
Dish, beef Burgundy	5 oz	167	20	5	1	3	6.8	5.7	214
Dish, beef cube steak, lean, battered, fried	5 oz	366	37	11	0	3	18.3	5.3	268
Dish, beef cube steak, lean, breaded, fried	5 oz	390	38	16	1	1	18.6	4.2	476
Dish, beef curry	5 oz	259	16	8	2	1	18.6	9.8	208
Dish, beefsteak, battered, fried	5 oz	441	33	11	0	3	28.3	9.3	262
Dish, beefsteak, breaded, fried	5 oz	464	34	16	1	1	28.4	5.7	214

ENTRÉES AND SIDE DISHES continued

Item	Serving Size	Calories	Protein	Carb	Fiber	Sugar	Total Fat	Sat Fat	Sodium
Dish, beef steak, lean, battered, fried, diced	5 oz	366	37	11	0	3	18.3	8.3	97
Dish, beets, with Harvard sauce	5 oz	166	2	32	2	28	4.6	0.6	16
Dish, broccoli, batter-dipped, fried	5 oz	201	6	15	4	3	14.5	1.6	220
Dish, carrots, glazed	5 oz	189	1	24	4	18	10.2	4.4	284
Dish, cauliflower, batter-dipped, fried	5 oz	284	6	18	3	6	21.3	9.2	372
Dish, chicken, almond	5 oz	162	13	10	2	2	8.4	4.5	784
Dish, chicken & rice	5 oz	244	17	28	2	1	7.1	0.2	1015
Dish, chili beans, ranch style barbecue, cooked	5 oz	136	7	24	6	7	1.4	3.8	510
Dish, Chinese pressed duck	5 oz	268	10	27	1	17	13.9	1.1	508
Dish, corned beef & potatoes, with tortilla, Apache	5 oz	314	11	41	2	3	11.6	4.5	584
Dish, cornmeal mush, prepared with milk	5 oz	193	9	30	2	1	4.3	2.6	364
Dish, crab, soft shell, breaded, fried	5 oz	468	29	24	1	1	28.0	2.6	364
Dish, creamed eggs	5 oz	211	11	8	0	4	14.9	1.5	188
Dish, creamed onion	5 oz	115	3	14	1	7	5.7	2.4	203
Dish, eggplant, batter-dipped, fried	5 oz	210	3	17	3	5	15.0	5.6	226
Dish, eggs, deviled	5 oz	283	16	2	0	2	22.9	2.2	232
Dish, empanadas, beef	5 oz	469	16	44	3	3	25.7	3.9	745
Dish, fried rice	5 oz	228	7	43	2	1	3.2	0.6	734
Dish, lamb curry	5 oz	152	17	2	1	1	8.2	1.3	130
Dish, loaf, lentil	5 oz	247	12	28	9	3	10.5	3.8	675
Dish, lobster, battered, fried	5 oz	296	27	11	0	1	15.5	16.2	674
Dish, lobster Newberg	5 oz	351	17	7	0	3	28.6	17.0	371
Dish, lobster Thermidor	5 oz	351	17	7	0	3	28.6	3.1	493
Dish, mushrooms, batter-dipped, fried	5 oz	311	4	22	2	5	23.6	6.3	868
Dish, mushrooms, stuffed	5 oz	402	15	38	3	8	21.4	0.6	869
Dish, olives, green, stuffed	5 oz	144	2	3	2	0	15.3	4.8	442

ENTRÉES AND SIDE DISHES continued

Item	Serving Size	Calories	Protein	Carb	Fiber	Sugar	Total Fat	Sat Fat	Sodium
Dish, oysters Rockefeller	5 oz	188	10	13	2	2	10.7	2.0	383
Dish, pork chop, breaded, broiled or baked	5 oz	363	36	9	0	1	19.6	5.1	583
Dish, pork chop, breaded, lean, broiled or baked	5 oz	322	37	9	0	1	14.5	2.7	1139
Dish, pork steak or cutlet, breaded, fried	5 oz	393	32	13	0	1	22.3	5.4	252
Dish, pork steak or cutlet, breaded, lean, fried	5 oz	366	33	14	0	1	18.8	1.3	519
Dish, pork, sweet & sour	5 oz	143	9	16	1	12	5.1	2.5	388
Dish, rice & red beans	5 oz	199	6	33	4	0	4.8	3.7	650
Dish, shrimp, sweet & sour	5 oz	383	10	36	1	31	23.8	1.8	359
Dish, steak, Swiss	5 oz	146	16	5	1	1	6.3	9.1	168
Dish, sweet potatoes, with fruit, mashed	5 oz	159	1	39	2	30	0.3	0.4	2162
Dish, turkey, breaded, batter-fried	5 oz	396	20	22	1	0	25.2	6.6	1120
Dish, veal leg, top round steak, breaded, fried	5 oz	333	38	14	0	1	12.9	2.2	637
Dish, veal leg, top round steak, lean, breaded, fried	5 oz	302	40	14	0	1	8.8	3.0	655
Dish, vegetables, tempura battered, fried	5 oz	228	6	20	2	3	14.2	2.4	251
Dish, venison steak, breaded/floured, fried	5 oz	291	31	16	1	1	10.5	1.9	390
Dish, winter squash, mashed with fat & sugar	5 oz	104	1	20	4	11	3.2	6.1	73
Egg roll, assorted	5 oz	350	12	38	4	5	16.7	1.3	784
Egg roll, chicken, cooked	5 oz	276	15	40	3	8	6.3	2.2	735
Egg roll, pork, cooked	5 oz	311	14	41	3	7	10.0	1.1	785
Egg roll, vegetable, cooked	5 oz	274	9	45	4	10	6.5	3.3	412
Fried chicken, breast, broiler or fryer, with skin, batter-fried	3 oz	221	21	8	0	0	11.2	2.1	65
Fried chicken, broiler or fryer, whole, with skin, batter-fried	3 oz	246	19	8	0	0	14.7	3.5	71
Fried chicken, broiler or fryer, whole, with skin, flour-fried	3 oz	229	24	3	0	0	12.7	3.9	76

ENTRÉES AND SIDE DISHES continued

Item	Serving Size	Calories	Protein	Carb	Fiber	Sugar	Total Fat	Sat Fat	Sodium
Fried chicken, dark meat, broiler or fryer, with skin, flour-fried	3 oz	242	23	3	0	0	14.4	4.2	251
Fried chicken, light meat, broiler or fryer, with skin, flour-fried	3 oz	209	26	2	0	0	10.3	5.3	235
Goulash, beef	5 oz	152	19	4	1	2	6.5	2.0	73
Macaroni & cheese, prepared from dry with 2% milk & margarine	5 oz	242	8	34	2	8	8.1	4.5	230
Mashed potatoes, flakes, prepared from dry with milk & butter	5 oz	136	2	15	1	2	7.2	2.0	465
Mashed potatoes, granules with milk, prepared with water & margarine	5 oz	162	3	23	2	2	6.7	1.8	368
Mashed potatoes, prepared from recipe with whole milk	5 oz	116	3	25	2	2	0.8	3.7	444
Mashed potatoes, prepared from recipe with whole milk & butter	5 oz	158	3	24	2	2	5.9	1.2	588
Mashed potatoes, prepared from recipe with whole milk & margarine	5 oz	158	3	24	2	2	5.9	0.4	423
Meal, turkey, stuffing potatoes, gravy and vegetables, microwaved from frozen	10 oz	358	20	46	4	13	10.9	1.2	5225
Patty, corn flour, fried	5 oz	307	6	58	6	6	6.5	4.3	599
Salad, fruit, canned, with heavy syrup	5 oz	102	0	27	1	25	0.1	0.0	7
Soup, bean & bacon, prepared from canned with water	1 cup	151	7	20	7	4	5.2	0.9	840
Soup, bean & bacon, prepared from dehydrated with water	1 cup	96	5	15	8	1	1.9	0.6	449
Soup, bean & ham, reduced sodium, prepared with water from canned	1 cup	178	10	33	10	8	2.5	2.7	1702

ENTRÉES AND SIDE DISHES continued

Item	Serving Size	Calories	Protein	Carb	Fiber	Sugar	Total Fat	Sat Fat	Sodium
Soup, bean & pork, condensed, canned	1 cup	310	14	41	14	7	10.6	3.9	1994
Soup, beef, chunky, ready to serve	1 cup	158	10	24	1	2	2.7	1.2	881
Soup, beef & mushroom, chunky, low sodium, canned	1 cup	166	10	23	0	2	5.5	2.9	1702
Soup, beef noodle, prepared with water	1 cup	82	5	9	1	2	3.0	5.6	1044
Soup, beef Stroganoff, chunky, ready to serve, canned	1 cup	235	12	22	1	4	11.0	1.3	862
Soup, black bean, condensed, canned	1 cup	218	12	37	16	6	3.2	0.4	1169
Soup, black bean, prepared with water, canned	1 cup	110	6	19	8	3	1.6	3.8	1639
Soup, cheese, condensed, canned	1 cup	290	10	20	2	1	19.6	8.7	974
Soup, chicken, chunky, ready to serve, canned	1 cup	170	12	17	1	2	6.3	0.8	1757
Soup, chicken dumplings, condensed, canned	1 cup	190	11	12	1	1	10.8	1.3	857
Soup, chicken dumplings, prepared with water	1 cup	96	6	6	0	1	5.5	0.6	1663
Soup, chicken gumbo, prepared from canned with water	1 cup	55	3	8	2	2	1.4	0.3	938
Soup, chicken gumbo, prepared with water	1 cup	55	3	8	2	2	1.4	4.6	1586
Soup, chicken mushroom, condensed, canned	1 cup	262	8	18	0	3	17.5	2.4	926
Soup, chicken noodle, chunky, ready to serve	1 cup	89	8	10	1	2	2.2	1.0	823
Soup, chicken noodle, chunky, ready to serve, canned	1 cup	89	8	10	1	2	2.2	1.3	1291
Soup, chicken noodle, condensed	1 cup	125	6	14	1	1	4.7	1.3	1291
Soup, chicken noodle, low sodium, canned	1 cup	60	3	7	0	1	2.3	0.6	636

ENTRÉES AND SIDE DISHES continued

Item	Serving Size	Calories	Protein	Carb	Fiber	Sugar	Total Fat	Sat Fat	Sodium
Soup, chicken noodle, prepared from canned with water	1 cup	60	3	7	0	1	2.3	0.3	550
Soup, chicken noodle, prepared from dehydrated with water	1 cup	55	2	9	0	1	1.3	1.0	888
Soup, chicken rice, chunky, ready to serve	1 cup	127	12	13	1	1	3.2	1.0	888
Soup, chicken rice, chunky, ready to serve, canned	1 cup	127	12	13	1	1	3.2	0.9	1596
Soup, chicken rice, condensed	1 cup	118	7	14	1	0	3.7	0.9	1596
Soup, chicken rice, prepared from canned with water	1 cup	58	3	7	1	0	1.9	0.3	461
Soup, chicken vegetable, prepared from canned with water	1 cup	74	4	9	1	1	2.8	0.2	773
Soup, chicken vegetable, with potato & cheese, chunky, ready to serve, canned	1 cup	156	3	12	1	2	10.7	1.9	850
Soup, cream of asparagus, condensed	1 cup	166	4	20	1	2	7.8	2.0	1586
Soup, cream of chicken, condensed, canned	1 cup	216	6	17	0	1	13.8	3.9	1891
Soup, cream of chicken, prepared from dehydrated with water	1 cup	98	2	12	0	4	4.9	4.5	1013
Soup, cream of chicken, reduced sodium, condensed, canned	1 cup	139	4	23	1	1	3.1	3.3	1548
Soup, cream of mushroom, condensed, canned	1 cup	204	4	16	0	4	14.1	3.2	797
Soup, cream of mushroom, prepared from canned with milk	1 cup	161	6	14	0	8	9.3	1.6	763
Soup, cream of mushroom, prepared from canned with water	1 cup	101	2	8	0	2	6.9	1.3	919

ENTRÉES AND SIDE DISHES continued

Item	Serving Size	Calories	Protein	Carb	Fiber	Sugar	Total Fat	Sat Fat	Sodium
Soup, cream of mushroom, ready to serve, low sodium, canned	1 cup	127	2	11	0	4	8.9	2.4	48
Soup, cream of mushroom, reduced sodium, condensed, canned	1 cup	125	3	19	1	5	4.1	2.4	48
Soup, cream of onion, condensed, canned	1 cup	211	5	25	1	9	10.1	3.9	972
Soup, cream of shrimp, prepared from canned with milk	1 cup	146	7	14	0	6	7.8	3.1	938
Soup, cream of shrimp, prepared from canned with water	1 cup	86	3	8	0	1	5.0	4.6	850
Soup, cream of shrimp, prepared with milk	1 cup	146	7	14	0	6	7.8	3.1	938
Soup, cream of vegetable, dehydrated	1 cup	1070	19	125	7	42	57.8	1.3	1080
Soup, cream of vegetable, prepared from dry with water	1 cup	98	2	11	0	0	5.3	1.3	1080
Soup, leek, prepared from dehydrated with water	1 cup	70	2	11	1	2	2.1	1.1	1277
Soup, minestrone, ready to serve, reduced sodium, canned	1 cup	120	5	22	6	5	1.9	0.8	1375
Soup, mushroom, prepared from dehydrated with water	1 cup	79	2	11	0	0	4.4	0.8	967
Soup, mushroom, with beef stock, condensed	1 cup	163	6	18	0	5	7.7	3.0	1855
Soup, onion, dehydrated	1 cup	703	18	156	16	11	0.8	0.0	830
Soup, pea, green, prepared from canned with water	1 cup	146	8	24	5	8	2.6	0.4	1085
Soup, pepper pot, prepared with water	1 cup	98	6	9	0	0	4.4	1.5	1469
Soup, potato, instant	1 cup	823	22	183	18	24	7.4	18.1	4886

ENTRÉES AND SIDE DISHES continued

Item	Serving Size	Calories	Protein	Carb	Fiber	Sugar	Total Fat	Sat Fat	Sodium
Soup, ramen noodle, reduced fat & sodium, assorted flavors, dry	1 cup	840	26	170	6	2	6.0	2.2	1718
Soup, Scotch broth, prepared with water	1 cup	79	5	9	1	1	2.6	3.2	866
Soup, split pea, reduced sodium, canned	1 cup	170	9	28	5	12	2.2	1.6	1750
Soup, split pea, with ham, chunky, ready to serve	1 cup	185	11	27	4	5	4.0	1.6	965
Soup, tomato, prepared from canned with milk	1 cup	132	6	21	1	16	3.1	0.2	653
Soup, tomato, prepared from canned with water	1 cup	72	2	16	1	10	0.7	1.7	696
Soup, tomato, prepared with milk	1 cup	132	6	21	1	16	3.1	0.4	53
Soup, tomato, reduced sodium, condensed	1 cup	156	4	32	3	19	1.3	0.4	53
Soup, tomato beef, with noodle, prepared with water	1 cup	134	4	20	1	2	4.1	1.0	1644
Soup, tomato rice, condensed	1 cup	223	4	41	3	14	5.1	0.5	766
Soup, tomato rice, prepared from canned with water	1 cup	113	2	20	2	7	2.5	0.5	766
Soup, tomato vegetable, dehydrated	1 cup	780	28	144	7	9	12.2	0.4	1322
Soup, turkey noodle, condensed	1 cup	132	7	17	1	1	3.8	1.1	1560
Soup, turkey vegetable, condensed	1 cup	144	6	17	1	3	5.9	1.8	1774
Soup, turkey vegetable, condensed, canned	1 cup	144	6	17	1	3	5.9	0.9	902
Soup, vegetable, chunky, ready to serve	1 cup	122	4	19	1	4	3.7	0.4	924
Soup, vegetable, low sodium, condensed, canned	1 cup	156	5	29	5	10	2.2	0.6	1613

ENTRÉES AND SIDE DISHES continued

Item	Serving Size	Calories	Protein	Carb	Fiber	Sugar	Total Fat	Sat Fat	Sodium
Soup, vegetable, low sodium, prepared from dry mix	1 cup	53	2	10	0	1	0.7	2.3	541
Soup, vegetable, vegetarian, condensed	1 cup	142	4	23	1	8	3.8	0.6	1613
Soup, vegetable, vegetarian, prepared with water	1 cup	67	2	12	1	4	1.9	0.9	1586
Soup, vegetable, with beef broth, condensed	1 cup	158	6	26	3	4	3.7	0.9	1586
Soup, vegetable, with beef broth, prepared with water	1 cup	79	3	13	2	2	1.9	3.6	1027
Soup, vegetable beef, condensed	1 cup	151	11	19	4	2	3.6	0.6	1332
Soup, vegetable beef, prepared from canned with water	1 cup	74	5	10	2	1	1.8	0.5	749
Soup, vegetable beef, prepared from dry with water	1 cup	50	3	8	1	1	1.1	0.8	761
Soup, vegetable beef, prepared with water	1 cup	74	5	10	2	1	1.8	0.5	902
Stew, beef, canned	1 cup	243	11	19	2	4	13.5	5.0	1813
Tamales, Navajo	5 oz	214	9	25	4	1	8.6	5.0	482
Tart, corn flour, fried	5 oz	307	6	58	6	6	6.5	3.9	401
Tortellini, cheese-filled	5 oz	430	19	66	3	1	10.1	5.3	428

FATS AND OILS

Item	Serving Size	Calories	Protein	Carb	Fiber	Sugar	Total Fat	Sat Fat	Sodium
Bacon fat, rendered from cooking	1 tbsp	135	0	0	0	0	14.9	4.8	4
Bacon grease	1 tbsp	135	0	0	0	0	14.9	5.9	23
Beef fat, tallow	1 tbsp	135	0	0	0	0	15.0	7.5	0
Butter, clarified, Odell's	1 tbsp	130	0	0	0	0	14.0	9.0	0
Butter, honey, Land O Lakes	1 tbsp	90	0	4	0	3	8.0	4.0	35
Butter, light, salted	1 tbsp	76	0	0	0	0	8.3	5.1	68
Butter, light, salted, whipped	1 tbsp	45	0	1	0	0	5.0	3.0	80
Butter, light, unsalted	1 tbsp	75	0	0	0	0	8.3	5.1	5
Butter, light, with canola oil, tub, Land O Lakes	1 tbsp	50	0	0	0	0	5.0	2.0	95
Butter, popcorn, Odell's	1 tbsp	130	0	0	0	0	14.0	9.0	0
Butter, garlic, Land O Lakes	1 tbsp	100	0	0	0	0	11.0	5.0	110
Butter, salted	1 tbsp	108	0	0	0	0	12.2	7.7	86
Butter, unsalted	1 tbsp	108	0	0	0	0	12.2	7.7	2
Butter & margarine, blend, 80%, unsalted, stick	1 tbsp	108	0	0	0	0	12.1	4.0	4
Chicken fat	1 tbsp	135	0	0	0	0	15.0	4.5	0
Duck fat	1 tbsp	132	0	0	0	0	15.0	5.0	0
Fat replacer, prune paste, Mariani	1 tbsp	6	0	2	0	1	0.0	0.0	1
Goose fat	1 tbsp	135	0	0	0	0	15.0	4.2	0
Lard	1 tbsp	135	0	0	0	0	15.0	5.9	0
Margarine, 80% unsalted	1 tbsp	108	0	0	0	0	12.1	2.3	0
Margarine, 80% unsalted, tub	1 tbsp	107	0	0	0	0	12.0	2.1	4
Margarine, 80% salted, with vitamin D, stick	1 tbsp	108	0	0	0	0	12.1	2.3	141
Margarine, 80% unsalted, with vitamin D, stick	1 tbsp	108	0	0	0	0	12.1	2.3	0
Margarine, 80% salted, with vitamin D, tub	1 tbsp	107	0	0	0	0	12.0	2.1	99

FATS AND OILS continued

Item	Serving Size	Calories	Protein	Carb	Fiber	Sugar	Total Fat	Sat Fat	Sodium
Margarine, 80% salted, stick	1 tbsp	108	0	0	0	0	12.1	2.3	141
Margarine, 80% salted, tub	1 tbsp	107	0	0	0	0	12.0	2.1	99
Margarine, hard, hydrogenated soybean oil, stick	1 tbsp	108	0	0	0	0	12.1	2.5	141
Margarine & butter, blend, with soybean oil	1 tbsp	107	0	0	0	0	12.0	2.1	95
Meat drippings, lard, beef fat & mutton tallow	1 tbsp	133	0	0	0	0	14.8	6.7	82
Mutton tallow	1 tbsp	135	0	0	0	0	15.0	7.1	0
Oil, almond	1 tbsp	133	0	0	0	0	15.0	1.2	0
Oil, apricot kernel	1 tbsp	133	0	0	0	0	15.0	0.9	0
Oil, avocado	1 tbsp	133	0	0	0	0	15.0	1.7	0
Oil, babassu	1 tbsp	133	0	0	0	0	15.0	12.2	0
Oil, bearded seal, Alaskan	1 tbsp	135	0	0	0	0	14.9	1.6	0
Oil, beluga whale, Alaskan	1 tbsp	135	0	0	0	0	15.0	2.2	0
Oil, canola	1 tbsp	133	0	0	0	0	15.0	1.1	0
Oil, cocoa butter	1 tbsp	133	0	0	0	0	15.0	9.0	0
Oil, coconut	1 tbsp	129	0	0	0	0	15.0	13.0	0
Oil, corn & canola	1 tbsp	133	0	0	0	0	15.0	1.2	0
Oil, corn, peanut, & olive	1 tbsp	133	0	0	0	0	15.0	2.2	0
Oil, corn, salad or cooking	1 tbsp	133	0	0	0	0	15.0	1.9	0
Oil, cottonseed, salad or cooking	1 tbsp	133	0	0	0	0	15.0	3.9	0
Oil, fish, cod liver	1 tbsp	135	0	0	0	0	15.0	3.4	0
Oil, fish, herring	1 tbsp	135	0	0	0	0	15.0	3.2	0
Oil, fish, menhaden	1 tbsp	135	0	0	0	0	15.0	4.6	0
Oil, fish, salmon	1 tbsp	135	0	0	0	0	15.0	3.0	0
Oil, fish, sardine	1 tbsp	135	0	0	0	0	15.0	4.5	0
Oil, flaxseed	1 tbsp	133	0	0	0	0	15.0	1.4	0
Oil, grapeseed	1 tbsp	133	0	0	0	0	15.0	1.4	0
Oil, hazelnut	1 tbsp	133	0	0	0	0	15.0	1.1	0

FATS AND OILS continued

Item	Serving Size	Calories	Protein	Carb	Fiber	Sugar	Total Fat	Sat Fat	Sodium
Oil, mustard	1 tbsp	133	0	0	0	0	15.0	1.7	0
Oil, nutmeg butter	1 tbsp	133	0	0	0	0	15.0	13.5	0
Oil, oat	1 tbsp	133	0	0	0	0	15.0	2.9	0
Oil, olive, salad or cooking	1 tbsp	133	0	0	0	0	15.0	2.1	0
Oil, oogruk, Alaskan	1 tbsp	135	0	0	0	0	14.9	1.6	0
Oil, palm	1 tbsp	133	0	0	0	0	15.0	7.4	0
Oil, palm kernel	1 tbsp	129	0	0	0	0	15.0	12.2	0
Oil, peanut, salad or cooking	1 tbsp	133	0	0	0	0	15.0	2.5	0
Oil, poppy seed	1 tbsp	133	0	0	0	0	15.0	2.0	0
Oil, rice bran	1 tbsp	133	0	0	0	0	15.0	3.0	0
Oil, safflower, salad or cooking	1 tbsp	133	0	0	0	0	15.0	0.9	0
Oil, sesame, salad or cooking	1 tbsp	133	0	0	0	0	15.0	2.1	0
Oil, shea nut	1 tbsp	133	0	0	0	0	15.0	7.0	0
Oil, soybean lecithin	1 tbsp	114	0	0	0	0	15.0	2.3	0
Oil, soybean, salad or cooking	1 tbsp	133	0	0	0	0	15.0	2.3	0
Oil, soybean, salad or cooking, partially hydrogenated	1 tbsp	133	0	0	0	0	15.0	2.2	
Oil, soybean, salad or cooking, partially hydrogenated, with cottonseed oil	1 tbsp	133	0	0	0	0	15.0	2.7	0
Oil, spotted seal, Alaskan	1 tbsp	134	0	0	0	0	14.9	2.2	0
Oil, sunflower, 65% linoleic acid	1 tbsp	133	0	0	0	0	15.0	1.5	0
Oil, sunflower, more than 70% oleic acid	1 tbsp	133	0	0	0	0	15.0	1.5	0
Oil, sunflower, less than 60% linoleic acid	1 tbsp	133	0	0	0	0	15.0	1.5	0
Oil, sunflower, partially hydrogenated, linoleic acid	1 tbsp	133	0	0	0	0	15.0	2.0	0
Oil, tea seed	1 tbsp	133	0	0	0	0	15.0	3.2	0
Oil, tomato seed	1 tbsp	133	0	0	0	0	15.0	3.0	0
Oil, ucuhuba butter	1 tbsp	133	0	0	0	0	15.0	12.8	0

FATS AND OILS continued

Item	Serving Size	Calories	Protein	Carb	Fiber	Sugar	Total Fat	Sat Fat	Sodium
Oil, walnut	1 tbsp	133	0	0	0	0	15.0	1.4	0
Oil, wheat germ	1 tbsp	133	0	0	0	0	15.0	2.8	0
Shortening, all purpose, partially hydrogenated soy & cottonseed oil	1 tbsp	133	0	0	0	0	15.0	3.5	0
Shortening, baking, palm, cottonseed, & hydrogenated soy oil	1 tbsp	133	0	0	0	0	15.0	4.3	0
Shortening, bread, cottonseed & hydrogenated soy oil	1 tbsp	133	0	0	0	0	15.0	3.3	0
Shortening, cake & frosting, hydrogenated soybean	1 tbsp	133	0	0	0	0	15.0	3.0	0
Shortening, cake mix, hydrogenated soy & cottonseed oil	1 tbsp	133	0	0	0	0	15.0	4.1	0
Shortening, confectionery, fractionated palm oil	1 tbsp	133	0	0	0	0	15.0	9.8	0
Shortening, confectionery, hydrogenated coconut & palm oil	1 tbsp	133	0	0	0	0	15.0	13.7	0
Shortening, frying, heavy duty, beef fat tallow & cottonseed oil	1 tbsp	135	0	0	0	0	15.0	6.7	0
Shortening, frying, heavy duty, hydrogenated palm oil	1 tbsp	133	0	0	0	0	15.0	7.1	0
Shortening, frying, heavy duty, hydrogenated soy oil, <1% linoleic acid	1 tbsp	133	0	0	0	0	15.0	3.2	0
Shortening, household, hydrogenated soybean & cottonseed oil	1 tbsp	133	0	0	0	0	15.0	3.8	0
Shortening, household, lard & vegetable oil	1 tbsp	135	0	0	0	0	15.0	6.0	0
Shortening, household, palm & hydrogenated soybean oil	1 tbsp	133	0	0	0	0	15.0	3.8	0

FATS AND OILS continued

Item	Serving Size	Calories	Protein	Carb	Fiber	Sugar	Total Fat	Sat Fat	Sodium
Shortening, household, vegetable oil	1 tbsp	133	0	0	0	0	15.0	3.7	1
Shortening, institutional	1 tbsp	134	0	0	0	0	15.0	3.6	0
Shortening, multipurpose, hydrogenated soybean & palm oil	1 tbsp	133	0	0	0	0	15.0	4.6	0
Shortening, soybean & partially hydrogenated soybean	1 tbsp	133	0	0	0	0	15.0	2.6	0
Spread, 37% vegetable oil, with vitamin D	1 tbsp	51	0	0	0	0	5.7	1.3	88
Spread, 60% vegetable oil, unsalted, with vitamin D, bottle	10-second spray	1	0	0	0	0	0.1	0.0	0
Spread, 60% vegetable oil, unsalted, with vitamin D, stick	1 tbsp	81	0	0	0	0	9.0	1.8	0
Spread, 60% vegetable oil, unsalted, with vitamin D, tub	1 tbsp	81	0	0	0	0	9.0	1.8	0
Spread, 60% vegetable oil, with vitamin D, stick	1 tbsp	81	0	0	0	0	9.1	1.6	118
Spread, 60% vegetable oil, with vitamin D, tub	1 tbsp	80	0	0	0	0	9.0	1.8	118
Spread, buttery, whipped, Smart Balance	1 tbsp	80	0	0	0	0	9.0	2.5	100
Spread, buttery, omega-3 Smart Balance	1 tbsp	91	0	0	0	0	10.6	3.0	109
Spread, margarine, 60% vegetable oil, with vitamin D, bottle	10-second spray	1	0	0	0	0	0.1	0.0	2
Spread, margarine, 60% vegetable oil, with vitamin D, stick	1 tbsp	80	0	0	0	0	8.9	1.5	118
Spread, margarine, 60% vegetable oil, with vitamin D, tub	1 tbsp	80	0	0	0	0	8.9	1.5	118
Spread, margarine, reduced calorie, unspecified oil, 37% fat	1 tbsp	51	0	0	0	0	5.7	1.3	88
Spread, sweetened	1 tbsp	80	0	3	0	3	7.8	1.3	81

FATS AND OILS continued

Item	Serving Size	Calories	Protein	Carb	Fiber	Sugar	Total Fat	Sat Fat	Sodium
Spread, vegetable oil & butter, reduced calorie	1 tbsp	70	0	0	0	0	8.0	2.7	87
Spread, vegetable oil, 20% fat	1 tbsp	26	0	0	0	0	2.9	0.4	110
Spread, vegetable oil, 20% unsalted	1 tbsp	26	0	0	0	0	2.9	0.4	0
Spread, vegetable oil, 60% bottle	10-second spray	1	0	0	0	0	0.1	0.0	2
Spread, vegetable oil, 60% fat	1 tbsp	79	0	0	0	0	8.9	1.5	118
Spread, vegetable oil, 60% stick	1 tbsp	81	0	0	0	0	9.1	1.6	118
Spread, vegetable oil, 60% tub	1 tbsp	80	0	0	0	0	9.0	1.8	118
Spread, vegetable oil, 60% unsalted, bottle	10-second spray	1	0	0	0	0	0.1	0.0	0
Spread, vegetable oil, 60% unsalted, stick	1 tbsp	80	0	0	0	0	9.0	1.8	0
Spread, vegetable oil, 60% unsalted, tub	1 tbsp	80	0	0	0	0	9.0	1.8	0
Spread, vegetable oil, fat-free, tub	1 tbsp	7	0	1	0	0	0.5	0.3	87
Spread, vegetable oil, reduced calorie, tub	1 tbsp	68	0	0	0	0	7.5	2.5	91
Spread, vegetable oil, tub	1 tbsp	54	0	0	0	0	6.0	1.1	118
Spread, made with yogurt, Brummel & Brown	1 tbsp	45	0	0	0	0	5.0	1.0	90
Spread, yogurt, 40% reduced calorie, tub	1 tbsp	50	0	0	0	0	5.3	1.1	95
Spread, yogurt, 70% stick	1 tbsp	95	0	0	0	0	10.5	2.0	89

FISH

Item	Serving Size	Calories	Protein	Carb	Fiber	Sugar	Total Fat	Sat Fat	Sodium
Fish, anchovies, European, canned, with oil, drained	3 oz	179	25	0	0	0	8.3	1.1	88
Fish, anchovies, European, raw	3 oz	111	17	0	0	0	4.1	1.9	3118
Fish, anchovies, European, with oil, drained	3 oz	179	25	0	0	0	8.3	0.9	77
Fish, bass, freshwater, mixed species, fillet, baked or broiled	3 oz	124	21	0	0	0	4.0	0.7	60
Fish, bass, freshwater, mixed species, fillet, raw	3 oz	97	16	0	0	0	3.1	0.6	74
Fish, bass, sea, mixed species, fillet, baked or broiled	3 oz	105	20	0	0	0	2.2	0.4	58
Fish, bass, sea, mixed species, fillet, raw	3 oz	82	16	0	0	0	1.7	0.6	75
Fish, bass, striped, fillet, baked or broiled	3 oz	105	19	0	0	0	2.5	0.6	75
Fish, blackfish, whole, Alaskan	3 oz	70	13	0	0	0	1.5	1.0	65
Fish, bluefish, fillet, baked or broiled	3 oz	135	22	0	0	0	4.6	1.0	65
Fish, bluefish, fillet, raw	3 oz	105	17	0	0	0	3.6	0.2	105
Fish, burbot, fillet, baked or broiled	3 oz	98	21	0	0	0	0.9	0.1	82
Fish, butterfish, fillet, baked or broiled	3 oz	159	19	0	0	0	8.7	2.9	76
Fish, butterfish, fillet, raw	3 oz	124	15	0	0	0	6.8	1.2	54
Fish, carp, fillet, baked or broiled	3 oz	138	19	0	0	0	6.1	1.2	54
Fish, carp, fillet, raw	3 oz	108	15	0	0	0	4.8	1.5	68
Fish, catfish, channel, farmed, fillet, baked or broiled	3 oz	129	16	0	0	0	6.8	1.5	45
Fish, catfish, channel, farmed, fillet, raw	3 oz	115	13	0	0	0	6.5	0.6	37
Fish, catfish, channel, fillet, raw, wild	3 oz	81	14	0	0	0	2.4	0.6	43
Fish, catfish, channel, wild, fillet, baked or broiled	3 oz	89	16	0	0	0	2.4	0.4	47

FISH continued

Item	Serving Size	Calories	Protein	Carb	Fiber	Sugar	Total Fat	Sat Fat	Sodium
Fish, catfish, fillet, cooked	3 oz	130	17	0	0	0	6.0	0.0	65
Fish, cisco, fillet, raw	3 oz	83	16	0	0	0	1.6	1.5	409
Fish, cisco, smoked	3 oz	150	14	0	0	0	10.1	0.1	185
Fish, cod, Atlantic, canned, with liquid	3 oz	89	19	0	0	0	0.7	0.4	5973
Fish, cod, Atlantic, dried & salted	3 oz	247	53	0	0	0	2.0	0.1	66
Fish, cod, Atlantic, fillet, baked or broiled	3 oz	89	19	0	0	0	0.7	0.1	46
Fish, cod, Atlantic, fillet, raw	3 oz	70	15	0	0	0	0.6	0.1	77
Fish, cod, cooked	3 oz	90	20	0	0	0	1.0	0.0	100
Fish, cod, Pacific, fillet, baked or broiled	3 oz	89	20	0	0	0	0.7	0.1	60
Fish, cod, Pacific, fillet, raw	3 oz	70	15	0	0	0	0.5	0.9	48
Fish, cusk, fillet, baked or broiled	3 oz	95	21	0	0	0	0.7	0.1	26
Fish, devilfish, Alaskan	3 oz	82	10	0	0	0	4.5	0.2	96
Fish, dolphin fish, fillet, baked or broiled	3 oz	93	20	0	0	0	0.8	0.2	75
Fish, dolphin fish, fillet, raw	3 oz	72	16	0	0	0	0.6	1.2	82
Fish, drum, fillet, baked or broiled	3 oz	130	19	0	0	0	5.4	1.0	64
Fish, drum, freshwater, fillet, raw	3 oz	101	15	0	0	0	4.2	0.3	89
Fish, flounder, cooked	3 oz	100	19	0	0	0	1.5	0.0	85
Fish, flounder, fillet, baked or broiled	3 oz	99	21	0	0	0	1.3	0.2	69
Fish, flounder, fillet, raw	3 oz	77	16	0	0	0	1.0	0.3	45
Fish, grouper, mixed species, fillet, baked or broiled	3 oz	100	21	0	0	0	1.1	0.3	45
Fish, grouper, mixed species, fillet, raw	3 oz	78	16	0	0	0	0.9	0.1	74
Fish, haddock, fillet, baked or broiled	3 oz	95	21	0	0	0	0.8	0.1	58
Fish, haddock, fillet, cooked	3 oz	100	21	0	0	0	1.0	0.0	60
Fish, haddock, fillet, raw	3 oz	74	16	0	0	0	0.6	0.1	649
Fish, haddock, smoked	3 oz	99	21	0	0	0	0.8	0.4	59
Fish, halibut, Atlantic or Pacific, fillet, baked or broiled	3 oz	119	23	0	0	0	2.5	0.3	46

FISH continued

Item	Serving Size	Calories	Protein	Carb	Fiber	Sugar	Total Fat	Sat Fat	Sodium
Fish, halibut, Atlantic or Pacific, fillet, raw	3 oz	94	18	0	0	0	1.9	2.6	88
Fish, halibut, fillet, cooked	3 oz	120	23	0	0	0	2.0	0.0	70
Fish, halibut, Greenland, fillet, baked or broiled	3 oz	203	16	0	0	0	15.1	2.1	68
Fish, halibut, Greenland, fillet, raw	3 oz	158	12	0	0	0	11.8	0.4	73
Fish, halibut, with skin, cooked, Alaskan	3 oz	96	19	0	0	0	2.3	0.6	67
Fish, herring, Atlantic smoked kippered fillet	3 oz	184	21	0	0	0	10.5	2.2	98
Fish, herring, Atlantic, fillet, baked/broiled	3 oz	173	20	0	0	0	9.9	1.7	77
Fish, herring, Atlantic, fillet, raw	3 oz	134	15	0	0	0	7.7	2.0	740
Fish, herring, Atlantic, pickled	3 oz	223	12	8	0	7	15.3	2.0	740
Fish, herring, Atlantic, smoked, kippered	3 oz	184	21	0	0	0	10.5	3.5	81
Fish, herring, Pacific, fillet, baked or broiled	3 oz	213	18	0	0	0	15.1	2.8	63
Fish, hoki, grilled	3 oz	0	0	0	0	0	1.0	0.9	255
Fish, ling, fillet, baked or broiled	3 oz	94	21	0	0	0	0.7	0.1	115
Fish, ling, fillet, raw	3 oz	74	16	0	0	0	0.5	0.2	65
Fish, lingcod, fillet, baked or broiled	3 oz	93	19	0	0	0	1.2	0.2	50
Fish, lingcod, raw, Alaskan	3 oz	67	15	0	0	0	0.7	3.6	71
Fish, mackerel, Atlantic, fillet, baked or broiled	3 oz	223	20	0	0	0	15.1	2.8	77
Fish, mackerel, Atlantic, fillet, raw	3 oz	174	16	0	0	0	11.8	1.6	322
Fish, mackerel, dried	3 oz	259	16	0	0	0	21.3	1.9	4254
Fish, mackerel, jack, canned, drained	3 oz	133	20	0	0	0	5.4	1.6	322
Fish, mackerel, king, fillet, baked or broiled	3 oz	114	22	0	0	0	2.2	0.3	134
Fish, mackerel, king, fillet, raw	3 oz	89	17	0	0	0	1.7	2.4	94

FISH continued

Item	Serving Size	Calories	Protein	Carb	Fiber	Sugar	Total Fat	Sat Fat	Sodium
Fish, mackerel, Pacific & jack fillet, baked or broiled mixed	3 oz	171	22	0	0	0	8.6	2.4	94
Fish, mackerel, Spanish, fillet, baked or broiled	3 oz	134	20	0	0	0	5.4	1.6	50
Fish, mackerel, Spanish, fillet, raw	3 oz	118	16	0	0	0	5.4	0.2	96
Fish, mahi mahi, fillet, baked or broiled	3 oz	93	20	0	0	0	0.8	0.2	96
Fish, milkfish, fillet, baked or broiled	3 oz	162	22	0	0	0	7.3	1.4	61
Fish, monkfish, baked or broiled	3 oz	82	16	0	0	0	1.7	0.3	15
Fish, monkfish, raw	3 oz	65	12	0	0	0	1.3	0.3	15
Fish, moochim, Korean style, dried	3 oz	289	32	10	1	9	13.3	2.4	780
Fish, mullet, striped, fillet, baked or broiled	3 oz	128	21	0	0	0	4.1	1.0	55
Fish, mullet, striped, fillet, raw	3 oz	99	16	0	0	0	3.2	0.0	59
Fish, orange roughy, fillet, baked/broiled	3 oz	89	19	0	0	0	0.8	0.0	61
Fish, orange roughy, fillet, cooked	3 oz	80	16	0	0	0	1.0	0.5	95
Fish, orange roughy, fillet, raw	3 oz	65	14	0	0	0	0.6	0.2	67
Fish, perch, mixed species, fillet, baked/broiled	3 oz	99	21	0	0	0	1.0	0.2	53
Fish, perch, mixed species, fillet, raw	3 oz	77	16	0	0	0	0.8	0.3	82
Fish, perch, ocean, Atlantic, fillet, baked/broiled	3 oz	103	20	0	0	0	1.8	0.2	64
Fish, perch, ocean, Atlantic, fillet, raw	3 oz	80	16	0	0	0	1.4	0.1	42
Fish, perch, ocean, cooked	3 oz	110	21	0	0	0	2.0	0.0	110
Fish, pike, northern, fillet, baked/broiled	3 oz	96	21	0	0	0	0.7	0.1	33
Fish, pike, walleye, fillet, baked/broiled	3 oz	101	21	0	0	0	1.3	0.2	43

FISH continued

Item	Serving Size	Calories	Protein	Carb	Fiber	Sugar	Total Fat	Sat Fat	Sodium
Fish, pike, walleye, fillet, raw	3 oz	79	16	0	0	0	1.0	0.1	94
Fish, pollock, Atlantic, fillet, baked/broiled	3 oz	100	21	0	0	0	1.1	0.1	73
Fish, pollock, Atlantic, fillet, raw	3 oz	78	17	0	0	0	0.8	0.2	99
Fish, pollock, walleye, fillet, baked/broiled	3 oz	96	20	0	0	0	1.0	0.1	84
Fish, pollock, walleye, fillet, raw	3 oz	69	15	0	0	0	0.7	3.8	65
Fish, pompano, Florida, fillet, baked/broiled	3 oz	179	20	0	0	0	10.3	3.0	55
Fish, pompano, Florida, fillet, raw	3 oz	139	16	0	0	0	8.0	0.3	66
Fish, pout, ocean, fillet, baked/broiled	3 oz	87	18	0	0	0	1.0	0.3	52
Fish, pout, ocean, fillet, raw	3 oz	67	14	0	0	0	0.8	0.2	88
Fish, pumpkinseed sunfish, fillet, baked/broiled	3 oz	97	21	0	0	0	0.8	0.1	68
Fish, pumpkinseed sunfish, fillet, raw	3 oz	76	16	0	0	0	0.6	0.4	65
Fish, rockfish, Pacific, mixed species, fillet, baked/broiled	3 oz	103	20	0	0	0	1.7	0.3	51
Fish, rockfish, Pacific, mixed species, fillet, raw	3 oz	80	16	0	0	0	1.3	3.5	61
Fish, sablefish, fillet, baked/broiled	3 oz	213	15	0	0	0	16.7	2.7	48
Fish, sablefish, fillet, raw	3 oz	166	11	0	0	0	13.0	3.6	626
Fish, sablefish, smoked	3 oz	218	15	0	0	0	17.1	2.1	52
Fish, salmon, Atlantic, farmed, fillet, baked/broiled	3 oz	175	19	0	0	0	10.5	2.6	50
Fish, salmon, Atlantic, farmed, fillet, raw	3 oz	177	17	0	0	0	11.4	1.1	48
Fish, salmon, Atlantic, wild, fillet, baked/broiled	3 oz	155	22	0	0	0	6.9	0.8	37
Fish, salmon, Atlantic, wild, fillet, raw	3 oz	121	17	0	0	0	5.4	2.7	51

FISH continued

Item	Serving Size	Calories	Protein	Carb	Fiber	Sugar	Total Fat	Sat Fat	Sodium
Fish, salmon, chinook, fillet, baked/broiled	3 oz	196	22	0	0	0	11.4	2.6	40
Fish, salmon, chinook, fillet, raw	3 oz	152	17	0	0	0	8.9	1.6	41
Fish, salmon, chinook, lox	3 oz	99	16	0	0	0	3.7	0.8	666
Fish, salmon, chinook, smoked	3 oz	99	16	0	0	0	3.7	0.8	666
Fish, salmon, chinook, smoked, canned, Alaskan	3 oz	128	20	0	0	0	5.0	5.9	589
Fish, salmon, chinook, smoked, with brine, Alaskan	3 oz	366	34	0	0	0	25.5	2.0	162
Fish, salmon, chum, dried, Alaskan	3 oz	321	53	0	0	0	12.2	0.9	54
Fish, salmon, chum, fillet, baked/broiled	3 oz	131	22	0	0	0	4.1	0.7	43
Fish, salmon, chum, fillet, raw	3 oz	102	17	0	0	0	3.2	0.5	50
Fish, salmon, chum, pink, fillet, cooked	3 oz	130	22	0	0	0	4.0	2.0	55
Fish, salmon, chum, with bone, canned, drained	3 oz	120	18	0	0	0	4.7	1.3	64
Fish, salmon, chum, with bone, canned, drained, unsalted	3 oz	120	18	0	0	0	4.7	1.6	44
Fish, salmon, coho, Atlantic, fillet, cooked	3 oz	200	24	0	0	0	10.0	2.0	55
Fish, salmon, coho, farmed, fillet, baked/broiled	3 oz	151	21	0	0	0	7.0	1.5	40
Fish, salmon, coho, farmed, fillet, raw	3 oz	136	18	0	0	0	6.5	0.8	49
Fish, salmon, coho, fillet, raw, Alaskan	3 oz	119	19	0	0	0	4.7	0.9	49
Fish, salmon, coho, wild, fillet, baked/broiled	3 oz	118	20	0	0	0	3.7	1.1	39
Fish, salmon, coho, wild, fillet, raw	3 oz	124	18	0	0	0	5.0	1.4	45
Fish, salmon, coho, wild, fillet, steamed	3 oz	156	23	0	0	0	6.4	1.6	41

FISH continued

Item	Serving Size	Calories	Protein	Carb	Fiber	Sugar	Total Fat	Sat Fat	Sodium
Fish, salmon, king, smoked, canned, Alaskan	3 oz	128	20	0	0	0	5.0	5.9	589
Fish, salmon, king, smoked, with brine, Alaskan	3 oz	366	34	0	0	0	25.5	2.1	740
Fish, salmon, king, with skin, kippered, Alaskan	3 oz	178	20	0	0	0	11.0	0.6	73
Fish, salmon, pink, fillet, baked/broiled	3 oz	127	22	0	0	0	3.8	0.5	57
Fish, salmon, pink, fillet, raw	3 oz	99	17	0	0	0	2.9	0.7	339
Fish, salmon, pink, with bone, canned, drained	3 oz	116	20	0	0	0	4.1	1.3	471
Fish, salmon, pink, with bone, canned, with liquid	3 oz	118	17	0	0	0	5.1	1.3	64
Fish, salmon, pink, with bone, unsalted, canned, with liquid	3 oz	118	17	0	0	0	5.1	0.9	51
Fish, salmon, red, fillet, raw, Alaskan	3 oz	130	19	0	0	0	6.2	0.7	391
Fish, salmon, red, kippered, Alaskan	3 oz	120	21	0	0	0	4.0	2.2	43
Fish, salmon, red, smoked, Alaskan	3 oz	293	52	0	0	0	9.7	1.3	510
Fish, salmon, red, smoked, canned, Alaskan	3 oz	175	30	0	0	0	6.2	0.8	332
Fish, salmon, red, without bone, canned, Alaskan	3 oz	137	23	0	0	0	4.9	0.8	49
Fish, salmon, silver, fillet, raw, Alaskan	3 oz	119	19	0	0	0	4.7	1.6	56
Fish, salmon, sockeye, fillet, baked/broiled	3 oz	184	23	0	0	0	9.3	1.3	40
Fish, salmon, sockeye, fillet, cooked	3 oz	200	24	0	0	0	10.0	0.0	100
Fish, salmon, sockeye, fillet, raw	3 oz	143	18	0	0	0	7.3	0.9	51
Fish, salmon, sockeye, fillet, raw, Alaskan	3 oz	130	19	0	0	0	6.2	0.7	391
Fish, salmon, sockeye, kippered, Alaskan	3 oz	120	21	0	0	0	4.0	2.2	43

FISH continued

Item	Serving Size	Calories	Protein	Carb	Fiber	Sugar	Total Fat	Sat Fat	Sodium
Fish, salmon, sockeye, smoked, Alaskan	3 oz	293	52	0	0	0	9.7	1.3	510
Fish, salmon, sockeye, smoked, canned, Alaskan	3 oz	175	30	0	0	0	6.2	1.3	306
Fish, salmon, sockeye, with bone, canned, drained	3 oz	141	20	0	0	0	6.2	1.4	64
Fish, salmon, tipnuk, fermented, Alaskan	3 oz	135	14	0	0	0	9.0	1.3	429
Fish, sardines, Atlantic, with bones, canned, with oil, drained	3 oz	177	21	0	0	0	9.7	1.3	429
Fish, sardines, without skin & bone, with water	3 oz	184	21	0	0	0	10.5	1.4	108
Fish, scup, fillet, baked/broiled	3 oz	115	21	0	0	0	3.0	0.5	36
Fish, scup, fillet, raw	3 oz	89	16	0	0	0	2.3	1.1	63
Fish, sea trout, mixed species, fillet, baked/broiled	3 oz	113	18	0	0	0	3.9	0.9	49
Fish, shad, American, fillet, baked/broiled	3 oz	214	18	0	0	0	15.0	2.7	43
Fish, shad, American, fillet, raw	3 oz	167	14	0	0	0	11.7	0.8	67
Fish, shark, mixed species, raw	3 oz	111	18	0	0	0	3.8	0.4	44
Fish, sheefish, dried, Alaskan	3 oz	98	19	0	0	0	2.4	0.3	62
Fish, sheepshead, fillet, baked/broiled	3 oz	107	22	0	0	0	1.4	0.5	60
Fish, sheepshead, fillet, raw	3 oz	92	17	0	0	0	2.0	3.1	357
Fish, smelt, dried, Alaskan	3 oz	328	48	0	0	0	15.2	0.5	65
Fish, smelt, rainbow, baked/broiled	3 oz	105	19	0	0	0	2.6	0.4	51
Fish, smelt, rainbow, raw	3 oz	82	15	0	0	0	2.1	0.3	48
Fish, snapper, mixed species, fillet, baked/broiled	3 oz	109	22	0	0	0	1.5	0.3	48
Fish, snapper, mixed species, fillet, raw	3 oz	85	17	0	0	0	1.1	0.3	89
Fish, sole, cooked	3 oz	100	19	0	0	0	1.5	1.5	100

FISH continued

Item	Serving Size	Calories	Protein	Carb	Fiber	Sugar	Total Fat	Sat Fat	Sodium
Fish, sole, fillet, baked/broiled	3 oz	99	21	0	0	0	1.3	0.2	69
Fish, sole, fillet, raw	3 oz	77	16	0	0	0	1.0	1.6	31
Fish, spot, fillet, baked/broiled	3 oz	134	20	0	0	0	5.3	1.2	25
Fish, spot, fillet, raw	3 oz	105	16	0	0	0	4.2	1.0	59
Fish, sprat, dried	3 oz	0	0	0	0	0	1.5	2.6	697
Fish, sturgeon, mixed species, baked/broiled	3 oz	115	18	0	0	0	4.4	1.0	59
Fish, sturgeon, mixed species, fillet, raw	3 oz	89	14	0	0	0	3.4	0.9	628
Fish, sturgeon, mixed species, smoked	3 oz	147	27	0	0	0	3.7	0.5	43
Fish, sucker, white, fillet, baked/broiled	3 oz	101	18	0	0	0	2.5	0.4	34
Fish, sucker, white, fillet, raw	3 oz	78	14	0	0	0	2.0	0.2	122
Fish, surimi	3 oz	84	13	6	0	0	0.8	1.2	98
Fish, swordfish, fillet, baked/broiled	3 oz	132	22	0	0	0	4.4	0.9	77
Fish, tilapia, baked/broiled	3 oz	109	22	0	0	0	2.3	0.6	44
Fish, tilapia, raw	3 oz	82	17	0	0	0	1.4	0.7	50
Fish, tilefish, fillet, baked/broiled	3 oz	125	21	0	0	0	4.0	0.4	45
Fish, tilefish, fillet, raw	3 oz	82	15	0	0	0	2.0	1.2	57
Fish, trout, mixed species, fillet, baked/broiled	3 oz	162	23	0	0	0	7.2	1.0	44
Fish, trout, mixed species, fillet, raw	3 oz	126	18	0	0	0	5.6	1.8	36
Fish, trout, rainbow, farmed, fillet, baked/broiled	3 oz	144	21	0	0	0	6.1	1.3	30
Fish, trout, rainbow, farmed, fillet, raw	3 oz	117	18	0	0	0	4.6	1.4	48
Fish, trout, rainbow, wild, fillet, baked/broiled	3 oz	128	19	0	0	0	4.9	0.6	26
Fish, trout, rainbow, wild, fillet, raw	3 oz	101	17	0	0	0	2.9	1.3	100

FISH continued

Item	Serving Size	Calories	Protein	Carb	Fiber	Sugar	Total Fat	Sat Fat	Sodium
Fish, trout, steelhead, cooked, canned, Alaskan	3 oz	135	18	0	0	0	7.0	0.7	2423
Fish, trout, steelhead, dried, Shoshone Bannock	3 oz	325	66	0	0	0	6.9	1.4	43
Fish, tuna, bluefin, fillet, baked/broiled	3 oz	156	25	0	0	0	5.3	1.4	43
Fish, tuna, bluefin, raw	3 oz	122	20	0	0	0	4.2	1.3	43
Fish, tuna, cooked	3 oz	130	26	0	0	0	1.5	0.0	320
Fish, tuna, dried	3 oz	153	25	0	0	0	5.2	2.4	94
Fish, tuna, light, canned, with oil, drained	3 oz	168	25	0	0	0	7.0	0.2	287
Fish, tuna, light, canned, with water, drained	3 oz	99	22	0	0	0	0.7	0.4	40
Fish, tuna, light, unsalted, canned, with oil, drained	3 oz	168	25	0	0	0	7.0	0.2	43
Fish, tuna, light, unsalted, canned, with water, drained	3 oz	99	22	0	0	0	0.7	1.3	301
Fish, tuna, skipjack, fillet, baked/broiled	3 oz	112	24	0	0	0	1.1	0.3	31
Fish, tuna, skipjack, fillet, raw	3 oz	88	19	0	0	0	0.9	1.1	337
Fish, tuna, smoked	3 oz	171	22	0	0	0	8.6	0.2	8237
Fish, tuna, white, canned, with oil, drained	3 oz	158	23	0	0	0	6.9	1.4	43
Fish, tuna, white, unsalted, canned, with oil, drained	3 oz	158	23	0	0	0	6.9	0.7	43
Fish, tuna, white, unsalted, canned, with water, drained	3 oz	109	20	0	0	0	2.5	0.7	320
Fish, tuna, white, with water, drained, can	3 oz	109	20	0	0	0	2.5	0.3	40
Fish, tuna, yellowfin, fillet, baked/broiled	3 oz	118	25	0	0	0	1.0	0.2	31
Fish, turbot, European, fillet, baked/broiled	3 oz	104	17	0	0	0	3.2	0.0	163
Fish, turbot, European, fillet, raw	3 oz	81	14	0	0	0	2.5	0.4	136
Fish, whitefish, dried, Alaskan	3 oz	315	53	0	0	0	11.4	1.0	55

FISH continued

Item	Serving Size	Calories	Protein	Carb	Fiber	Sugar	Total Fat	Sat Fat	Sodium
Fish, whitefish, mixed species, fillet, baked/broiled	3 oz	146	21	0	0	0	6.4	1.0	55
Fish, whitefish, mixed species, fillet, raw	3 oz	114	16	0	0	0	5.0	1.2	43
Fish, whitefish, mixed species, raw, Alaskan	3 oz	111	16	0	0	0	5.2	0.2	866
Fish, whitefish, mixed species, smoked, flaked	3 oz	92	20	0	0	0	0.8	0.3	112
Fish, whiting, mixed species, fillet, baked/broiled	3 oz	99	20	0	0	0	1.4	0.2	61
Fish, whiting, mixed species, fillet, raw	3 oz	77	16	0	0	0	1.1	0.4	93
Fish, wolffish, Atlantic, fillet, baked/broiled	3 oz	105	19	0	0	0	2.6	0.3	72
Fish, yellowtail, mixed species, fillet, baked/broiled	3 oz	159	25	0	0	0	5.7	1.1	33
Fish, yellowtail, mixed species, fillet, raw	3 oz	124	20	0	0	0	4.5	0.2	8237
Sashimi, mackerel, Pacific & jack, mixed species, fillet	3 oz	134	17	0	0	0	6.7	2.6	40
Sashimi, salmon, chinook, fillet	3 oz	152	17	0	0	0	8.9	0.2	54
Sashimi, snapper, mixed species, fillet	3 oz	85	17	0	0	0	1.1	1.1	33
Sashimi, tuna, bluefin	3 oz	122	20	0	0	0	4.2	0.3	31
Sashimi, tuna, skipjack, fillet	3 oz	88	19	0	0	0	0.9	0.2	31
Sashimi, tuna, yellowfin, fillet, without bone	3 oz	92	20	0	0	0	0.8	1.1	33
Sashimi, yellowtail, mixed species, fillet	3 oz	124	20	0	0	0	4.5	0.1	676

FRUITS

Item	Serving Size	Calories	Protein	Carb	Fiber	Sugar	Total Fat	Sat Fat	Sodium
Adam's fig, fresh	5 oz	171	2	45	3	21	0.5	0.2	6
Apples, fresh	5 oz	73	0	19	3	15	0.2	0.0	1
Apples, fresh, peeled	5 oz	67	0	18	2	14	0.2	0.0	0
Apples, fresh, quartered	5 oz	73	0	19	3	15	0.2	0.0	1
Apples, peeled, cooked from fresh	5 oz	74	0	19	3	15	0.5	0.1	1
Apples, peeled, microwaved	5 oz	78	0	20	4	16	0.6	0.1	1
Apples, sulfured, dehydrated	1.5 oz	138	1	37	5	32	0.2	0.0	50
Apples, sulfured, rings, dried	1.5 oz	97	0	26	3	23	0.1	0.0	35
Apples, sulfured, stewed from dehydrated	1.5 oz	30	0	8	1	7	0.0	0.0	10
Apples, sulfured, stewed from dried, with added sugar	1.5 oz	33	0	8	1	7	0.0	0.0	8
Apples, sulfured, stewed from dried, without added sugar	1.5 oz	23	0	6	1	5	0.0	0.0	8
Apples, sweetened, drained, canned, cooked	5 oz	94	0	24	3	21	0.6	0.1	4
Apricots, canned, with heavy syrup, drained	5 oz	116	1	30	4	26	0.2	0.0	6
Apricots, fresh	5 oz	67	2	16	3	13	0.5	0.0	1
Apricots, sulfured, dried	5 oz	337	5	88	10	75	0.7	0.0	14
Apricots, sulfured, stewed from dried, without added sugar	5 oz	119	2	31	4	27	0.3	0.0	6
Apricots, whole, with skin, canned, with heavy syrup	5 oz	116	1	30	2	28	0.1	0.0	6
Apricots, with skin, canned, with juice	5 oz	67	1	17	2	15	0.1	0.0	6
Apricots, with skin, canned, with light syrup	5 oz	88	1	23	2	21	0.1	0.0	6
Apricots, with skin, canned, with water	5 oz	38	1	9	2	7	0.2	0.0	4
Avocadoes, California, fresh	5 oz	234	3	12	10	0	21.6	3.0	11
Avocadoes, Florida, fresh	5 oz	168	3	11	8	3	14.1	2.7	3
Bananas, dehydrated	1.5 oz	138	2	35	4	19	0.7	0.3	1
Bananas, fresh	5 oz	125	2	32	4	17	0.5	0.2	1

FRUITS continued

Item	Serving Size	Calories	Protein	Carb	Fiber	Sugar	Total Fat	Sat Fat	Sodium
Blackberries, canned, with heavy syrup	5 oz	129	2	32	5	28	0.2	0.0	4
Blackberries, fresh	5 oz	60	2	13	7	6	0.7	0.0	1
Blackberries, unsweetened, frozen	5 oz	90	2	22	7	15	0.6	0.0	1
Blueberries, canned, with heavy syrup	5 oz	123	1	31	2	29	0.5	0.0	4
Blueberries, fresh	5 oz	80	1	20	3	14	0.5	0.0	1
Blueberries, sweetened, frozen	5 oz	113	1	31	3	28	0.2	0.0	1
Blueberries, wild, frozen	5 oz	71	0	19	6	10	0.2	0.0	4
Boysenberries, unsweetened, frozen	5 oz	70	2	17	7	10	0.4	0.0	1
Breadfruits, fresh	5 oz	144	1	38	7	15	0.3	0.1	3
Carambolas, fresh	5 oz	43	1	9	4	6	0.5	0.0	3
Cherimoyas, fresh	5 oz	105	2	25	4	18	1.0	0.3	10
Cherries, maraschino, canned, drained	1 oz	50	0	13	1	12	0.1	0.0	1
Cherries, red, sour, canned, with heavy syrup	5 oz	127	1	33	2	31	0.1	0.0	10
Cherries, red, sour, canned, with water	5 oz	50	1	13	2	11	0.1	0.0	10
Cherries, red, sour, fresh	5 oz	70	1	17	2	12	0.4	0.1	4
Cherries, red, sour, unsweetened, frozen	5 oz	64	1	15	2	13	0.6	0.1	1
Cherries, red, tart, canned, with water	5 oz	50	1	13	2	11	0.1	0.0	10
Cherries, sweet, canned, with extra heavy syrup	5 oz	143	1	37	2	34	0.2	0.0	4
Cherries, sweet, canned, with heavy syrup	5 oz	116	1	30	2	23	0.2	0.0	4
Cherries, sweet, canned, with light syrup	5 oz	94	1	24	2	22	0.2	0.0	4
Cherries, sweet, canned, with water	5 oz	64	1	16	2	14	0.2	0.0	1
Cherries, sweet, fresh	5 oz	88	1	22	3	18	0.3	0.1	0
Cherries, sweet, sweetened, frozen	5 oz	125	2	31	3	28	0.2	0.0	1
Cherries, sweetened, canned, with juice	5 oz	76	1	19	2	17	0.0	0.0	4

FRUITS continued

Item	Serving Size	Calories	Protein	Carb	Fiber	Sugar	Total Fat	Sat Fat	Sodium
Chinese gooseberries, fresh	5 oz	85	2	21	4	13	0.7	0.0	4
Chinese gooseberries, gold, fresh	5 oz	84	2	20	3	15	0.8	0.2	4
Cranberries, dried, sweetened	1.5 oz	123	0	33	2	26	0.5	0.0	1
Cranberries, fresh	5 oz	64	1	17	6	6	0.2	0.0	3
Cranberry sauce, sweetened, canned, slice	5 oz	211	0	54	1	53	0.2	0.0	41
Currants, red, fresh	5 oz	78	2	19	6	10	0.3	0.0	1
Currants, white, fresh	5 oz	78	2	19	6	10	0.3	0.0	1
Currants, Zante, dried	1.5 oz	113	2	30	3	27	0.1	0.0	3
Date plums, fresh	5 oz	98	1	26	5	18	0.3	0.0	1
Dates, Deglet Noor, whole	1.5 oz	118.4	1.0	31.5	3.4	26.6	0.2	0.0	0.8
Figs, canned, with heavy syrup	5 oz	123	1	32	3	29	0.1	0.0	1
Figs, canned, with light syrup	5 oz	97	1	25	3	23	0.1	0.0	1
Figs, canned, with water	5 oz	74	1	20	3	17	0.1	0.0	1
Figs, dried	1.5 oz	100	1	26	4	19	0.4	0.1	4
Figs, fresh	5 oz	104	1	27	4	23	0.4	0.1	1
Figs, stewed from dried	1.5 oz	43	1	11	2	9	0.2	0.0	2
Fruit, peach, pear, grape, canned, with lite syrup	5 oz	77	1	20	2	16	0.1	0.0	8
Fruit, peach, pear, grape, canned, with lite syrup, drained	5 oz	80	1	21	2	16	0.1	0.0	7
Fruits, candied	5 oz	451	0	116	2	113	0.1	0.0	137
Fruit cocktail, canned, with heavy syrup	5 oz	102	1	26	1	25	0.1	0.0	8
Fruit cocktail, canned, with heavy syrup, drained	5 oz	98	1	26	2	24	0.1	0.0	8
Fruit cocktail, canned, with juice	5 oz	64	1	17	1	15	0.0	0.0	6
Fruit cocktail, canned, with light syrup	5 oz	80	1	21	1	20	0.1	0.0	8
Fruit cocktail, canned, with water	5 oz	45	1	12	1	11	0.1	0.0	6

FRUITS continued

Item	Serving Size	Calories	Protein	Carb	Fiber	Sugar	Total Fat	Sat Fat	Sodium
Granadillas, purple, fresh	5 oz	136	3	33	15	16	1.0	0.1	39
Grapefruit, canned, with juice, sectioned	5 oz	52	1	13	1	12	0.1	0.0	10
Grapefruit, canned, with light syrup, sectioned	5 oz	84	1	22	1	21	0.1	0.0	3
Grapefruit, canned, with water, sectioned	5 oz	50	1	13	1	12	0.1	0.0	3
Grapefruit, pink, fresh	5 oz	59	1	15	2	10	0.2	0.0	0
Grapefruit, red, fresh	5 oz	59	1	15	2	10	0.2	0.0	0
Grapefruit, white, fresh	5 oz	45	1	11	2	10	0.1	0.0	0
Grapes, Concord, fresh	5 oz	94	1	24	1	23	0.5	0.2	3
Grapes, green European-type varieties, fresh	5 oz	97	1	25	1	22	0.2	0.1	3
Grapes, red European-type varieties, fresh	5 oz	97	1	25	1	22	0.2	0.1	3
Grapes, slip skin, fresh	5 oz	94	1	24	1	23	0.5	0.2	3
Grapes, Thompson seedless, canned, with heavy syrup	5 oz	106	1	28	1	27	0.1	0.0	7
Grapes, Thompson seedless, canned, with water	5 oz	56	1	14	1	14	0.2	0.1	8
Grapes, Thompson seedless, fresh	5 oz	97	1	25	1	22	0.2	0.1	3
Guanabanas, fresh	5 oz	92	1	24	5	19	0.4	0.1	20
Guavas, fresh	5 oz	95	4	20	8	12	1.3	0.4	3
Indian dates, fresh	5 oz	335	4	88	7	80	0.8	0.4	39
Kaki fruits, fresh	5 oz	98	1	26	5	18	0.3	0.0	1
Kiwis, fresh	5 oz	85	2	21	4	13	0.7	0.0	4
Kiwis, gold, fresh	5 oz	84	2	20	3	15	0.8	0.2	4
Kumquats, fresh	5 oz	99	3	22	9	13	1.2	0.1	14
Limes, peeled, fresh	5 oz	42	1	15	4	2	0.3	0.0	3
Loganberries, frozen	5 oz	77	2	18	7	11	0.4	0.0	1
Lychees, dried	1.5 oz	111	2	28	2	26	0.5	0.1	2
Lychees, fresh	5 oz	92	1	23	2	21	0.6	0.1	1
Mandarin oranges, canned, with juice	5 oz	52	1	13	1	12	0.0	0.0	7
Mandarin oranges, canned, with juice, drained	5 oz	53	1	13	2	12	0.1	0.0	7
Mandarin oranges, canned, with light syrup	5 oz	85	1	23	1	22	0.1	0.0	8

FRUITS continued

Item	Serving Size	Calories	Protein	Carb	Fiber	Sugar	Total Fat	Sat Fat	Sodium
Mandarin oranges, fresh	5 oz	74	1	19	3	15	0.4	0.1	3
Mangos, fresh	5 oz	91	1	24	3	21	0.4	0.1	3
Maracujas, fresh	5 oz	136	3	33	15	16	1.0	0.1	39
Melons, cantaloupe, fresh	5 oz	48	1	11	1	10	0.3	0.1	22
Melons, casaba, fresh	5 oz	39	2	9	1	8	0.1	0.0	13
Melons, honeydew, fresh	5 oz	50	1	13	1	11	0.2	0.1	25
Mulberries, fresh	5 oz	60	2	14	2	11	0.5	0.0	14
Nectarines, fresh	5 oz	62	1	15	2	11	0.4	0.0	0
Oranges, all types, fresh	5 oz	66	1	16	3	13	0.2	0.0	0
Papayas, fresh	5 oz	55	1	14	3	8	0.2	0.1	4
Passion fruits, purple, fresh	5 oz	136	3	33	15	16	1.0	0.1	39
Peaches, canned, with extra heavy syrup	5 oz	134	1	36	1	35	0.0	0.0	11
Peaches, canned, with extra light syrup	5 oz	59	1	16	1	14	0.1	0.0	7
Peaches, canned, with heavy syrup	5 oz	104	1	28	2	26	0.1	0.0	8
Peaches, canned, with heavy syrup, drained	5 oz	108	1	28	3	25	0.2	0.0	8
Peaches, canned, with juice	5 oz	62	1	16	2	14	0.0	0.0	6
Peaches, canned, with light syrup	5 oz	76	1	20	2	19	0.0	0.0	7
Peaches, canned, with water	5 oz	34	1	9	2	7	0.1	0.0	4
Peaches, fresh, without skin	5 oz	55	1	13	2	11	0.4	0.0	0
Peaches, spiced, canned, with heavy syrup	5 oz	105	1	28	2	26	0.1	0.0	6
Peaches, sulfured, dehydrated	1.5 oz	130	2	33	4	28	0.4	0.0	4
Peaches, sulfured, dried	1.5 oz	96	1	25	3	17	0.3	0.0	3
Peaches, sulfured, stewed from dehydrated	1.5 oz	53	1	14	2	11	0.2	0.0	2
Peaches, sulfured, stewed from dried without added sugar	1.5 oz	31	0	8	1	7	0.1	0.0	1
Peaches, sweetened, frozen	5 oz	132	1	34	3	31	0.2	0.0	8

FRUITS continued

Item	Serving Size	Calories	Protein	Carb	Fiber	Sugar	Total Fat	Sat Fat	Sodium
Pears, canned, with extra heavy syrup	5 oz	136	0	35	2	30	0.2	0.0	7
Pears, canned, with extra light syrup	5 oz	66	0	17	2	12	0.1	0.0	3
Pears, canned, with heavy syrup	5 oz	104	0	27	2	21	0.2	0.0	7
Pears, canned, with juice	5 oz	70	0	18	2	14	0.1	0.0	6
Pears, canned, with light syrup	5 oz	80	0	21	2	17	0.0	0.0	7
Pears, canned, with water	5 oz	41	0	11	2	9	0.0	0.0	3
Pears, fresh, Asian	5 oz	59	1	15	5	10	0.3	0.0	0
Pears, fresh, cubed	5 oz	81	1	22	4	14	0.2	0.0	1
Pears, sulfured, dried	1.5 oz	105	1	28	3	25	0.3	0.0	3
Pears, sulfured, stewed from dried without added sugar	1.5 oz	51	0	14	3	11	0.1	0.0	2
Persimmons, Japanese, fresh	5 oz	98	1	26	5	18	0.3	0.0	1
Pineapple, canned, with heavy syrup	5 oz	109	0	28	1	24	0.2	0.0	1
Pineapple, canned, with juice	5 oz	84	1	22	1	20	0.1	0.0	1
Pineapple, canned, with light syrup	5 oz	73	1	19	1	18	0.2	0.0	1
Pineapple, canned, with water	5 oz	45	1	12	1	11	0.1	0.0	1
Pineapple, fresh	5 oz	70	1	18	2	14	0.2	0.0	1
Pineapple chunks, canned, with heavy syrup	5 oz	109	0	28	1	24	0.2	0.0	1
Pineapple chunks, canned, with juice	5 oz	84	1	22	1	20	0.1	0.0	1
Pineapple chunks, canned, with water	5 oz	45	1	12	1	11	0.1	0.0	1
Pineapple chunks, sweetened, frozen	5 oz	120	1	31	2	30	0.1	0.0	3
Pineapple spears, canned, with juice, drained	5 oz	84	1	22	2	20	0.2	0.0	1
Plantains, cooked	1 oz	35	0	9	1	4	0.1	0.0	2
Plantains, fresh	5 oz	171	2	45	3	21	0.5	0.2	6
Plantains, green, fried	1 oz	93	0	15	1	1	3.5	1.1	6

FRUITS continued

Item	Serving Size	Calories	Protein	Carb	Fiber	Sugar	Total Fat	Sat Fat	Sodium
Plantains, yellow, fried	1 oz	71	0	12	1	7	2.3	0.5	2
Plums, canned, with heavy syrup, drained	5 oz	125	1	32	2	30	0.2	0.0	27
Plums, fresh	5 oz	64	1	16	2	14	0.4	0.0	0
Plums, purple, canned, with extra heavy syrup	5 oz	141	1	37	1	34	0.1	0.0	27
Plums, purple, canned, with heavy syrup	5 oz	125	1	33	1	31	0.1	0.0	27
Plums, purple, canned, with juice	5 oz	81	1	21	1	20	0.0	0.0	1
Plums, purple, canned, with light syrup	5 oz	88	1	23	1	21	0.0	0.0	28
Plums, purple, canned, with water	5 oz	57	1	15	1	14	0.0	0.0	1
Pomegranates, fresh	5 oz	116	2	26	6	19	1.6	0.2	4
Prunes, dehydrated	1.5 oz	136	1	36	4	24	0.3	0.0	2
Prunes, dried	1.5 oz	96	1	26	3	15	0.2	0.0	1
Prunes, pureed	1.5 oz	103	1	26	1	16	0.1	0.0	9
Prunes, stewed from dehydrated	1.5 oz	45	0	12	3	7	0.1	0.0	1
Prunes, stewed from dried with added sugar	1.5 oz	50	0	13	2	9	0.1	0.0	1
Prunes, stewed from dried without added sugar	1.5 oz	43	0	11	1	10	0.1	0.0	0
Raisins, golden, seedless	1.5 oz	121	1	32	2	24	0.2	0.1	5
Raisins, seedless	1.5 oz	120	1	32	1	24	0.2	0.0	4
Raspberries, fresh	1 cup	73	2	17	9	6	0.9	0.0	1
Raspberries, red, canned, with heavy syrup	1 cup	127	1	33	5	28	0.2	0.0	4
Rhubarb, cooked from frozen with sugar	1 oz	35	0	9	1	9	0.0	0.0	0
Rhubarb, fresh	1 cup	29	1	6	3	2	0.3	0.1	6
Rhubarb, frozen	1 cup	29	1	7	3	2	0.2	0.0	3
Rowals, fresh	1 cup	155	3	33	9	20	2.8	0.4	6
Sharon fruits, fresh	1 cup	98	1	26	5	18	0.3	0.0	1
Soursops, fresh	1 cup	92	1	24	5	19	0.4	0.1	20
Star fruits, fresh	1 cup	43	1	9	4	6	0.5	0.0	3

FRUITS continued

Item	Serving Size	Calories	Protein	Carb	Fiber	Sugar	Total Fat	Sat Fat	Sodium
Strawberries, canned, with heavy syrup	1 cup	129	1	33	2	31	0.4	0.0	6
Strawberries, fresh	1 cup	45	1	11	3	7	0.4	0.0	1
Strawberries, sweetened, frozen	1 cup	134	1	36	3	34	0.2	0.0	4
Strawberries, sweetened, frozen, thawed, whole	1 cup	109	1	29	3	26	0.2	0.0	1
Strawberries, unsweetened, frozen	1 cup	49	1	13	3	6	0.2	0.0	3
Tamarinds, fresh	1 cup	335	4	88	7	80	0.8	0.4	39
Tangerines, canned, with juice	1 cup	52	1	13	1	12	0.0	0.0	7
Tangerines, canned, with juice, drained	1 cup	53	1	13	2	12	0.1	0.0	7
Tangerines, canned, with light syrup	1 cup	85	1	23	1	22	0.1	0.0	8
Tangerines, fresh	1 cup	74	1	19	3	15	0.4	0.1	3
Watermelons, fresh	1 wedge	84	2	21	1	17	0.4	0.1	3

GELATINS AND PUDDINGS, Prepared

Item	Serving Size	Calories	Protein	Carb	Fiber	Sugar	Total Fat	Sat Fat	Sodium
Custard, egg, prepared from dry mix with 2% milk	3 oz	95	4	15	0	4	2.4	1.3	74
Custard, egg, prepared from dry mix with whole milk	3 oz	104	3	15	0	4	3.4	1.7	71
Dessert, arroz con leche	3 oz	124	3	21	0	13	3.1	1.6	90
Dessert, egg custard, baked, prepared from recipe	3 oz	88	4	9	0	9	3.9	1.8	52
Dessert, flan, caramel custard, prepared from recipe	3 oz	123	4	19	0	19	3.4	1.5	45
Dessert, mousse, chocolate, prepared from recipe	3 oz	191	4	14	1	13	13.6	7.8	32
Dessert, rice pudding	3 oz	124	3	21	0	13	3.1	1.6	90
Gelatin, black cherry, sugar-free, snack cup	3 oz	9	1	0	0	0	0.0	0.0	42

GELATINS AND PUDDINGS, Prepared continued

Item	Serving Size	Calories	Protein	Carb	Fiber	Sugar	Total Fat	Sat Fat	Sodium
Gelatin, cherry, sugar-free, snack cup	3 oz	9	1	0	0	0	0.0	0.0	42
Gelatin, cotton candy, ready to eat, sticks	2 1/4 oz	60	0	16	0	15	0.0	0.0	35
Gelatin, green apple, snack cup	3 oz	86	0	21	0	21	0.0	0.0	39
Gelatin, lemon-lime, sugar-free, snack cup	3 oz	9	1	0	0	0	0.0	0.0	42
Gelatin, lime, with pineapple	3 oz	62	0	16	0	15	0.0	0.0	66
Gelatin, orange, snack cup	3 oz	60	1	15	0	15	0.0	0.0	34
Gelatin, orange, sugar-free, snack cup	3 oz	9	1	0	0	0	0.0	0.0	42
Gelatin, orange, with mandarins	3 oz	62	0	16	0	15	0.0	0.0	62
Gelatin, peach, sugar-free, snack cup	3 oz	9	1	0	0	0	0.0	0.0	42
Gelatin, prepared from dry mix with water	3 oz	53	1	12	0	11	0.0	0.0	64
Gelatin, raspberry, ready to eat, sticks	2 1/4 oz	60	0	16	0	15	0.0	0.0	35
Gelatin, raspberry, snack cup	3 oz	60	1	15	0	15	0.0	0.0	34
Gelatin, raspberry, sugar-free, snack cup	3 oz	9	1	0	0	0	0.0	0.0	42
Gelatin, reduced calorie, with aspartame, prepared with water	3 oz	17	1	4	0	0	0.0	0.0	41
Gelatin, strawberry kiwi, sugar-free, snack cup	3 oz	9	1	0	0	0	0.0	0.0	42
Gelatin, strawberry, ready to eat, sticks	2 1/4 oz	60	0	16	0	15	0.0	0.0	35
Gelatin, strawberry, snack cup	3 oz	60	1	15	0	15	0.0	0.0	34
Gelatin, strawberry, with peaches	3 oz	62	0	16	0	15	0.0	0.0	62
Gelatin, tropical berry, sugar-free, snack cup	3 oz	9	1	0	0	0	0.0	0.0	42
Gelatin, variety pack, ready to eat, sticks	2 1/4 oz	60	0	16	0	15	0.0	0.0	35

GELATINS AND PUDDINGS, Prepared continued

Item	Serving Size	Calories	Protein	Carb	Fiber	Sugar	Total Fat	Sat Fat	Sodium
Gelatin, watermelon, snack cup	3 oz	86	0	21	0	21	0.0	0.0	39
Gelatin, watermelon, sugar-free, snack cup	3 oz	9	1	0	0	0	0.0	0.0	42
Gelatin substitute, cherry tropical punch, Kool-Aid Gels	3 oz	77	0	19	0	19	0.0	0.0	39
Gelatin substitute, Groovalicious Grape, Kool-Aid Gels	3 oz	86	0	21	0	21	0.0	0.0	39
Gelatin substitute, Ice Blue Raspberry, Kool-Aid Gels	3 oz	77	0	19	0	19	0.0	0.0	39
Gelatin substitute, Oh Yeah Orange, Kool-Aid Gels	3 oz	69	0	17	0	17	0.0	0.0	39
Gelatin substitute, Soarin' Strawberry, Kool-Aid Gels	3 oz	86	0	21	0	21	0.0	0.0	39
Pie filling, apple, canned	3 oz	85	0	22	1	12	0.1	0.0	40
Pie filling, blueberry, canned	3 oz	154	0	38	2	32	0.2	0.0	10
Pie filling, cherry, low calorie	3 oz	45	1	10	1	8	0.1	0.0	10
Pie filling, pumpkin, canned	3 oz	90	1	20	2	17	0.5	0.0	115
Pudding, banana, instant, prepared with whole milk	3 oz	98	2	17	0	15	2.4	1.3	247
Pudding, banana, prepared from dry mix with whole milk	3 oz	94	2	16	0	14	2.5	1.4	134
Pudding, bubble gum, snack cup	3 oz	105	1	18	0	14	2.6	1.1	120
Pudding, chocolate, fat-free, ready to eat	3 oz	79	2	18	0	13	0.3	0.0	94
Pudding, chocolate, prepared from dry mix with 2% milk	3 oz	94	3	17	1	10	1.8	1.1	87
Pudding, chocolate, prepared from dry mix with whole milk	3 oz	102	3	17	1	10	2.7	1.5	83
Pudding, chocolate, ready to eat	3 oz	118	2	20	1	17	3.1	1.2	142

GELATINS AND PUDDINGS, Prepared continued

Item	Serving Size	Calories	Protein	Carb	Fiber	Sugar	Total Fat	Sat Fat	Sodium
Pudding, chocolate, ready to eat, sticks	2 1/4 oz	80	1	16	1	12	2.0	1.0	100
Pudding, chocolate, sugar-free, snack cup	3 oz	48	2	11	1	0	1.2	0.8	144
Pudding, chocolate & caramel cream swirled, snack cup	3 oz	120	2	21	0	17	3.8	1.5	143
Pudding, chocolate chip cookie, snack cup	3 oz	103	2	19	1	14	3.4	0.9	137
Pudding, chocolate fudge sundae, snack cup	3 oz	105	2	19	0	15	2.6	1.1	128
Pudding, chocolate vanilla swirl, fat-free, snack cup	3 oz	75	2	17	1	13	0.0	0.0	150
Pudding, chocolate vanilla swirl, snack cup	3 oz	105	2	20	1	15	3.0	1.1	128
Pudding, chocolate vanilla swirl, sugar-free, snack cup	3 oz	48	2	10	1	0	1.2	0.8	152
Pudding, chocolate vanilla, doubles, snack cup	3 oz	103	1	19	0	14	3.0	0.9	129
Pudding, cotton candy, snack cup	3 oz	105	1	18	0	14	2.6	1.1	120
Pudding, devil's food, fat-free, snack cup	3 oz	75	2	17	1	12	0.0	0.0	143
Pudding, no sugar added, vanilla, prepared from dry mix, with water	3 oz	43	1	6	0	10	1.2	0.3	77
Pudding, orange & cream swirled, snack cup	3 oz	98	2	19	0	15	2.3	1.5	64
Pudding, rice, snack cup	3 oz	120	3	16	0	9	5.2	0.9	112
Pudding, soy, banana	3 oz	75	2	16	1	11	0.8	0.0	56
Pudding, soy, chocolate	3 oz	83	2	17	1	11	1.5	0.0	98
Pudding, soy, chocolate, ZenSoy	3 oz	98	2	22	2	16	0.8	0.0	56
Pudding, soy, vanilla	3 oz	83	2	17	1	11	0.8	0.0	45
Pudding, soy, vanilla, ZenSoy	3 oz	83	2	17	1	11	0.8	0.0	56
Pudding, strawberries & cream swirled, snack cup	3 oz	98	2	19	0	15	2.3	1.5	64
Pudding, strawberry cheesecake, with topping, snack cup	3 oz	129	2	21	0	19	3.9	1.7	103

GELATINS AND PUDDINGS, Prepared continued

Item	Serving Size	Calories	Protein	Carb	Fiber	Sugar	Total Fat	Sat Fat	Sodium
Pudding, tapioca, fat-free, ready to eat	3 oz	80	1	18	0	12	0.3	0.1	159
Pudding, tapioca, fat-free, snack cup	3 oz	75	1	17	0	13	0.0	0.0	173
Pudding, tapioca, French cream, snack cup	3 oz	94	1	18	1	16	0.0	0.0	29
Pudding, tapioca, snack cup	3 oz	98	1	19	0	14	2.3	0.8	113
Pudding, vanilla caramel sundae, fat-free, snack cup	3 oz	75	1	17	0	12	0.0	0.0	173
Pudding, vanilla, fat-free, ready to eat	3 oz	76	2	17	0	13	0.0	0.0	162
Pudding, vanilla, instant, prepared with whole milk	3 oz	97	2	17	0	15	2.5	1.5	243
Pudding, vanilla, prepared from dry mix with whole milk	3 oz	96	2	16	0	15	2.5	1.4	133

GELATINS AND PUDDINGS, Dry Mix

Item	Serving Size	Calories	Protein	Carb	Fiber	Sugar	Total Fat	Sat Fat	Sodium
Custard, flan, with caramel sauce	22 g	80	0	20	0	20	0.0	0.0	5
Gelatin, apricot	22 g	80	2	19	0	19	0.0	0.0	80
Gelatin, berry blue	22 g	80	2	19	0	19	0.0	0.0	80
Gelatin, black cherry	22 g	80	2	19	0	19	0.0	0.0	80
Gelatin, cherry	22 g	80	2	19	0	19	0.0	0.0	100
Gelatin, chocolate, dry mix, prepared with milk	16 g	60	2	14	0	14	0.0	0.0	0
Gelatin, cranberry	22 g	80	2	19	0	19	0.0	0.0	75
Gelatin, cranberry raspberry	22 g	80	2	19	0	19	0.0	0.0	75
Gelatin, grape	22 g	80	2	19	0	19	0.0	0.0	80
Gelatin, island pineapple	22 g	80	2	19	0	19	0.0	0.0	80
Gelatin, lemon	22 g	80	2	19	0	19	0.0	0.0	120
Gelatin, lime	22 g	80	2	19	0	19	0.0	0.0	100
Gelatin, Mystery Magical Twist	22 g	80	2	19	0	19	0.0	0.0	80
Gelatin, orange	22 g	80	2	19	0	19	0.0	0.0	80
Gelatin, peach	22 g	80	2	19	0	19	0.0	0.0	80

GELATINS AND PUDDINGS, Dry Mix continued

Item	Serving Size	Calories	Protein	Carb	Fiber	Sugar	Total Fat	Sat Fat	Sodium
Gelatin, raspberry	22 g	80	2	19	0	19	0.0	0.0	80
Gelatin, strawberry	22 g	80	2	19	0	19	0.0	0.0	90
Gelatin, strawberry banana	22 g	80	2	19	0	19	0.0	0.0	80
Gelatin, strawberry, for milk	16 g	60	2	14	0	14	0.0	0.0	0
Gelatin, strawberry kiwi	22 g	80	2	19	0	19	0.0	0.0	80
Gelatin, vanilla, for milk	16 g	60	2	14	0	14	0.0	0.0	0
Gelatin, wild strawberry	22 g	80	2	19	0	19	0.0	0.0	120
Pudding, banana cream	22 g	80	0	20	0	15	0.0	0.0	180
Pudding, banana cream, fat- & sugar-free, instant	8 g	25	0	6	0	0	0.0	0.0	320
Pudding, banana cream, instant	25 g	90	0	23	0	18	0.0	0.0	360
Pudding, butter cream, instant	25 g	90	0	23	0	18	0.0	0.0	360
Pudding, butterscotch, dry	26 g	100	1	24	1	19	0.0	0.0	130
Pudding, butterscotch, fat- & sugar-free, instant	8 g	25	0	6	0	0	0.0	0.0	320
Pudding, butterscotch, instant	25 g	90	0	23	0	18	0.0	0.0	390
Pudding, cheesecake, instant	26 g	100	0	24	0	20	0.0	0.0	360
Pudding, chocolate, fat- & sugar-free, instant	11 g	35	1	8	1	0	0.0	0.0	300
Pudding, chocolate cherry, instant	1 oz	100	1	25	1	19	0.0	0.0	420
Pudding, chocolate fudge	25 g	90	1	22	1	15	0.0	0.0	115
Pudding, chocolate fudge, fat- & sugar-free, instant	11 g	35	1	8	1	0	0.0	0.0	300

GELATINS AND PUDDINGS, Dry Mix continued

Item	Serving Size	Calories	Protein	Carb	Fiber	Sugar	Total Fat	Sat Fat	Sodium
Pudding, chocolate fudge, instant	1 oz	100	1	25	1	17	0.0	0.0	380
Pudding, chocolate mint, instant	1 oz	100	1	25	1	17	0.0	0.0	380
Pudding, coconut cream	22 g	90	0	18	1	14	2.5	2.5	150
Pudding, French vanilla, instant	25 g	90	0	23	0	18	0.0	0.0	350
Pudding, lemon	14 g	50	0	12	0	6	0.0	0.0	70
Pudding, lemon, instant	25 g	90	0	24	0	19	0.0	0.0	310
Pudding, milk chocolate	25 g	90	0	22	0	16	0.0	0.0	125
Pudding, Oreo cookies 'n' cream, instant	31 g	120	0	28	0	21	1.0	0.0	390
Pudding, pistachio, fat- & sugar-free, instant	8 g	30	0	6	0	0	0.0	0.0	300
Pudding, pistachio, instant	25 g	100	0	23	0	18	0.5	0.0	360
Pudding, rice, fat-free	25 g	90	1	23	0	13	0.0	0.0	100
Pudding, tapioca, fat-free	23 g	90	0	22	0	15	0.0	0.0	115
Pudding, vanilla	22 g	80	0	20	0	16	0.0	0.0	135
Pudding, vanilla, fat- & sugar-free, instant	8 g	25	0	6	0	0	0.0	0.0	320
Pudding, white chocolate, fat- & sugar-free, instant	8 g	25	0	6	0	0	0.0	0.0	320
Pudding, white chocolate, instant	25 g	90	0	23	0	19	0.0	0.0	350

GRAINS AND RICES

Item	Serving Size	Calories	Protein	Carb	Fiber	Sugar	Total Fat	Sat Fat	Sodium
All-purpose flour, self-rising, white, enriched	2 tbsp	106	3	22	1	0	0.3	0.0	381
All-purpose flour, white, bleached, enriched	2 tbsp	109	3	23	1	0	0.3	0.0	1
All-purpose flour, white, calcium fortified, enriched	2 tbsp	109	3	23	1	0	0.3	0.0	1
All-purpose flour, white, unbleached, enriched	2 tbsp	109	3	23	1	0	0.3	0.0	1
All-purpose flour, white, unenriched	2 tbsp	109	3	23	1	0	0.3	0.0	1
Amaranth, dry	1/4 cup	167	6	29	3	1	3.2	0.7	2
Bakery-mix flour, low fat	2 tbsp	108	3	21	1	0	1.4	0.3	408
Bakery-mix flour	2 tbsp	120	3	19	2	0	3.9	0.9	423
Barley flour	2 tbsp	104	3	22	3	0	0.5	0.1	1
Barley flour, malt	2 tbsp	108	3	23	2	0	0.6	0.1	3
Barley, hulled, dry	1/4 cup	159	6	33	8	0	1.0	0.2	5
Barley, pearled, cooked	1 cup	172	3	40	5	0	0.6	0.1	4
Barley, pearled, dry	1/4 cup	158	4	35	7	0	0.5	0.1	4
Bran, corn, crude	1 cup	314	12	120	111	0	1.3	0.2	10
Bran, oat, dry	15 g	37	3	10	2	0	1.0	0.2	1
Bran, rice, crude	15 g	47	2	7	3	0	3.1	0.6	1
Bran, wheat, crude	15 g	32	2	10	6	0	0.6	0.1	0
Brown rice flour	2 tbsp	109	2	23	1	0	0.8	0.2	2
Buckwheat flour, whole groat	2 tbsp	101	4	21	3	1	0.9	0.2	3
Buckwheat, groats, roasted, cooked	1 cup	129	5	28	4	1	0.9	0.2	6
Carob flour	2 tbsp	67	1	27	12	15	0.2	0.0	11
Chickpea flour, besan	2 tbsp	116	7	17	3	3	2.0	0.2	19
Corn flour, masa, white, enriched	2 tbsp	110	3	23	3	0	1.1	0.2	2
Corn flour, white, whole grain	2 tbsp	108	2	23	2	0	1.2	0.2	2
Corn flour, yellow, degermed, unenriched	2 tbsp	113	2	25	1	0	0.4	0.1	0
Corn flour, yellow, whole grain	2 tbsp	108	2	23	2	0	1.2	0.2	2
Cornmeal, blue, Navajo	2 tbsp	119	3	23	3	1	1.6	0.3	2

GRAINS AND RICES continued

Item	Serving Size	Calories	Protein	Carb	Fiber	Sugar	Total Fat	Sat Fat	Sodium
Cornmeal, white, bolted, enriched, self-rising	2 tbsp	100	2	21	2	0	1.0	0.1	374
Cornmeal, white, degermed, enriched	2 tbsp	111	2	24	1	0	0.5	0.1	2
Cornmeal, white, degermed, enriched, self-rising	2 tbsp	107	3	22	2	0	0.5	0.1	404
Cornmeal, white, degermed, unenriched	2 tbsp	111	2	24	1	0	0.5	0.1	2
Cornmeal, white, Navajo	2 tbsp	119	3	23	3	0	1.5	0.3	1
Cornmeal, white, whole grain	2 tbsp	109	2	23	2	0	1.1	0.2	11
Cornmeal, yellow, degermed, enriched	2 tbsp	111	2	24	1	0	0.5	0.1	2
Cornmeal, yellow, degermed, unenriched	2 tbsp	111	2	24	1	0	0.5	0.1	2
Cornmeal, yellow, Navajo	2 tbsp	115	3	22	3	0	1.8	0.3	1
Cornmeal, yellow, whole grain	2 tbsp	109	2	23	2	0	1.1	0.2	11
Flour, bread, unenriched	2 tbsp	108	4	22	1	0	0.5	0.1	1
Flour, bread, white, enriched	2 tbsp	108	4	22	1	0	0.5	0.1	1
Flour, cake, white, enriched, unsifted	2 tbsp	109	2	23	1	0	0.3	0.0	1
Grits, corn, yellow, quick, enriched, dry	1/4 cup	147	3	32	2	0	0.6	0.1	1
Grits, corn, yellow, regular, enriched, dry	1/4 cup	147	3	32	2	0	0.6	0.1	1
Kasha, roasted, cooked	1 cup	129	5	28	4	1	0.9	0.2	6
Millet, cooked	1 cup	167	5	33	2	0	1.4	0.2	3
Oat flour, partially debranned	2 tbsp	121	4	20	2	0	2.7	0.5	6
Potato flour	2 tbsp	107	2	25	2	1	0.1	0.0	17
Quinoa, cooked	1 cup	168	6	30	0	0	0.0	1.0	7
Rice, brown, long grain, cooked	1 cup	155	4	32	3	0	1.3	0.3	7
Rice, white, glutinous, cooked	1 cup	136	3	30	1	0	0.3	0.1	7
Rice, white, long grain, cooked	1 cup	182	4	39	1	0	0.4	0.1	1

GRAINS AND RICES continued

Item	Serving Size	Calories	Protein	Carb	Fiber	Sugar	Total Fat	Sat Fat	Sodium
Rice, white, long grain, enriched, cooked	1 cup	182	4	39	1	0	0.4	0.1	0
Rice, white, long grain, enriched, cooked with salt	1 cup	182	4	39	1	0	0.4	0.1	535
Rice, white, long grain, enriched, parboiled, cooked	1 cup	172	4	36	1	0	0.5	0.1	3
Rice, white, long grain, enriched, prepared from instant	1 cup	164	3	35	1	0	0.7	0.0	6
Rice, white, long grain, unenriched, cooked	1 cup	182	4	39	1	0	0.4	0.1	1
Rice, white, long grain, unenriched, cooked with salt	1 cup	182	4	39	1	0	0.4	0.1	535
Rice, white, long grain, unenriched, parboiled, cooked	1 cup	172	4	36	1	0	0.5	0.1	3
Rice, white, medium grain, cooked	1 cup	182	3	40	0	1	0.3	0.1	0
Rice, white, medium grain, unenriched, cooked	1 cup	182	3	40	0	0	0.3	0.1	0
Rice, white, short grain, unenriched, cooked	1 cup	182	3	40	0	0	0.3	0.1	0
Rice, wild, cooked	1 cup	141	6	30	3	1	0.5	0.1	4
Rye flour, dark	2 tbsp	98	5	21	7	1	0.7	0.1	1
Rye flour, light	2 tbsp	107	3	23	2	0	0.4	0.0	1
Rye flour, medium	2 tbsp	105	3	23	4	0	0.5	0.1	1
Semolina flour, enriched	2 tbsp	108	4	22	1	1	0.3	0.0	0
Semolina flour, unenriched	2 tbsp	108	4	22	1	1	0.3	0.0	0
Soy flour, defatted	2 tbsp	112	15	9	5	4	2.7	0.4	3
Soy flour, defatted, stirred	2 tbsp	99	14	12	5	6	0.4	0.0	6
Soy flour, full fat, stirred, raw	2 tbsp	131	10	11	3	2	6.2	0.9	4
Soy flour, full fat, stirred, roasted	2 tbsp	132	10	10	3	2	6.6	0.9	4
Soy flour, low fat, stirred	2 tbsp	113	14	10	5	3	2.7	0.4	3
Triticale flour, whole grain	2 tbsp	101	4	22	4	1	0.5	0.1	1
Wheat, bulgur, cooked	1 cup	116	4	26	6	0	0.3	0.1	7
White rice flour	2 tbsp	110	2	24	1	0	0.4	0.1	0
Whole-wheat flour	2 tbsp	102	4	22	4	0	0.6	0.1	2

HERBS AND SPICES

Item	Serving Size	Calories	Protein	Carb	Fiber	Sugar	Total Fat	Sat Fat	Sodium
Alfalfa, dried	1/4 tsp	2	0	0	0	0	0.0	0.0	0
Apple, dried	1/4 tsp	2	0	0	0	0	0.1	0.1	2
Asparagus root, dried	1/4 tsp	2	0	0	0	0	0.0	0.0	0
Basil, dried, ground	1/4 tsp	1	0	0	0	0	0.0	0.0	0
Basil, fresh	1/4 tsp	0	0	0	0	0	0.0	0.0	0
Black walnut, hulls, rind, dried	1/4 tsp	2	0	0	0	0	0.0	0.0	0
Broccoli, dried	1/4 tsp	2	0	0	0	0	0.0	0.0	2
Carrots, dried	1/4 tsp	2	0	0	0	0	0.0	0.0	1
Caraway, seed	1/4 tsp	2	0	0	0	0	0.1	0.0	0
Cayenne chili pepper, dried	1/4 tsp	2	0	0	0	0	0.1	0.0	0
Celery, seed	1/4 tsp	2	0	0	0	0	0.1	0.0	1
Celery, seed, dried	1/4 tsp	2	0	0	0	0	0.0	0.0	1
Chamomile, flower, dried	1/4 tsp	2	0	0	0	0	0.0	0.0	1
Chapparal, dried	1/4 tsp	2	0	0	0	0	0.0	0.0	0
Chili pepper, powder	1/4 tsp	2	0	0	0	0	0.1	0.0	5
Chili pepper, powder, light	1/4 tsp	2	0	0	0	0	0.1	0.0	7
Chives, fresh	1/4 tsp	0	0	0	0	0	0.0	0.0	0
Cilantro, dried	1/4 tsp	1	0	0	0	0	0.0	0.0	1
Cilantro, fresh	1/4 tsp	0	0	0	0	0	0.0	0.0	0
Cinnamon, ground	1/4 tsp	1	0	0	0	0	0.0	0.0	0
Clove, ground	1/4 tsp	2	0	0	0	0	0.1	0.0	1
Coriander, dried	1/4 tsp	1	0	0	0	0	0.0	0.0	1
Coriander, fresh	1/4 tsp	0	0	0	0	0	0.0	0.0	0
Cumin, seed	1/4 tsp	2	0	0	0	0	0.1	0.0	1
Curry, blend, powder	1/4 tsp	2	0	0	0	0	0.1	0.0	0
Dandelion, root, dried	1/4 tsp	2	0	0	0	0	0.0	0.0	1
Fennel, seed, dried	1/4 tsp	2	0	0	0	0	0.1	0.1	0
Fenugreek, seed, dried	1/4 tsp	2	0	0	0	0	0.0	0.0	0
Garlic, bulb, dried	1/4 tsp	2	0	0	0	0	0.0	0.0	0
Garlic, powder	1/4 tsp	2	0	0	0	0	0.0	0.0	0
Garlic, soluble	1/4 tsp	1	0	0	0	0	0.0	0.0	0
Ginger, root, dried	1/4 tsp	2	0	0	0	0	0.0	0.0	0

HERBS AND SPICES continued

Item	Serving Size	Calories	Protein	Carb	Fiber	Sugar	Total Fat	Sat Fat	Sodium
Ginger root, fresh	1/4 tsp	0	0	0	0	0	0.0	0.0	0
Ginger, ground	1/4 tsp	2	0	0	0	0	0.0	0.0	0
Grapefruit, dried	1/4 tsp	2	0	0	0	0	0.1	0.1	2
Hibiscus flower, dried	1/4 tsp	2	0	0	0	0	0.0	0.0	0
Horseradish root, dried	1/4 tsp	2	0	0	0	0	0.0	0.0	1
Lemon grass, dried	1/4 tsp	2	0	0	0	0	0.0	0.0	2
Lemon, dried	1/4 tsp	2	0	0	0	0	0.1	0.1	2
Licorice root, dried	1/4 tsp	2	0	0	0	0	0.0	0.0	4
Marjoram, dried	1/4 tsp	1	0	0	0	0	0.0	0.0	0
Mustard seed, yellow, ground	1/4 tsp	3	0	0	0	0	0.2	0.0	0
Mustard seed, choice ground	1/4 tsp	3	0	0	0	0	0.2	0.0	0
Mustard seed, special ground	1/4 tsp	3	0	0	0	0	0.2	0.0	0
Nutmeg, ground	1/4 tsp	3	0	0	0	0	0.2	0.1	0
Oat grass, dried	1/4 tsp	2	0	0	0	0	0.0	0.0	2
Onion, dehydrated	1/4 tsp	2	0	0	0	0	0.0	0.0	0
Onion, dried	1/4 tsp	2	0	0	0	0	0.0	0.0	1
Onion, powder	1/4 tsp	2	0	0	0	0	0.0	0.0	0
Orange, dried	1/4 tsp	2	0	0	0	0	0.1	0.1	2
Oregano, dried	1/4 tsp	1	0	0	0	0	0.0	0.0	0
Papaya, dried	1/4 tsp	2	0	0	0	0	0.0	0.0	0
Paprika	1/4 tsp	1	0	0	0	0	0.1	0.0	0
Parsley, dried	1/4 tsp	1	0	0	0	0	0.0	0.0	2
Parsley, fresh	1/4 tsp	0	0	0	0	0	0.0	0.0	0
Passionflower, dried	1/4 tsp	2	0	0	0	0	0.0	0.0	0
Pepper, black	1/4 tsp	1	0	0	0	0	0.0	0.0	0
Peppermint, dried	1/4 tsp	2	0	0	0	0	0.0	0.0	1
Pineapple, dried	1/4 tsp	2	0	0	0	0	0.1	0.1	2
Poppy, seed	1/4 tsp	3	0	0	0	0	0.2	0.0	0
Psyllium, seed, dried	1/4 tsp	2	0	0	0	0	0.0	0.0	0
Pumpkin pie, blend	1/4 tsp	2	0	0	0	0	0.1	0.0	0
Red clover, flower, dried	1/4 tsp	2	0	0	0	0	0.0	0.0	0
Red raspberry, dried	1/4 tsp	2	0	0	0	0	0.0	0.0	0
Rose hips, dried	1/4 tsp	2	0	0	0	0	0.0	0.0	22
Safflower, flower, dried	1/4 tsp	2	0	0	0	0	0.0	0.0	1

HERBS AND SPICES continued

Item	Serving Size	Calories	Protein	Carb	Fiber	Sugar	Total Fat	Sat Fat	Sodium
Sage, dried	1/4 tsp	2	0	0	0	0	0.1	0.1	1
Sarsaparilla, root, dried	1/4 tsp	2	0	0	0	0	0.0	0.0	0
Spice, red chili pepper, dried	1/4 tsp	2	0	0	0	0	0.1	0.0	0
Spirulina, dried	1/4 tsp	2	0	0	0	0	0.0	0.0	0
Thyme, dried	1/4 tsp	1	0	0	0	0	0.0	0.0	0
Turmeric, ground	1/4 tsp	2	0	0	0	0	0.0	0.0	0

MEATS, Beef

Item	Serving Size	Calories	Protein	Carb	Fiber	Sugar	Total Fat	Sat Fat	Sodium
Beef, average of all cuts, cooked	3 oz	232	23	0	0	0	15	6	53
Beef, average of all cuts, cooked, 1/4" trim	3 oz	259	22	0	0	0	18	7	53
Beef, average of all cuts, cooked, 1/8" trim	3 oz	247	22	0	0	0	17	7	54
Beef, average of all cuts, cooked, choice, 0" trim	3 oz	241	23	0	0	0	16	6	53
Beef, average of all cuts, cooked, choice, 1/4" trim	3 oz	274	22	0	0	0	20	8	52
Beef, average of all cuts, cooked, choice, 1/8" trim	3 oz	256	22	0	0	0	18	7	53
Beef, average of all cuts, cooked, prime, 1/2" trim	3 oz	344	20	0	0	0	29	12	48
Beef, average of all cuts, cooked, prime, 1/4" trim	3 oz	274	22	0	0	0	20	8	53
Beef, average of all cuts, cooked, prime, 1/8" trim	3 oz	254	22	0	0	0	18	7	54
Beef, average of all cuts, cooked, select	3 oz	222	23	0	0	0	14	5	54
Beef, average of all cuts, cooked, select, 1/4" trim	3 oz	247	22	0	0	0	17	7	53
Beef, average of all cuts, cooked, select, 1/8" trim	3 oz	236	23	0	0	0	15	6	54
Beef, average of all cuts, lean, cooked	3 oz	179	25	0	0	0	8	3	56
Beef, average of all cuts, lean, cooked, 1/4" trim	3 oz	184	25	0	0	0	8	3	57

MEATS, Beef continued

Item	Serving Size	Calories	Protein	Carb	Fiber	Sugar	Total Fat	Sat Fat	Sodium
Beef, average of all cuts, lean, cooked, choice	3 oz	186	25	0	0	0	9	3	56
Beef, average of all cuts, lean, cooked, choice, 1/4" trim	3 oz	189	25	0	0	0	9	3	57
Beef, average of all cuts, lean, cooked, prime, 1/2" trim	3 oz	214	26	0	0	0	11	4	55
Beef, average of all cuts, lean, cooked, prime, 1/4" trim	3 oz	205	25	0	0	0	11	4	57
Beef, average of all cuts, lean, cooked, select	3 oz	171	25	0	0	0	7	3	56
Beef, average of all cuts, lean, cooked, select, 1/4" trim	3 oz	174	25	0	0	0	7	3	57
Beef, bottom round outside steak, grilled	3 oz	155	23	0	0	0	6	2	49
Beef, bottom round outside steak, grilled, choice, 0" trim	3 oz	162	23	0	0	0	7	3	48
Beef, bottom round outside steak, grilled, select	3 oz	141	24	0	0	0	4	1	51
Beef, bottom round steak, braised	3 oz	190	29	0	0	0	8	3	37
Beef, bottom round steak, braised, choice	3 oz	196	28	0	0	0	9	3	36
Beef, bottom round steak, braised, select	3 oz	184	29	0	0	0	7	2	38
Beef, breakfast strips, cured, cooked	3 oz	382	27	1	0	0	29	12	1915
Beef, brisket, corned, cured, cooked	3 oz	213	15	0	0	0	16	5	964
Beef, canned	3 oz	209	17	0	0	0	15	7	159
Beef, chuck arm pot roast, braised	3 oz	252	25	0	0	0	16	6	40
Beef, chuck arm pot roast, braised, select	3 oz	241	25	0	0	0	15	6	41
Beef, chuck arm pot roast, lean, braised, choice	3 oz	180	28	0	0	0	7	2	46
Beef, chuck blade roast, braised, choice	3 oz	296	23	0	0	0	22	9	55
Beef, chuck blade roast, braised, select	3 oz	266	23	0	0	0	18	7	56

MEATS, Beef continued

Item	Serving Size	Calories	Protein	Carb	Fiber	Sugar	Total Fat	Sat Fat	Sodium
Beef, chuck clod roast, lean, roasted	3 oz	146	23	0	0	0	5	2	63
Beef, chuck clod roast, lean, roasted, choice	3 oz	145	22	0	0	0	6	2	63
Beef, chuck clod roast, lean, roasted, select	3 oz	146	24	0	0	0	5	2	63
Beef, chuck tender steak, broiled	3 oz	136	22	0	0	0	5	2	60
Beef, chuck tender steak, broiled, choice	3 oz	137	22	0	0	0	5	1	62
Beef, chuck tender steak, broiled, select	3 oz	135	22	0	0	0	4	2	58
Beef, chuck top blade, broiled	3 oz	184	22	0	0	0	10	3	57
Beef, chuck top blade, broiled, choice	3 oz	193	22	0	0	0	11	4	58
Beef, chuck top blade, broiled, select	3 oz	170	22	0	0	0	8	3	57
Beef, corned, cured, canned	3 oz	213	23	0	0	0	13	5	855
Beef, cured, dried, slices	3 oz	130	26	2	0	2	2	1	2372
Beef, cured, thin slices	3 oz	150	24	5	0	0	3	1	1223
Beef, flank steak, London broil, broiled	3 oz	163	24	0	0	0	7	3	48
Beef, flank steak, London broil, broiled, choice	3 oz	172	23	0	0	0	8	3	45
Beef, flank steak, London broil, broiled, select	3 oz	156	24	0	0	0	6	3	49
Beef, ground, bulk or coarse, cooked from frozen	3 oz	220	22	0	0	0	14	5	81
Beef, ground, hamburger patty, broiled, 5% fat	3 oz	145	22	0	0	0	6	3	55
Beef, ground, hamburger patty, broiled, 10% fat	3 oz	184	22	0	0	0	10	4	58
Beef, ground, hamburger patty, broiled, 15% fat	3 oz	213	22	0	0	0	13	5	61
Beef, ground, hamburger patty, broiled, 20% fat	3 oz	230	22	0	0	0	15	6	64
Beef, ground, hamburger patty, broiled, 25% fat	3 oz	236	22	0	0	0	16	6	66

MEATS, Beef continued

Item	Serving Size	Calories	Protein	Carb	Fiber	Sugar	Total Fat	Sat Fat	Sodium
Beef, ground, hamburger patty, broiled, 30% fat	3 oz	232	22	0	0	0	15	6	69
Beef, jerky	1 oz	115	9	3	1	3	7	3	627
Beef, porterhouse steak, broiled	3 oz	235	20	0	0	0	16	6	55
Beef, porterhouse steak, broiled, choice	3 oz	241	20	0	0	0	17	6	55
Beef, porterhouse steak, broiled, select	3 oz	227	21	0	0	0	15	6	55
Beef, rib eye steak, broiled	3 oz	210	23	0	0	0	13	5	48
Beef, rib eye steak, broiled, choice	3 oz	225	23	0	0	0	14	6	45
Beef, rib eye steak, broiled, select	3 oz	196	24	0	0	0	11	4	50
Beef, rib pot roast, lean, roasted	3 oz	202	23	0	0	0	11	5	62
Beef, rib pot roast, lean, roasted, choice	3 oz	215	23	0	0	0	13	5	62
Beef, rib pot roast, lean, roasted, select	3 oz	187	23	0	0	0	10	4	62
Beef, rib steak, broiled	3 oz	212	23	0	0	0	13	5	48
Beef, rib steak, broiled, choice	3 oz	265	21	0	0	0	19	8	54
Beef, rib steak, broiled, select	3 oz	242	21	0	0	0	17	7	54
Beef, round eye roast, lean, roasted	3 oz	138	25	0	0	0	3	1	32
Beef, round eye roast, lean, roasted, choice	3 oz	138	24	0	0	0	4	1	32
Beef, round eye roast, lean, roasted, select	3 oz	139	25	0	0	0	3	1	33
Beef, round knuckle center steak, grilled	3 oz	150	23	0	0	0	6	2	44
Beef, round knuckle center steak, grilled, choice	3 oz	160	23	0	0	0	7	2	43
Beef, round knuckle center steak, grilled, select	3 oz	138	23	0	0	0	5	2	45
Beef, round tip roast, lean, roasted	3 oz	148	23	0	0	0	5	2	31

MEATS, Beef continued

Item	Serving Size	Calories	Protein	Carb	Fiber	Sugar	Total Fat	Sat Fat	Sodium
Beef, round tip roast, lean, roasted, choice	3 oz	150	24	0	0	0	5	2	31
Beef, round tip roast, lean, roasted, select	3 oz	127	23	0	0	0	4	1	31
Beef, skirt steak, broiled	3 oz	187	22	0	0	0	10	4	64
Beef, skirt steak, inside, lean, broiled	3 oz	174	23	0	0	0	9	3	65
Beef, skirt steak, outside, broiled	3 oz	217	20	0	0	0	15	6	78
Beef, skirt steak, outside,lean, broiled	3 oz	198	21	0	0	0	12	5	80
Beef, T-bone steak, broiled	3 oz	210	21	0	0	0	14	5	57
Beef, T-bone steak, broiled, choice	3 oz	219	20	0	0	0	15	5	57
Beef, T-bone steak, broiled, select	3 oz	196	21	0	0	0	12	5	58
Beef, T-bone steak, lean, broiled,	3 oz	161	22	0	0	0	7	3	60
Beef, tenderloin, filet mignon, broiled	3 oz	185	23	0	0	0	9	4	48
Beef, tenderloin, filet mignon, broiled, choice	3 oz	196	24	0	0	0	11	4	47
Beef, tenderloin, filet mignon, broiled, select	3 oz	174	23	0	0	0	8	3	49
Beef, tenderloin, filet mignon, lean, broiled	3 oz	164	24	0	0	0	7	3	50
Beef, top loin, strip steak, broiled	3 oz	164	25	0	0	0	7	3	50
Beef, top loin, strip steak, broiled, choice	3 oz	174	24	0	0	0	8	3	48
Beef, top loin, strip steak, broiled, select	3 oz	153	25	0	0	0	5	2	52
Beef, top round steak, braised	3 oz	178	30	0	0	0	5	2	38
Beef, top round steak, braised, 1/4" trim	3 oz	211	29	0	0	0	10	4	38
Beef, top round steak, braised, 1/8" trim	3 oz	202	29	0	0	0	9	3	38

MEATS, Beef continued

Item	Serving Size	Calories	Protein	Carb	Fiber	Sugar	Total Fat	Sat Fat	Sodium
Beef, top round steak, braised, choice	3 oz	184	30	0	0	0	6	2	38
Beef, top round steak, braised, choice, 1/4" trim	3 oz	221	29	0	0	0	11	4	38
Beef, top round steak, braised, choice, 1/8" trim	3 oz	213	29	0	0	0	10	4	38
Beef, top round steak, braised, select	3 oz	170	30	0	0	0	5	2	38
Beef, top round steak, braised, select, 1/4" trim	3 oz	199	29	0	0	0	8	3	38
Beef, top round steak, braised, select, 1/8" trim	3 oz	191	29	0	0	0	7	3	38
Beef, top round steak, broiled	3 oz	160	27	0	0	0	5	2	35
Beef, top round steak, broiled, choice	3 oz	170	27	0	0	0	6	2	36
Beef, top round steak, broiled, select	3 oz	150	27	0	0	0	4	1	36
Beef, top sirloin steak, broiled	3 oz	180	25	0	0	0	8	3	52
Beef, top sirloin steak, broiled, choice	3 oz	186	25	0	0	0	9	3	49
Beef, top sirloin steak, broiled, select	3 oz	175	25	0	0	0	7	3	54
Beef, tri-tip roast, loin, lean, roasted	3 oz	155	23	0	0	0	7	3	47
Beef, tri-tip roast, sirloin, roasted	3 oz	179	22	0	0	0	9	3	45
Beef, tri-tip roast, sirloin, roasted, choice	3 oz	188	22	0	0	0	11	4	43
Beef, tri-tip roast, sirloin, roasted, select	3 oz	171	22	0	0	0	8	3	48
Beef, tri-tip steak, loin, broiled	3 oz	225	25	0	0	0	13	5	61
Beef, tri-tip steak, loin, lean, broiled	3 oz	213	26	0	0	0	11	4	62
Beef, tri-tip steak, sirloin, lean, roasted, choice	3 oz	164	22	0	0	0	8	3	46
Beef, tri-tip steak, sirloin, lean, roasted, select	3 oz	152	23	0	0	0	6	2	49

MEATS, Beef continued

Item	Serving Size	Calories	Protein	Carb	Fiber	Sugar	Total Fat	Sat Fat	Sodium
Beef, whole rib, broiled, 1/8" trim	3 oz	286	19	0	0	0	23	9	54
Beef, whole rib, broiled, choice, 1/8" trim	3 oz	299	19	0	0	0	24	10	54
Beef, whole rib, broiled, prime, 1/8" trim	3 oz	328	19	0	0	0	28	11	53
Beef, whole rib, broiled, select, 1/8" trim	3 oz	268	19	0	0	0	21	8	54
Frankfurter, beef	3 oz	281	10	3	0	3	25	10	969
Frankfurter, beef, cooked	3 oz	277	10	3	0	3	25	10	981
Frankfurter, beef, low fat	3 oz	196	10	1	0	0	17	7	885
Frankfurter, cheese pork beef, cheesefurter smokies	3 oz	279	12	1	0	1	25	9	920
Pastrami, beef, 98% fat-free, slices	3 oz	81	17	1	0	0	1	0	859
Pastrami, beef, cured	3 oz	125	19	0	0	0	5	2	752
Salami, beef, cooked, slice	3 oz	222	11	2	0	1	19	8	969
Sausage, beef, cooked from fresh	3 oz	282	15	0	0	0	24	9	554
Sausage, beef, precooked	3 oz	344	13	0	0	0	32	13	774

MEATS, Game

Item	Serving Size	Calories	Protein	Carb	Fiber	Sugar	Total Fat	Sat Fat	Sodium
Antelope, roasted	3 oz	128	25	0	0	0	2	1	46
Bear, cooked	3 oz	220	28	0	0	0	11	3	60
Beaver, roasted	3 oz	180	30	0	0	0	6	2	50
Beefalo, roasted	3 oz	160	26	0	0	0	5	2	70
Bison, grass fed, cooked	3 oz	152	22	0	0	0	7	3	65
Bison, ground, pan-broiled	3 oz	202	20	0	0	0	13	5	62
Bison, rib eye steak, lean, 1" thick, broiled	3 oz	150	25	0	0	0	5	2	44
Bison, roasted	3 oz	122	24	0	0	0	2	1	48
Bison, shoulder clod roast, lean, braised	3 oz	164	29	0	0	0	5	2	48
Bison, top round steak, lean, 1" thick, broiled	3 oz	148	26	0	0	0	4	2	35
Boar, wild, roasted	3 oz	136	24	0	0	0	4	1	51

MEATS, Game continued

Item	Serving Size	Calories	Protein	Carb	Fiber	Sugar	Total Fat	Sat Fat	Sodium
Buffalo, grass fed, cooked	3 oz	152	22	0	0	0	7	3	65
Caribou, hind quarter, cooked, Alaskan	3 oz	135	24	0	0	0	4	2	38
Caribou, roasted	3 oz	142	25	0	0	0	4	1	51
Caribou, rump, partially dried, Alaskan	3 oz	217	44	0	0	0	4	1	332
Caribou, shoulder, dried, Alaskan	3 oz	230	50	0	0	0	3	1	808
Cornish game hen, whole, with skin, roasted	3 oz	220	19	0	0	0	15	4	54
Cornish game hen, whole, without skin, roasted	3 oz	114	20	0	0	0	3	1	54
Deer, ground, pan-broiled	3 oz	159	22	0	0	0	7	3	66
Deer, loin, lean, 1" thick steak, broiled	3 oz	128	26	0	0	0	2	1	48
Deer, roasted	3 oz	134	26	0	0	0	3	1	46
Deer, shoulder clod roast, lean, braised	3 oz	162	31	0	0	0	3	2	44
Deer, tenderloin, lean, broiled	3 oz	127	25	0	0	0	2	1	48
Deer, top round steak, lean, 1" thick, broiled	3 oz	129	27	0	0	0	2	1	38
Dove, whole, cooked	3 oz	181	20	0	0	0	11	3	48
Duck, domesticated, whole, with skin, roasted	3 oz	286	16	0	0	0	24	8	50
Duck, domesticated, whole, without skin, roasted	3 oz	171	20	0	0	0	10	3	55
Duckling, white Pekin, breast, with skin, roasted	3 oz	172	21	0	0	0	9	2	71
Duckling, white Pekin, breast, without skin, broiled	3 oz	119	23	0	0	0	2	0	89
Duckling, white Pekin, leg, with skin, roasted	3 oz	184	23	0	0	0	10	3	94
Duckling, white Pekin, leg, without skin, braised	3 oz	151	25	0	0	0	5	1	92
Elk, free range, ground, patty, cooked, Shoshone Bannock	3 oz	122	25	0	0	0	2	1	48
Elk, free range, round eye roast, cooked, Shoshone Bannock	3 oz	126	26	0	0	0	2	1	43

MEATS, Game continued

Item	Serving Size	Calories	Protein	Carb	Fiber	Sugar	Total Fat	Sat Fat	Sodium
Elk, ground, pan broiled	3 oz	164	23	0	0	0	7	3	72
Elk, loin, lean, broiled	3 oz	142	26	0	0	0	3	1	46
Elk, roasted	3 oz	124	26	0	0	0	2	1	52
Elk, round, lean, broiled	3 oz	133	26	0	0	0	2	1	43
Elk, tenderloin, lean, broiled	3 oz	138	26	0	0	0	3	1	43
Emu, fan fillet, broiled	3 oz	131	27	0	0	0	2	0	45
Emu, full rump, broiled	3 oz	143	29	0	0	0	2	1	94
Emu, ground, broiled	3 oz	139	24	0	0	0	4	1	55
Emu, inside drum, broiled	3 oz	133	28	0	0	0	2	1	100
Emu, patty, broiled	3 oz	139	24	0	0	0	4	1	55
Emu, top loin, broiled	3 oz	129	25	0	0	0	3	1	49
Goat, roasted	3 oz	122	23	0	0	0	3	1	73
Goose, whole, with skin, roasted	3 oz	259	21	0	0	0	19	6	60
Goose, whole, without skin, roasted	3 oz	202	25	0	0	0	11	4	65
Horse, roasted	3 oz	149	24	0	0	0	5	2	47
Moose, roasted	3 oz	114	25	0	0	0	1	0	59
Opossum, roasted	3 oz	188	26	0	0	0	9	1	49
Ostrich, ground, broiled	3 oz	149	22	0	0	0	6	2	68
Ostrich, inside leg, cooked	3 oz	120	25	0	0	0	2	1	71
Ostrich, inside strip, cooked	3 oz	139	25	0	0	0	4	1	62
Ostrich, outside strip, cooked	3 oz	133	24	0	0	0	3	1	61
Ostrich, oyster, cooked	3 oz	135	24	0	0	0	3	1	69
Ostrich, patty, broiled	3 oz	149	22	0	0	0	6	2	68
Ostrich, tip, cooked	3 oz	123	24	0	0	0	2	1	68
Ostrich, top loin, cooked	3 oz	132	24	0	0	0	3	1	65
Pheasant, whole, cooked	3 oz	203	28	0	0	0	10	3	37
Quail, whole, cooked	3 oz	193	21	0	0	0	12	3	44
Rabbit, domestic, roasted	3 oz	167	25	0	0	0	7	2	40
Rabbit, domestic, stewed	3 oz	175	26	0	0	0	7	2	31
Rabbit, wild, stewed	3 oz	147	28	0	0	0	3	1	38
Raccoon, roasted	3 oz	217	25	0	0	0	12	3	67
Seal, bearded, dried, with oil, Alaskan	3 oz	312	30	0	0	0	21	3	102
Seal, oogruk, dried, with oil, Alaskan	3 oz	312	30	0	0	0	21	3	102

MEATS, Game continued

Item	Serving Size	Calories	Protein	Carb	Fiber	Sugar	Total Fat	Sat Fat	Sodium
Seal, ringed, meat, Alaskan	3 oz	121	24	0	0	0	3	1	94
Squab, whole, cooked	3 oz	181	20	0	0	0	11	3	48
Squirrel, roasted	3 oz	147	26	0	0	0	4	1	101
Venison, roasted	3 oz	134	26	0	0	0	3	1	46
Water buffalo, roasted	3 oz	111	23	0	0	0	2	1	48
Whale, beluga, dried, Alaskan	3 oz	278	59	0	0	0	5	1	187

MEATS, Lamb

Item	Serving Size	Calories	Protein	Carb	Fiber	Sugar	Total Fat	Sat Fat	Sodium
Lamb, Australian, average of all cuts, cooked, 1/8" trim	3 oz	218	21	0	0	0	14	7	65
Lamb, Australian, average of all cuts, lean, cooked, 1/8" trim	3 oz	171	23	0	0	0	8	3	68
Lamb, Australian, center slice, lean, broiled, 1/8" trim	3 oz	156	23	0	0	0	7	3	56
Lamb, Australian, foreshank, lean, braised, 1/8" trim	3 oz	140	23	0	0	0	4	2	85
Lamb, Australian, leg, shank half, lean, roasted, 1/8" trim	3 oz	155	23	0	0	0	6	2	59
Lamb, Australian, leg, sirloin half, lean, roasted, 1/8" trim	3 oz	183	24	0	0	0	9	4	71
Lamb, Australian, leg, whole, lean, roasted, 1/8" trim	3 oz	162	23	0	0	0	7	3	61
Lamb, Australian, loin, lean, broiled, 1/8" trim	3 oz	163	23	0	0	0	7	3	68
Lamb, Australian, rib, lean, roasted, 1/8" trim	3 oz	179	21	0	0	0	10	4	70
Lamb, Australian, shoulder, arm chop, lean, braised, 1/8" trim	3 oz	202	29	0	0	0	9	4	66
Lamb, Australian, shoulder, blade chop, lean, broiled, 1/8" trim	3 oz	196	20	0	0	0	12	5	80
Lamb, Australian, shoulder, whole, lean, cooked, 1/8" trim	3 oz	198	22	0	0	0	11	5	77

MEATS, Lamb continued

Item	Serving Size	Calories	Protein	Carb	Fiber	Sugar	Total Fat	Sat Fat	Sodium
Lamb, Australian, sirloin chop, lean, broiled, 1/8" trim	3 oz	160	23	0	0	0	7	3	56
Lamb, average of all cuts, cooked, choice, 1/4" trim	3 oz	250	21	0	0	0	18	8	61
Lamb, average of all cuts, cooked, choice, 1/8" trim	3 oz	230	22	0	0	0	15	6	61
Lamb, average of all cuts, lean, cooked, choice, 1/4" trim	3 oz	175	24	0	0	0	8	3	65
Lamb, ground, broiled, 20% fat	3 oz	241	21	0	0	0	17	7	69
Lamb, kabob meat, lean, braised, choice, 1/4" trim	3 oz	190	29	0	0	0	7	3	60
Lamb, leg, shank half, lean, roasted, choice, 1/4" trim	3 oz	153	24	0	0	0	6	2	56
Lamb, leg, shank half, roasted, choice, 1/8" trim	3 oz	184	23	0	0	0	10	4	55
Lamb, leg, sirloin half, roasted, choice, 1/8" trim	3 oz	241	21	0	0	0	17	7	58
Lamb, leg, whole, roasted, choice, 1/8" trim	3 oz	206	22	0	0	0	12	5	57
Lamb, loin, broiled, choice, 1/8" trim	3 oz	252	22	0	0	0	18	7	66
Lamb, loin, roasted, choice, 1/8" trim	3 oz	247	20	0	0	0	18	8	54
Lamb, New Zealand, average of all cuts, cooked from frozen	3 oz	259	21	0	0	0	19	9	39
Lamb, New Zealand, average of all cuts, cooked from frozen, 1/8" trim	3 oz	230	21	0	0	0	15	7	39
Lamb, New Zealand, average of all cuts, lean, cooked from frozen	3 oz	175	25	0	0	0	8	3	43
Lamb, rib, broiled, choice, 1/8" trim	3 oz	289	20	0	0	0	23	10	65
Lamb, rib, roasted, choice, 1/8" trim	3 oz	290	19	0	0	0	23	10	63
Lamb, shoulder, arm chop, braised, choice, 1/8" trim	3 oz	286	26	0	0	0	19	8	61

MEATS, Lamb continued

Item	Serving Size	Calories	Protein	Carb	Fiber	Sugar	Total Fat	Sat Fat	Sodium
Lamb, shoulder, arm chop, broiled, 1/8" trim	3 oz	229	21	0	0	0	15	7	66
Lamb, shoulder, arm chop, roasted, choice, 1/8" trim	3 oz	227	19	0	0	0	16	7	55
Lamb, shoulder, blade chop, braised, choice, 1/8" trim	3 oz	288	25	0	0	0	20	8	64
Lamb, shoulder, blade chop, broiled, choice, 1/8" trim	3 oz	227	20	0	0	0	16	6	71
Lamb, shoulder, blade chop, roasted, choice, 1/8" trim	3 oz	230	19	0	0	0	16	7	57
Lamb, shoulder, whole, braised, 1/8" trim	3 oz	287	25	0	0	0	20	8	63
Lamb, shoulder, whole, broiled, choice, 1/8" trim	3 oz	228	20	0	0	0	16	6	70
Lamb, shoulder, whole, roasted, choice, 1/8" trim	3 oz	229	19	0	0	0	16	7	56

MEATS, Pork

Item	Serving Size	Calories	Protein	Carb	Fiber	Sugar	Total Fat	Sat Fat	Sodium
Bacon, broiled/pan fried/roasted	3 oz	460	31	1	0	0	36	12	1964
Bacon, cured, reduced sodium, cooked	3 oz	460	31	1	0	0	36	12	876
Canadian bacon, cured, grilled	3 oz	157	21	1	0	0	7	2	1314
Frankfurter, pork	3 oz	229	11	0	0	0	20	7	694
Lunchmeat, ham	3 oz	153	14	4	0	0	9	3	1131
Lunchmeat, ham, extra lean, 5% fat	3 oz	91	16	1	0	0	2	1	901
Pork, average of retail cuts, leg, shoulder, & loin, lean, cooked	3 oz	171	23	0	0	0	8	3	47
Pork, average of retail cuts, leg, shoulder, loin, & sparerib, cooked	3 oz	202	22	0	0	0	12	4	48
Pork, average of retail cuts, loin & shoulder blade, cooked	3 oz	200	22	0	0	0	12	4	47

MEATS, Pork continued

Item	Serving Size	Calories	Protein	Carb	Fiber	Sugar	Total Fat	Sat Fat	Sodium
Pork, average of retail cuts, loin & shoulder blade, lean, cooked	3 oz	179	25	0	0	0	8	3	48
Pork, backribs, roasted	3 oz	315	21	0	0	0	25	9	86
Pork, breakfast strips, cured, cooked	3 oz	390	25	1	0	0	31	11	1784
Pork, chop, blade loin, broiled	3 oz	272	19	0	0	0	21	8	60
Pork, chop, blade loin, lean, braised	3 oz	191	21	0	0	0	11	4	53
Pork, chop, blade loin, lean, pan-fried	3 oz	205	21	0	0	0	13	4	66
Pork, chop, center loin, lean, braised	3 oz	172	25	0	0	0	7	3	53
Pork, chop, center loin, lean, with bone, broiled	3 oz	153	23	0	0	0	6	2	48
Pork, chop, center rib loin, braised	3 oz	217	22	0	0	0	13	5	34
Pork, chop, center rib loin, broiled	3 oz	221	23	0	0	0	13	5	53
Pork, chop, sirloin, braised	3 oz	161	23	0	0	0	7	3	39
Pork, chop, sirloin, broiled	3 oz	177	26	0	0	0	7	2	48
Pork, chop, sirloin, lean, braised	3 oz	149	23	0	0	0	6	2	39
Pork, chop, top loin, braised	3 oz	198	24	0	0	0	11	4	36
Pork, chop, top loin, broiled	3 oz	167	23	0	0	0	8	3	37
Pork, chop, whole loin, braised	3 oz	203	23	0	0	0	12	4	41
Pork, chop, whole loin, broiled	3 oz	206	23	0	0	0	12	4	53
Pork, chop, whole loin, lean, roasted	3 oz	178	24	0	0	0	8	3	49
Pork, chop, whole loin, roasted	3 oz	211	23	0	0	0	12	5	50
Pork, country-style ribs, braised	3 oz	232	23	0	0	0	15	5	49
Pork, country-style ribs, lean, braised	3 oz	210	24	0	0	0	12	4	51
Pork, cured ham & water product, lean, pan-broiled	3 oz	105	13	4	0	4	4	1	1182

MEATS, Pork continued

Item	Serving Size	Calories	Protein	Carb	Fiber	Sugar	Total Fat	Sat Fat	Sodium
Pork, cured ham & water product, lean, with bone, pan-broiled	3 oz	104	18	1	0	1	3	1	1051
Pork, cured ham & water product, rump, lean, with bone, roasted	3 oz	111	18	1	0	1	4	1	1077
Pork, cured ham & water product, shank, with bone, roasted	3 oz	199	15	1	0	1	15	5	803
Pork, ground, cooked	3 oz	252	22	0	0	0	18	7	62
Pork, ham, honey, smoked, cooked	3 oz	104	15	6	0	0	2	1	765
Pork, ham, shank half, lean, roasted, diced	3 oz	183	24	0	0	0	9	3	54
Pork, ham, whole, lean, roasted, diced	3 oz	179	25	0	0	0	8	3	54
Pork, ham, whole, roasted, diced	3 oz	232	23	0	0	0	15	5	51
Pork, hocks, pickled	3 oz	145	16	0	0	0	9	3	893
Pork, Oriental style, dehydrated	3 oz	523	10	1	0	0	53	20	582
Pork, roast, blade loin, lean, roasted	3 oz	210	23	0	0	0	13	5	25
Pork, roast, sirloin tip, braised	3 oz	133	26	0	0	0	2	1	37
Pork, roast, sirloin, lean, with bone, roasted	3 oz	173	24	0	0	0	8	2	50
Pork, roast, sirloin, roasted	3 oz	176	24	0	0	0	8	3	48
Pork, roast, top loin, lean, roasted	3 oz	147	23	0	0	0	5	2	40
Pork, shoulder, arm, lean, roasted	3 oz	194	23	0	0	0	11	4	68
Pork, shoulder, blade, Boston steak, lean, braised	3 oz	198	23	0	0	0	11	4	51
Pork, shoulder, breast, broiled	3 oz	138	24	0	0	0	4	1	46
Pork, shoulder, whole, roasted, diced	3 oz	248	20	0	0	0	18	7	58
Pork, smoked ham, lean, low sodium	3 oz	123	18	1	0	0	5	2	824

MEATS, Pork continued

Item	Serving Size	Calories	Protein	Carb	Fiber	Sugar	Total Fat	Sat Fat	Sodium
Pork, spare ribs, braised	3 oz	337	25	0	0	0	26	9	79
Pork, steak, leg cap, broiled	3 oz	134	23	0	0	0	4	1	65
Pork, tenderloin, chop, broiled	3 oz	171	25	0	0	0	7	2	54
Salami, Italian, pork	3 oz	361	18	1	0	1	31	11	1607
Sausage, bratwurst, pork, cooked	3 oz	283	12	2	0	0	25	9	719
Sausage, bratwurst, veal, cooked	3 oz	290	12	0	0	0	27	13	51
Sausage, braunschweiger, liver, pork	3 oz	278	12	3	0	0	24	8	986
Sausage, Italian, pork, link, cooked	3 oz	292	16	4	0	1	23	8	1026
Sausage, Italian, pork, link, cooked	3 oz	292	16	4	0	1	23	8	1026
Sausage, pork, smoked, link	3 oz	261	10	0	0	0	24	8	703

MEATS, Veal

Item	Serving Size	Calories	Protein	Carb	Fiber	Sugar	Total Fat	Sat Fat	Sodium
Veal, average of all cuts, cooked	3 oz	196	26	0	0	0	10	4	74
Veal, average of all cuts, lean, cooked	3 oz	167	27	0	0	0	6	2	76
Veal, breast, cooked	3 oz	443	8	0	0	0	45	18	42
Veal, breast, plate half, braised	3 oz	240	22	0	0	0	16	6	54
Veal, ground, broiled, 8% fat	3 oz	146	21	0	0	0	6	3	71
Veal, leg, top round steak, braised	3 oz	179	31	0	0	0	5	2	57
Veal, leg, top round steak, lean, roasted	3 oz	128	24	0	0	0	3	1	58
Veal, leg or shoulder, lean, braised, cubed	3 oz	160	30	0	0	0	4	1	79
Veal, loin chop, lean, braised	3 oz	192	29	0	0	0	8	2	71
Veal, loin, roasted	3 oz	184	21	0	0	0	10	4	79
Veal, rib chop, braised	3 oz	213	28	0	0	0	11	4	81

MEATS, Veal continued

Item	Serving Size	Calories	Protein	Carb	Fiber	Sugar	Total Fat	Sat Fat	Sodium
Veal, shank roast, braised	3 oz	162	27	0	0	0	5	2	79
Veal, short ribs, lean, roasted	3 oz	150	22	0	0	0	6	2	82
Veal, shoulder arm steak, roasted	3 oz	156	22	0	0	0	7	3	77
Veal, shoulder blade roast, roasted	3 oz	158	21	0	0	0	7	3	85
Veal, sirloin roast, lean, braised	3 oz	173	29	0	0	0	6	2	69
Veal, sirloin steak, lean, roasted	3 oz	143	22	0	0	0	5	2	72
Veal, whole shoulder roast, braised	3 oz	194	27	0	0	0	9	3	81

NUTS, SEEDS, AND BUTTERS

Item	Serving Size	Calories	Protein	Carb	Fiber	Sugar	Total Fat	Sat Fat	Sodium
Almond butter	2 tbsp	179	4	6	1	1	16.8	1.6	128
Almond butter, chocolate	2 tbsp	195	5	11	4	5	16.0	2.5	0
Almond butter, chocolate cherry haze	2 tbsp	190	4	7	3	3	17.0	2.5	0
Almond meal, stone ground	2 tbsp	160	6	6	3	1	14.0	1.0	10
Almonds	1 oz	163	6	6	3	1	14.0	1.1	0
Almonds, blanched	1 oz	581	22	20	10	5	50.6	3.9	28
Almonds, dry-roasted, salted	1 oz	169	6	5	3	1	15.0	1.1	96
Almonds, dry-roasted, unsalted	1 oz	169	6	5	3	1	15.0	1.1	0
Almonds, oil-roasted, salted	1 oz	172	6	5	3	1	15.6	1.2	96
Almonds, oil-roasted, unsalted	1 oz	172	6	5	3	1	15.6	1.2	0
Almonds, oven-roasted, cinnamon brown sugar	1 oz	160	6	7	3	3	14.0	1.0	30
Almonds, oven-roasted, sea salt	1 oz	170	6	5	3	1	15.0	1.0	135
Almonds, oven-roasted, vanilla bean	1 oz	160	6	7	3	3	14.0	1.0	25

NUTS, SEEDS, AND BUTTERS continued

Item	Serving Size	Calories	Protein	Carb	Fiber	Sugar	Total Fat	Sat Fat	Sodium
Almonds, paste, firmly packed cup	2 tbsp	130	3	14	1	10	7.9	0.7	3
Brazil nuts	1 oz	186	4	3	2	1	18.8	4.3	1
Cashew butter, plain	2 tbsp	166	5	8	1	1	14.0	2.8	174
Cashews	1 oz	157	5	9	1	2	12.4	2.2	3
Cashews, dry-roasted, salted	1 oz	163	4	9	1	1	13.1	2.6	181
Cashews, dry-roasted, unsalted	1 oz	163	4	9	1	1	13.1	2.6	5
Cashews, oil-roasted, salted	1 oz	165	5	9	1	1	13.5	2.4	87
Cashews, oil-roasted, unsalted	1 oz	164	5	8	1	1	13.5	2.4	4
Chestnuts, European	1 oz	60	1	13	2	3	0.6	0.1	1
Chestnuts, European, roasted	1 oz	69	1	15	1	3	0.6	0.1	1
Coconut, cream, canned	1 oz	101	0	15	0	15	4.6	4.4	10
Coconut, dried, flaked, sweetened	1 oz	129	1	15	3	10	7.9	7.5	81
Coconut, dried, shredded, sweetened	1 oz	142	1	14	1	12	10.1	8.9	74
Coconut, dried, unsweetened	1 oz	187	2	7	5	2	18.3	16.2	10
Coconut, toasted from dried	1 oz	168	2	13	2	11	13.3	11.8	10
Coconut, water, fresh	8 oz	46	2	9	3	6	0.5	0.4	252
Filberts	1 oz	178	4	5	3	1	17.2	1.3	0
Filberts, blanched	1 oz	178	4	5	3	1	17.3	1.3	0
Filberts, dry-roasted, unsalted	1 oz	183	4	5	3	1	17.7	1.3	0
Flax/linseed seeds	1 oz	151	5	8	8	0	12.0	1.0	9
Hazelnut butter, chocolate cherry haze, natural	2 tbsp	210	3	8	2	3	19.0	2.0	0
Hazelnut butter, chocolate haze, natural	2 tbsp	210	3	8	2	3	19.0	2.0	0
Hazelnuts	1 oz	178	4	5	3	1	17.2	1.3	0
Hazelnuts, dry-roasted, unsalted	1 oz	183	4	5	3	1	17.7	1.3	0
Macadamia nuts	1 oz	204	2	4	2	1	21.5	3.4	1
Macadamia nuts, dry-roasted, salted	1 oz	203	2	4	2	1	21.6	3.4	75

NUTS, SEEDS, AND BUTTERS continued

Item	Serving Size	Calories	Protein	Carb	Fiber	Sugar	Total Fat	Sat Fat	Sodium
Macadamia nuts, dry-roasted, unsalted	1 oz	204	2	4	2	1	21.6	3.4	1
Mixed nuts, with peanuts, dry-roasted, salted	1 oz	168	5	7	3	1	14.6	2.0	190
Mixed nuts, with peanuts, oil-roasted, salted	1 oz	175	5	6	3	1	16.0	2.5	119
Mixed nuts, with peanuts, oil-roasted, unsalted	1 oz	175	5	6	3	1	16.0	2.5	3
Mixed nuts, without peanuts, oil-roasted, salted	1 oz	174	4	6	2	1	15.9	2.6	87
Peanut butter, chunky	2 tbsp	167	7	6	2	2	14.2	2.3	138
Peanut butter, chunky, unsalted	2 tbsp	167	7	6	2	2	14.2	2.3	5
Peanut butter, chunky, vitamin- & mineral-fortified	2 tbsp	168	7	5	2	3	14.6	2.3	104
Peanut butter, creamy	2 tbsp	167	7	6	2	3	14.3	3.0	130
Peanut butter, creamy, reduced fat	2 tbsp	147	7	10	1	3	9.6	1.6	153
Peanut butter, creamy, unsalted	2 tbsp	167	7	6	2	3	14.3	2.9	5
Peanut butter, creamy, vitamin- & mineral-fortified	2 tbsp	168	7	5	2	3	14.4	2.9	119
Peanut butter, creamy, with omega 3	2 tbsp	172	7	5	2	1	15.4	2.7	101
Peanut butter, reduced sodium	2 tbsp	179	7	6	2	3	14.1	2.2	58
Peanut butter, reduced sugar	2 tbsp	184	7	4	2	1	15.6	2.9	127
Peanut butter, smooth	2 tbsp	167	6	7	2	2	14.0	2.7	135
Peanuts	1 oz	161	7	5	2	1	14.0	1.9	5
Peanuts, cooked with salt, in shell	1 oz	90	4	6	2	1	6.2	0.9	213
Peanuts, cooked with salt, shelled	1 oz	90	4	6	2	1	6.2	0.9	213
Peanuts, dry-roasted, salted	1 oz	166	7	6	2	1	14.1	2.0	230
Peanuts, dry-roasted, unsalted	1 oz	166	7	6	2	1	14.1	2.0	2
Peanuts, oil-roasted, salted	1 oz	170	8	4	3	1	14.9	2.5	91

NUTS, SEEDS, AND BUTTERS continued

Item	Serving Size	Calories	Protein	Carb	Fiber	Sugar	Total Fat	Sat Fat	Sodium
Peanuts, oil-roasted, unsalted	1 oz	165	7	5	2	1	14.0	1.9	2
Pecans	1 oz	196	3	4	3	1	20.4	1.8	0
Pecans, dry-roasted, salted	1 oz	201	3	4	3	1	21.1	1.8	109
Pecans, dry-roasted, unsalted	1 oz	201	3	4	3	1	21.1	1.8	0
Pecans, oil-roasted, salted	1 oz	203	3	4	3	1	21.3	2.1	111
Pecans, oil-roasted, unsalted	1 oz	203	3	4	3	1	21.3	2.1	0
Pine nuts, pignolia, dried	1 oz	191	4	4	1	1	19.4	1.4	1
Pine nuts, piñon/pinyon, roasted, Navajo	1 oz	153	2	14	12	1	9.7	0.9	88
Pistachios, dry-roasted, salted	1 oz	161	6	8	3	2	13.0	1.6	115
Pistachios, dry-roasted, unsalted	1 oz	162	6	8	3	2	13.0	1.6	3
Pistachios, salted	1 oz	159	6	8	3	2	12.9	1.6	0
Poppy seeds	1 oz	170	6	6	3	0	14.0	1.5	0
Pumpkin seeds, kernels, dried	1 oz	158	9	3	2	1	13.9	2.5	2
Pumpkin seeds, kernels, roasted, salted	1 oz	163	8	4	2	0	13.9	2.4	73
Pumpkin seeds, kernels, roasted, unsalted	1 oz	163	8	4	2	0	13.9	2.4	5
Safflower seeds, kernels, dried	1 oz	147	5	10	2	0	10.9	1.0	1
Sesame seed butter, from roasted & toasted kernels	1 oz	169	5	6	3	0	15.2	2.1	33
Sesame seeds, dried	1 oz	162	5	7	3	0	14.1	2.0	3
Sesame seeds, roasted & toasted	1 oz	160	5	7	4	0	13.6	1.9	3
Soy nuts, roasted, salted	1 oz	140	11	9	1	0	7.0	1.0	50
Soy nuts, roasted, unsalted	1 oz	140	11	9	1	0	7.0	1.0	0
Soy nuts, with wasabi	1 oz	140	10	11	5	2	7.0	1.0	110
Squash seeds, kernels, dried	1 oz	158	9	3	2	0	13.9	2.5	2
Squash seeds, kernels, roasted, salted	1 oz	163	8	4	2	0	13.9	2.4	73
Squash seeds, kernels, roasted, unsalted	1 oz	163	8	4	2	0	13.9	2.4	5

NUTS, SEEDS, AND BUTTERS continued

Item	Serving Size	Calories	Protein	Carb	Fiber	Sugar	Total Fat	Sat Fat	Sodium
Sunflower seeds, kernels, dried	1 oz	166	6	6	2	1	14.6	1.3	3
Sunflower seeds, kernels, dry-roasted, salted	1 oz	165	5	7	3	1	14.1	1.5	116
Sunflower seeds, kernels, dry-roasted, unsalted	1 oz	165	5	7	3	1	14.1	1.5	1
Sunflower seeds, kernels, oil-roasted, unsalted	1 oz	168	6	6	3	1	14.5	2.0	1
Sunflower seeds, kernels, toasted, salted	1 oz	175	5	6	3	1	16.1	1.7	174
Sunflower seeds, oil-roasted, salted	1 oz	168	6	6	3	1	14.5	2.0	116
Tahini, from roasted & toasted sesame seed kernels	1 oz	169	5	6	3	0	15.2	2.1	33
Walnuts, black, dried	1 oz	175	7	3	2	0	16.7	1.0	1
Walnuts, English, dried	1 oz	185	4	4	2	1	18.5	1.7	1
Yellow pond lily seeds, wocas, dried, Pacific Northwest	1 oz	102	2	23	5	0	0.3	0.0	7

PASTAS

Item	Serving Size	Calories	Protein	Carb	Fiber	Sugar	Total Fat	Sat Fat	Sodium
Acini di pepe, enriched, dry	2 oz	200	7	41	2	2	0.8	0.2	3
Alphabets, enriched, dry	2 oz	200	7	41	2	2	0.8	0.2	3
Angel hair, corn, dry	2 oz	210	4	46	0	0	1.5	0.0	15
Angel hair, garlic & parsley, dry	2 oz	210	7	42	2	1	1.0	0.0	15
Angel hair, rice, wheat free, dry	2 oz	210	4	46	1	0	0.5	0.0	15
Angel hair, semolina, dry	2 oz	210	7	43	1	2	1.0	0.0	5
Angel hair, semolina, tomato & basil, dry	2 oz	210	7	43	2	1	1.0	0.0	5
Angel hair, semolina, tomato & pesto, dry	2 oz	210	7	42	1	1	1.0	0.0	10
Angel hair, whole wheat, dry	2 oz	210	7	42	5	2	1.5	0.0	10

PASTAS continued

Item	Serving Size	Calories	Protein	Carb	Fiber	Sugar	Total Fat	Sat Fat	Sodium
Bow ties, enriched, dry	2 oz	200	7	41	2	2	0.8	0.2	3
Capellini, enriched, dry	2 oz	200	7	41	2	2	0.8	0.2	3
Cavatelli, enriched, dry	2 oz	200	7	41	2	2	0.8	0.2	3
Couscous, almondine, dry	2 oz	200	7	37	2	5	2.5	0.0	490
Couscous, dry	2 oz	190	7	43	7	0	1.0	0.0	5
Couscous, giant pearl, toasted, all natural, dry	2 oz	170	5	36	2	1	0.0	0.0	0
Couscous, whole wheat, dry	2 oz	210	8	45	7	0	1.0	0.0	0
Couscous, with roasted garlic & olive oil, low fat	2 oz	310	11	59	4	2	2.5	0.0	720
Ditalini, enriched, dry	2 oz	200	7	41	2	2	0.8	0.2	3
Egg, 1/2" wide, enriched, dry	2 oz	207	8	39	2	1	2.2	0.6	12
Egg, alphabets, enriched, dry	2 oz	206	8	38	2	1	2.2	0.6	12
Egg, bot boi, enriched, dry	2 oz	206	8	38	2	1	2.2	0.6	12
Egg, bow ties, enriched, dry	2 oz	206	8	38	2	1	2.2	0.6	12
Egg, dumpling, 1" wide, enriched, dry	2 oz	207	8	39	2	1	2.2	0.6	12
Egg, enriched, cooked	1 cup	193	6	35	2	1	2.9	0.6	7
Egg, enriched, dry	2 oz	211	8	39	2	1	2.4	0.6	12
Egg, enriched, kluski, dry	2 oz	207	8	39	1	1	1.9	0.7	130
Egg, extra wide, 3/4", enriched, dry	2 oz	207	8	39	2	1	2.2	0.6	12
Egg, fine, 1/16"wide, enriched, dry	2 oz	207	8	39	2	1	2.2	0.6	12
Egg, homestyle, 1" wide, enriched, dry	2 oz	207	8	39	2	1	2.2	0.6	12
Egg, medium, 1/4" wide, enriched, dry	2 oz	207	8	39	2	1	2.2	0.6	12

PASTAS continued

Item	Serving Size	Calories	Protein	Carb	Fiber	Sugar	Total Fat	Sat Fat	Sodium
Egg, medium, 5/16" wide, enriched, dry	2 oz	207	8	39	2	1	2.2	0.6	12
Egg, pot pie squares, enriched, dry	2 oz	206	8	38	2	1	2.2	0.6	12
Egg, spinach, enriched, cooked	1 cup	185	7	34	3	1	2.2	0.5	17
Egg, unenriched, cooked	1 cup	193	6	35	2	1	2.9	0.6	7
Egg, unenriched, dry	2 oz	211	8	39	2	1	2.4	0.6	12
Elbow, casserole, enriched, dry	2 oz	200	7	41	2	2	0.8	0.2	3
Elbow, corn, wheat-free, dry	2 oz	200	4	43	5	0	2.0	0.0	15
Elbow, dry	2 oz	210	7	43	1	2	1.0	0.0	5
Elbow, enriched, dry	2 oz	200	7	41	2	2	0.8	0.2	3
Farfalle, enriched, dry	2 oz	200	7	41	2	2	0.8	0.2	3
Fettuccine, enriched, dry	2 oz	200	7	41	2	2	0.8	0.2	3
Fettuccine, rice, dry	2 oz	210	4	46	1	0	0.5	0.0	15
Fettuccine, semolina, dry	2 oz	210	7	43	1	2	1.0	0.0	5
Fettuccine, semolina, spinach, dry	2 oz	210	7	43	3	1	1.0	0.0	20
Fettuccine, spinach, enriched, dry	2 oz	198	8	40	2	2	1.0	0.2	16
Fideo, coiled, enriched, dry	2 oz	200	7	41	2	2	0.8	0.2	3
Fideo, enriched, dry	2 oz	200	7	41	2	2	0.8	0.2	3
Fusilli, enriched, dry	2 oz	200	7	41	2	2	0.8	0.2	3
Fusilli, whole wheat, dry	2 oz	210	7	42	5	2	1.5	0.0	10
Gemelli twists, enriched, dry	2 oz	200	7	41	2	2	0.8	0.2	3
Lasagna, enriched, dry	2 oz	200	7	41	2	2	0.8	0.2	3
Lasagna, oven ready/no boil, dry	30.8	116	4	23	1	1	0.6	0.0	0
Linguine, enriched, dry	2 oz	200	7	41	2	2	0.8	0.2	3

PASTAS continued

Item	Serving Size	Calories	Protein	Carb	Fiber	Sugar	Total Fat	Sat Fat	Sodium
Linguine, semolina, dry	2 oz	210	7	43	1	2	1.0	0.0	5
Linguine, whole-wheat flax, dry	2 oz	208	9	36	8	3	3.5	0.5	15
Macaroni, enriched, cooked	1 cup	221	8	43	3	1	1.3	0.3	1
Macaroni, enriched, dry	2 oz	204	7	41	2	1	0.8	0.2	3
Macaroni, unenriched, cooked	1 cup	221	8	43	3	1	1.3	0.3	1
Macaroni, unenriched, dry	2 oz	204	7	41	2	1	0.8	0.2	3
Macaroni, whole wheat, cooked	1 cup	174	7	37	4	1	0.8	0.1	4
Manicotti, enriched, dry	2 oz	200	7	41	2	2	0.8	0.2	3
Mostaccioli rigati, enriched, dry	2 oz	200	7	41	2	2	0.8	0.2	3
Noodles, cellophane, dehydrated	2 oz	193	0	47	0	0	0.0	0.0	6
Noodles, crunchy, flat	2 oz	287	6	29	1	0	17.4	2.7	208
Noodles, long rice, dehydrated	2 oz	193	0	47	0	0	0.0	0.0	6
Noodles, mung bean, dehydrated	2 oz	193	0	47	0	0	0.0	0.0	6
Orzo, enriched, dry	2 oz	200	7	41	2	2	0.8	0.2	3
Pastina, enriched, dry	2 oz	200	7	41	2	2	0.8	0.2	3
Penne rigate, enriched, dry	2 oz	200	7	41	2	2	0.8	0.2	3
Penne, rice, dry	2 oz	210	4	46	1	0	0.5	0.0	15
Penne, semolina, dry	2 oz	210	7	43	1	2	1.0	0.0	5
Penne, whole-wheat flax, dry	2 oz	208	9	36	8	3	3.5	0.5	15
Penne, whole wheat, dry	2 oz	210	7	42	5	2	1.5	0.0	10
Radiatore, enriched, dry	2 oz	200	7	41	2	2	0.8	0.2	3
Ribbon, 1/2" wide, enriched, dry	2 oz	200	7	41	2	2	0.8	0.2	3
Ribbon, eggless, dry	2 oz	210	7	43	1	2	1.0	0.0	5

PASTAS continued

Item	Serving Size	Calories	Protein	Carb	Fiber	Sugar	Total Fat	Sat Fat	Sodium
Ribbons, yolk free, 1/2" wide, enriched, dry	2 oz	200	8	40	1	3	1.0	0.2	26
Rice paper	2 oz	200	7	41	0	2	1.0	0.0	60
Ziti, enriched, dry	2 oz	200	7	41	2	2	0.8	0.2	3
Rigatoni, enriched, dry	2 oz	200	7	41	2	2	0.8	0.2	3
Rigatoni, semolina, dry	2 oz	210	7	43	1	2	1.0	0.0	5
Rigatoni, whole wheat, dry	2 oz	210	7	42	5	2	1.5	0.0	10
Rotelle, enriched, dry	2 oz	200	7	41	2	2	0.8	0.2	3
Rotini, enriched, dry	2 oz	200	7	41	2	2	0.8	0.2	3
Rotini, rainbow, enriched, dry	2 oz	201	7	42	2	2	1.0	0.2	5
Rotini, semolina, dry	2 oz	210	7	43	1	2	1.0	0.0	5
Rotini, tricolor, enriched, dry	2 oz	201	7	42	2	2	1.0	0.2	5
Rotini, whole-wheat flax, dry	2 oz	208	9	36	8	3	3.5	0.5	15
Shells, jumbo, enriched, dry	2 oz	200	7	41	2	2	0.8	0.2	3
Shells, large, enriched, dry	2 oz	200	7	41	2	2	0.8	0.2	3
Shells, medium, enriched, dry	2 oz	200	7	41	2	2	0.8	0.2	3
Shells, semolina, dry	2 oz	210	7	43	1	2	1.0	0.0	5
Shells, small, enriched, cooked	1 cup	221	8	43	3	1	1.3	0.3	1
Shells, small, enriched, dry	2 oz	204	7	41	2	1	0.8	0.2	3
Shells, stuffing, enriched, dry	2 oz	200	7	41	2	2	0.8	0.2	3
Soba, 40% buckwheat, dry	2 oz	190	8	37	3	2	1.0	0.0	490
Soba, 100% buckwheat, dry	2 oz	200	6	43	3	2	1.0	0.0	5
Soba, cooked	1 cup	139	7	30	2	0	0.1	0.0	84
Soba, dry	2 oz	200	8	38	2	3	1.5	0.0	70
Soba, kamut, dry	2 oz	200	7	38	3	0	1.0	0.0	60
Soba, spelt, dry	2 oz	200	9	37	2	0	1.5	0.0	50

PASTAS continued

Item	Serving Size	Calories	Protein	Carb	Fiber	Sugar	Total Fat	Sat Fat	Sodium
Somen, cooked	1 cup	183	6	39	1	0	0.3	0.0	225
Somen, dry	2 oz	196	6	41	2	0	0.4	0.1	1012
Spaghetti, corn, wheat free, dry	2 oz	200	4	43	5	0	2.0	0.0	15
Spaghetti, enriched, cooked	1 cup	221	8	43	3	1	1.3	0.3	1
Spaghetti, enriched, cooked with salt	1 cup	220	8	43	3	1	1.3	0.3	183
Spaghetti, enriched, dry	2 oz	204	7	41	2	1	0.8	0.2	3
Spaghetti, rice, dry	2 oz	210	4	46	1	0	0.5	0.0	15
Spaghetti, semolina, dry	2 oz	210	7	43	1	2	1.0	0.0	5
Spaghetti, semolina, spinach, dry	2 oz	210	7	43	3	1	1.0	0.0	20
Spaghetti, spelt	2 oz	190	8	40	5	4	1.5	0.0	0
Spaghetti, spinach, dry	2 oz	180	9	38	8	1	2.0	0.0	20
Spaghetti, thin, enriched, dry	2 oz	200	7	41	2	2	0.8	0.2	3
Spaghetti, unenriched, cooked	1 cup	221	8	43	3	1	1.3	0.3	1
Spaghetti, unenriched, cooked with salt	1 cup	220	8	43	3	1	1.3	0.3	183
Spaghetti, unenriched, dry	2 oz	204	7	41	2	1	0.8	0.2	3
Spaghetti, whole-wheat flax, dry	2 oz	208	9	36	8	3	3.5	0.5	15
Spaghetti, whole wheat, cooked	1 cup	174	7	37	6	1	0.8	0.1	4
Spaghetti, whole wheat, dry	2 oz	191	8	41	7	2	0.8	0.1	4
Spiral, enriched, cooked	1 cup	221	8	43	3	1	1.3	0.3	1
Spiral, enriched, dry	2 oz	204	7	41	2	1	0.8	0.2	3
Spiral, vegetable, enriched, cooked	1 cup	179	6	37	6	2	0.2	0.0	8
Spiral, rice, dry	2 oz	210	4	46	1	0	0.5	0.0	15

PASTAS continued

Item	Serving Size	Calories	Protein	Carb	Fiber	Sugar	Total Fat	Sat Fat	Sodium
Tortiglioni, enriched, dry	2 oz	200	7	41	2	2	0.8	0.2	3
Tubettini, enriched, dry	2 oz	200	7	41	2	2	0.8	0.2	3
Udon, brown rice, dry	2 oz	200	8	38	3	1	2.0	0.0	80
Udon, dry	2 oz	200	8	38	3	1	1.5	0.0	80
Udon, kamut, dry	2 oz	200	10	37	3	0	1.5	0.0	55
Udon, spelt, dry	2 oz	200	8	39	2	1	1.0	0.0	75
Vermicelli, enriched, dry	2 oz	200	7	41	2	2	0.8	0.2	3
Vermicelli, soy, dry	2 oz	182	0	45	2	10	0.1	0.0	2
Wagon wheels, enriched, dry	2 oz	200	7	41	2	2	0.8	0.2	3
Ziti, rigate, enriched, dry	2 oz	200	7	41	2	2	0.8	0.2	3
Ziti, semolina, dry	2 oz	210	7	43	1	2	1.0	0.0	5

POULTRY

Item	Serving Size	Calories	Protein	Carb	Fiber	Sugar	Total Fat	Sat Fat	Sodium
Bacon, turkey, cooked	3 oz	325	25	3	0	0	23.7	7.0	1942
Chicken tenders, breast, cooked	3 oz	249	13	14	1	0	15.0	3.2	388
Chicken tenders, breast, microwaved	3 oz	214	14	15	0	0	11.0	2.7	379
Chicken, breast, fillet, mesquite, cooked frozen	3 oz	130	16	3	1	1	6.0	2.0	320
Chicken, breast, fillet, teriyaki, cooked frozen	3 oz	160	17	7	0	5	7.0	2.0	430
Chicken, breast, mesquite flavor, fat-free, sliced	3 oz	68	14	2	0	0	0.3	0.1	884
Chicken, breast, original recipe, fried	3 oz	188	19	5	0	0	10.2	2.3	501
Chicken, breast, oven roasted, fat-free, sliced	3 oz	67	14	2	0	0	0.3	0.1	924
Chicken, breast, Southwestern, grilled, strips	3 oz	110	19	1	0	0	3.5	1.0	770

POULTRY continued

Item	Serving Size	Calories	Protein	Carb	Fiber	Sugar	Total Fat	Sat Fat	Sodium
Chicken, broiler or fryer, back, with skin, raw	3 oz	271	12	0	0	0	24.4	7.1	54
Chicken, broiler or fryer, back, with skin, roasted	3 oz	255	22	0	0	0	17.8	4.9	74
Chicken, broiler or fryer, back, with skin, stewed	3 oz	219	19	0	0	0	15.4	4.3	54
Chicken, broiler or fryer, back, without skin, raw	3 oz	116	17	0	0	0	5.0	1.3	70
Chicken, broiler or fryer, back, without skin, roasted	3 oz	203	24	0	0	0	11.2	3.1	82
Chicken, broiler or fryer, back, without skin, stewed	3 oz	178	22	0	0	0	9.5	2.6	57
Chicken, broiler or fryer, back, with skin, seasoned, rotisserie	3 oz	221	20	0	0	0	15.8	4.2	496
Chicken, broiler or fryer, breast, enhanced, without skin, raw	3 oz	88	17	0	0	0	2.3	0.6	275
Chicken, broiler or fryer, breast, with skin, raw	3 oz	146	18	0	0	0	7.9	2.3	54
Chicken, broiler or fryer, breast, with skin, roasted	3 oz	167	25	0	0	0	6.6	1.9	60
Chicken, broiler or fryer, breast, with skin, seasoned, rotisserie	3 oz	156	23	0	0	0	7.0	1.8	295
Chicken, broiler or fryer, breast, with skin, stewed	3 oz	156	23	0	0	0	6.3	1.8	53
Chicken, broiler or fryer, breast, without skin, fried	3 oz	159	28	0	0	0	4.0	1.1	67
Chicken, broiler or fryer, breast, without skin, raw	3 oz	97	18	0	0	0	2.2	0.5	99
Chicken, broiler or fryer, breast, without skin, roasted	3 oz	140	26	0	0	0	3.0	0.9	63
Chicken, broiler or fryer, breast, without skin, season, rotisserie	3 oz	126	25	0	0	0	3.0	0.7	290
Chicken, broiler or fryer, breast, without skin, stewed	3 oz	128	25	0	0	0	2.6	0.7	54
Chicken, broiler or ryer, dark meat, with skin, raw	3 oz	201	14	0	0	0	15.6	4.5	62

POULTRY continued

Item	Serving Size	Calories	Protein	Carb	Fiber	Sugar	Total Fat	Sat Fat	Sodium
Chicken, broiler or fryer, dark meat, with skin, roasted	3 oz	215	22	0	0	0	13.4	3.7	74
Chicken, broiler or fryer, dark meat, with skin, stewed	3 oz	198	20	0	0	0	12.5	3.5	60
Chicken, broiler or fryer, dark meat, without skin, raw	3 oz	106	17	0	0	0	3.7	0.9	72
Chicken, broiler or fryer, dark meat, without skin, roasted	3 oz	174	23	0	0	0	8.3	2.3	79
Chicken, broiler or fryer, dark meat, without skin, stewed	3 oz	163	22	0	0	0	7.6	2.1	63
Chicken, broiler or fryer, drumstick, with skin, raw	3 oz	137	16	0	0	0	7.4	2.0	71
Chicken, broiler or fryer, drumstick, with skin, roasted	3 oz	184	23	0	0	0	9.5	2.6	77
Chicken, broiler or fryer, drumstick, with skin, season rotisserie	3 oz	183	23	0	0	0	10.2	2.6	349
Chicken, broiler or fryer, drumstick, with skin, stewed	3 oz	173	22	0	0	0	9.0	2.5	65
Chicken, broiler or fryer, drumstick, without skin, fried	3 oz	166	24	0	0	0	6.9	1.8	82
Chicken, broiler or fryer, drumstick, without skin, raw	3 oz	101	18	0	0	0	2.9	0.7	75
Chicken, broiler or fryer, drumstick, without skin, roasted	3 oz	146	24	0	0	0	4.8	1.3	81
Chicken, broiler or fryer, drumstick, without skin, seasoned, rotisserie	3 oz	150	24	0	0	0	5.8	1.4	354
Chicken, broiler or fryer, drumstick, without skin, stewed	3 oz	144	23	0	0	0	4.9	1.3	68
Chicken, broiler or fryer, leg, without skin, raw	3 oz	102	17	0	0	0	3.2	0.8	73
Chicken, broiler or fryer, leg, without skin, roasted	3 oz	162	23	0	0	0	7.2	1.9	77
Chicken, broiler or fryer, leg, without skin, stewed	3 oz	157	22	0	0	0	6.9	1.9	66
Chicken, broiler or fryer, whole, without skin, fried	3 oz	186	26	1	0	0	7.8	2.1	77

POULTRY continued

Item	Serving Size	Calories	Protein	Carb	Fiber	Sugar	Total Fat	Sat Fat	Sodium
Chicken, broiler or fryer, wing, without skin, fried	3 oz	179	26	0	0	0	7.8	2.1	77
Chicken, drumstick, extra crispy, without skin & breading, fried	3 oz	145	22	0	0	0	6.3	1.6	447
Chicken, drumstick, original recipe, without skin, fried	3 oz	203	19	5	0	0	12.1	2.8	531
Chicken, light & dark, chunk, with water, canned	2 oz	80	15	0	0	0	2.0	0.5	130
Chicken, light, chunk, premium, with water, canned	2 oz	70	15	0	0	0	1.0	0.0	180
Chicken, popcorn, fried	3 oz	298	15	18	1	0	18.5	3.4	969
Chicken, roasting, whole, with skin, raw	3 oz	184	15	0	0	0	13.5	3.9	58
Chicken, roasting, whole, with skin, roasted	3 oz	190	20	0	0	0	11.4	3.2	62
Chicken, roasting, whole, without skin, roasted	3 oz	142	21	0	0	0	5.6	1.5	64
Chicken, skin, extra crispy, with breading, fried	3 oz	394	9	19	1	0	31.1	6.4	704
Chicken, skin, original recipe, with breading, fried	3 oz	330	11	15	1	0	25.0	5.5	731
Chicken, stewing, dark meat, without skin, raw	3 oz	133	17	0	0	0	6.9	1.8	86
Chicken, stewing, dark meat, without skin, stewed	3 oz	219	24	0	0	0	13.0	3.5	81
Chicken, stewing, light meat, without skin, raw	3 oz	116	20	0	0	0	3.6	0.8	45
Chicken, stewing, light meat, without skin, stewed	3 oz	181	28	0	0	0	6.8	1.7	49
Chicken, stewing, whole, with giblet & neck, stewed	3 oz	182	21	0	0	0	10.1	2.8	57
Chicken, stewing, whole, with skin, raw	3 oz	219	15	0	0	0	17.3	4.9	60
Chicken, stewing, whole, with skin, stewed	3 oz	242	23	0	0	0	16.0	4.3	62
Chicken, stewing, whole, without skin, raw	3 oz	126	18	0	0	0	5.4	1.3	67
Chicken, stewing, whole, without skin, stewed	3 oz	201	26	0	0	0	10.1	2.6	66

POULTRY continued

Item	Serving Size	Calories	Protein	Carb	Fiber	Sugar	Total Fat	Sat Fat	Sodium
Chicken, thigh, extra crispy, without skin or breading, fried	3 oz	152	19	0	0	0	8.5	2.3	474
Chicken, wing, glazed, BBQ flavor, cooked from frozen in oven	3 oz	206	19	3	0	2	12.6	3.4	475
Chicken, wing, glazed, BBQ flavor, frozen	3 oz	179	17	3	1	2	10.8	2.8	523
Chicken, wing, glazed, BBQ flavor, microwaved from frozen	3 oz	211	22	3	1	2	11.8	3.1	711
Chicken, without skin, canned, drained	3 oz	138	23	0	0	0	4.9	1.3	230
Chicken, without skin, with broth, can	3 oz	140	19	0	0	0	6.8	1.9	428
Chicken, without skin, with water, canned	3 oz	110	19	0	0	0	3.9	1.1	213
Lunchmeat, chicken, breast, honey glazed	3 oz	93	17	3	0	3	1.3	0.3	1222
Nuggets, chicken, cooked from frozen	3 oz	252	13	12	2	0	16.8	3.4	473
Nuggets, chicken, frozen	3 oz	235	12	12	2	0	15.4	3.0	360
Turkey, average of back cuts, with skin, raw	3 oz	167	15	0	0	0	11.1	3.1	56
Turkey, average of back cuts, with skin, roasted	3 oz	207	23	0	0	0	12.2	3.6	62
Turkey, average of breast, with skin, raw	3 oz	133	19	0	0	0	6.0	1.6	50
Turkey, average of breast, with skin, roasted	3 oz	161	24	0	0	0	6.3	1.8	54
Turkey, average of dark meat, with skin, raw	3 oz	136	16	0	0	0	7.5	2.2	60
Turkey, average of dark meat, with skin, roasted	3 oz	188	23	0	0	0	9.8	3.0	65
Turkey, average of dark meat, without skin, raw	3 oz	106	17	0	0	0	3.7	1.2	65
Turkey, average of dark meat, without skin, roasted	3 oz	160	24	0	0	0	6.1	1.9	67
Turkey, average of leg, with skin, raw	3 oz	122	17	0	0	0	5.7	1.8	63

POULTRY continued

Item	Serving Size	Calories	Protein	Carb	Fiber	Sugar	Total Fat	Sat Fat	Sodium
Turkey, average of leg, with skin, roasted	3 oz	177	24	0	0	0	8.3	2.6	65
Turkey, average of light meat, with skin, raw	3 oz	135	18	0	0	0	6.3	1.7	50
Turkey, average of light meat, with skin, roasted	3 oz	167	24	0	0	0	7.1	2.0	54
Turkey, average of light meat, without skin, raw	3 oz	98	20	0	0	0	1.3	0.4	54
Turkey, average of light meat, without skin, roasted	3 oz	133	25	0	0	0	2.7	0.9	54
Turkey, average of skin cuts, raw	3 oz	331	11	0	0	0	31.4	8.2	31
Turkey, average of skin cuts, roasted	3 oz	377	17	0	0	0	33.7	8.8	45
Turkey, average of whole, with skin, raw	3 oz	136	17	0	0	0	6.8	1.9	55
Turkey, average of whole, with skin, roasted	3 oz	177	24	0	0	0	8.3	2.4	58
Turkey, average of whole, without skin, raw	3 oz	102	19	0	0	0	2.4	0.8	60
Turkey, average of wing, with skin, raw	3 oz	167	17	0	0	0	10.5	2.8	47
Turkey, average of wing, with skin, roasted	3 oz	195	23	0	0	0	10.6	2.9	52
Turkey, average of wing, without skin, roasted	3 oz	145	25	0	0	0	4.2	1.2	60
Turkey, breast, prebasted, with skin, roasted	3 oz	107	19	0	0	0	2.9	0.8	337
Turkey, breast, smoked, lemon pepper flavor, 97% fat-free sliced	3 oz	81	18	1	0	0	0.6	0.2	986
Turkey, dark meat, with skin, smoked	3 oz	170	24	0	0	0	8.2	2.4	847
Turkey, dark meat, without skin, smoked	3 oz	138	25	0	0	0	4.3	1.2	847
Turkey, drumstick, with skin, smoked	3 oz	170	24	0	0	0	8.3	2.6	847
Turkey, from turkey frames, mechanically deboned, raw	3 oz	171	11	0	0	0	13.6	4.5	41

POULTRY continued

Item	Serving Size	Calories	Protein	Carb	Fiber	Sugar	Total Fat	Sat Fat	Sodium
Turkey, fryer or roaster, back, with skin, raw	3 oz	128	17	0	0	0	6.2	1.8	51
Turkey, fryer or roaster, back, with skin, roasted	3 oz	173	22	0	0	0	8.7	2.5	60
Turkey, fryer or roaster, back, without skin, raw	3 oz	102	18	0	0	0	3.0	1.0	55
Turkey, fryer or roaster, back, without skin, roasted	3 oz	145	24	0	0	0	4.8	1.6	62
Turkey, fryer or roaster, breast, with skin, raw	3 oz	106	20	0	0	0	2.3	0.6	41
Turkey, fryer or roaster, breast, with skin, roasted	3 oz	130	25	0	0	0	2.7	0.7	45
Turkey, fryer or roaster, breast, without skin, raw	3 oz	94	21	0	0	0	0.6	0.2	42
Turkey, fryer or roaster, breast, without skin, roasted	3 oz	115	26	0	0	0	0.6	0.2	44
Turkey, fryer or roaster, dark meat, with skin, raw	3 oz	110	17	0	0	0	4.1	1.2	56
Turkey, fryer or roaster, dark meat, with skin, roasted	3 oz	155	24	0	0	0	6.0	1.8	65
Turkey, fryer or roaster, dark meat, without skin, raw	3 oz	94	17	0	0	0	2.3	0.8	59
Turkey, fryer or roaster, dark meat, without skin, roasted	3 oz	138	25	0	0	0	3.7	1.2	67
Turkey, fryer or roaster, leg, with skin, raw	3 oz	100	17	0	0	0	3.0	0.9	59
Turkey, fryer or roaster, leg, with skin, roasted	3 oz	145	24	0	0	0	4.6	1.4	68
Turkey, fryer or roaster, leg, without skin, raw	3 oz	92	17	0	0	0	2.0	0.7	60
Turkey, fryer or roaster, leg, without skin, roasted	3 oz	135	25	0	0	0	3.2	1.1	69
Turkey, fryer or roaster, light meat, with skin, raw	3 oz	113	20	0	0	0	3.2	0.9	43
Turkey, fryer or roaster, light meat, with skin, roasted	3 oz	139	24	0	0	0	3.9	1.1	48
Turkey, fryer or roaster, light meat, without skin, raw	3 oz	92	21	0	0	0	0.4	0.1	44
Turkey, fryer or roaster, light meat, without skin, roasted	3 oz	119	26	0	0	0	1.0	0.3	48

POULTRY continued

Item	Serving Size	Calories	Protein	Carb	Fiber	Sugar	Total Fat	Sat Fat	Sodium
Turkey, fryer or roaster, whole, with skin, raw	3 oz	114	19	0	0	0	3.6	1.0	49
Turkey, fryer or roaster, whole, with skin, roasted	3 oz	146	24	0	0	0	4.9	1.4	56
Turkey, fryer or roaster, whole, without skin, raw	3 oz	94	19	0	0	0	1.3	0.5	52
Turkey, fryer or roaster, whole, without skin, roasted	3 oz	128	25	0	0	0	2.2	0.7	57
Turkey, fryer or roaster, wing, with skin, raw	3 oz	135	18	0	0	0	6.6	1.8	48
Turkey, fryer or roaster, wing, with skin, roasted	3 oz	176	24	0	0	0	8.4	2.3	62
Turkey, fryer or roaster, wing, without skin, raw	3 oz	90	19	0	0	0	1.0	0.3	55
Turkey, fryer or roaster, wing, without skin, roasted	3 oz	139	26	0	0	0	2.9	0.8	66
Turkey, ground, 8% fat, raw	3 oz	127	15	0	0	0	7.0	1.9	80
Turkey, ground, patty, 13% fat, cooked, raw	3 oz	200	23	0	0	0	11.2	2.9	91
Turkey, ham, dark meat, smoked, frozen	3 oz	100	14	3	0	1	3.4	1.0	773
Turkey, hen, back, with skin, raw	3 oz	185	15	0	0	0	13.5	3.7	52
Turkey, hen, back, with skin, roasted	3 oz	216	22	0	0	0	13.3	3.9	59
Turkey, hen, breast, with skin, raw	3 oz	142	18	0	0	0	7.1	1.9	47
Turkey, hen, breast, with skin, roasted	3 oz	165	24	0	0	0	6.7	1.9	49
Turkey, hen, dark meat, with skin, raw	3 oz	146	16	0	0	0	8.7	2.5	57
Turkey, hen, dark meat, with skin, roasted	3 oz	197	23	0	0	0	10.9	3.3	61
Turkey, hen, dark meat, without skin, raw	3 oz	111	17	0	0	0	4.1	1.4	63
Turkey, hen, dark meat, without skin, roasted	3 oz	163	24	0	0	0	6.6	2.2	64
Turkey, hen, leg, with skin, raw	3 oz	128	17	0	0	0	6.4	1.9	60

POULTRY continued

Item	Serving Size	Calories	Protein	Carb	Fiber	Sugar	Total Fat	Sat Fat	Sodium
Turkey, hen, leg, with skin, roasted	3 oz	181	24	0	0	0	8.9	2.8	62
Turkey, hen, light meat, with skin, raw	3 oz	140	18	0	0	0	6.9	1.9	47
Turkey, hen, light meat, with skin, roasted	3 oz	176	24	0	0	0	8.0	2.3	49
Turkey, hen, light meat, without skin, raw	3 oz	99	20	0	0	0	1.4	0.5	51
Turkey, hen, light meat, without skin, roasted	3 oz	137	25	0	0	0	3.2	1.0	51
Turkey, hen, whole, with skin, raw	3 oz	143	17	0	0	0	7.7	2.2	52
Turkey, hen, whole, with skin, roasted	3 oz	185	24	0	0	0	9.2	2.7	54
Turkey, hen, whole, without skin, raw	3 oz	104	18	0	0	0	2.7	0.9	56
Turkey, hen, whole, without skin, roasted	3 oz	149	25	0	0	0	4.7	1.5	57
Turkey, hen, wing, with skin, raw	3 oz	179	17	0	0	0	11.8	3.1	43
Turkey, hen, wing, with skin, roasted	3 oz	202	23	0	0	0	11.4	3.1	48
Turkey, jerky, hot & spicy	1 oz	70	14	3	0	3	1.0	0.0	480
Turkey, jerky, original	1 oz	80	14	3	0	3	1.0	0.0	550
Turkey, jerky, teriyaki	1 oz	80	14	4	0	4	0.5	0.0	580
Turkey, light meat, with skin, smoked	3 oz	170	24	0	0	0	8.2	2.4	847
Turkey, light meat, without skin, smoked	3 oz	138	25	0	0	0	4.3	1.2	847
Turkey, light, chunk, premium, with water, canned	2 oz	80	16	0	0	0	1.5	0.5	150
Turkey, roast, light & dark meat, seasoned, roasted from frozen, box	3 oz	132	18	3	0	0	4.9	1.6	578
Turkey, taco meat, cooked from frozen	3 oz	126	14	3	0	0	6.4	1.5	537
Turkey, thigh, prebasted, with skin, without bone, roasted	3 oz	133	16	0	0	0	7.3	2.3	371

POULTRY continued

Item	Serving Size	Calories	Protein	Carb	Fiber	Sugar	Total Fat	Sat Fat	Sodium
Turkey, tom, back, with skin, raw	3 oz	152	16	0	0	0	9.5	2.7	60
Turkey, tom, back, with skin, roasted	3 oz	202	23	0	0	0	11.6	3.4	65
Turkey, tom, breast, with skin, raw	3 oz	128	19	0	0	0	5.4	1.5	54
Turkey, tom, breast, with skin, roasted	3 oz	161	24	0	0	0	6.3	1.8	57
Turkey, tom, dark meat, with skin, raw	3 oz	129	16	0	0	0	6.7	2.0	64
Turkey, tom, dark meat, with skin, roasted	3 oz	184	23	0	0	0	9.2	2.8	68
Turkey, tom, dark meat, without skin, raw	3 oz	105	17	0	0	0	3.5	1.2	68
Turkey, tom, dark meat, without skin, roasted	3 oz	157	24	0	0	0	5.9	2.0	70
Turkey, tom, leg, with skin, raw	3 oz	120	17	0	0	0	5.4	1.6	65
Turkey, tom, leg, with skin, roasted	3 oz	175	24	0	0	0	8.2	2.5	68
Turkey, tom, light meat, with skin, raw	3 oz	133	18	0	0	0	6.0	1.6	54
Turkey, tom, light meat, with skin, roasted	3 oz	162	24	0	0	0	6.5	1.8	57
Turkey, tom, light meat, without skin, raw	3 oz	97	20	0	0	0	1.3	0.4	57
Turkey, tom, light meat, without skin, roasted	3 oz	131	25	0	0	0	2.5	0.8	58
Turkey, tom, meat only, without skin, raw	3 oz	99	18	0	0	0	2.3	0.8	62
Turkey, tom, whole, with skin, raw	3 oz	131	17	0	0	0	6.3	1.8	58
Turkey, tom, whole, with skin, roasted	3 oz	172	24	0	0	0	7.7	2.2	61
Turkey, tom, whole, without skin, roasted	3 oz	143	25	0	0	0	4.0	1.3	63
Turkey, tom, wing, with skin, raw	3 oz	160	17	0	0	0	9.5	2.5	51
Turkey, tom, wing, with skin, roasted	3 oz	188	23	0	0	0	9.8	2.7	56
Turkey, with broth, canned	3 oz	144	20	1	0	0	5.8	1.7	397

SEAFOOD

Item	Serving Size	Calories	Protein	Carb	Fiber	Sugar	Total Fat	Sat Fat	Sodium
Calamari, mixed species, raw	3 oz	78	13	3	0	0	1.2	3.5	1275
Clams, cooked	3 oz	110	17	6	0	0	1.5	0.0	330
Clams, mixed species, canned, drained	3 oz	126	22	4	0	0	1.7	0.1	48
Clams, mixed species, raw	3 oz	63	11	2	0	0	0.8	0.1	48
Conchs, baked/broiled	3 oz	111	22	1	0	0	1.0	0.2	715
Crabs, Alaska king, imitation	3 oz	81	6	13	0	5	0.4	0.1	711
Crabs, Alaska king, leg, raw	3 oz	71	16	0	0	0	0.5	0.1	911
Crabs, Alaska king, leg, steamed	3 oz	82	16	0	0	0	1.3	0.1	911
Crabs, blue, canned, drained	3 oz	84	17	0	0	0	1.0	0.2	249
Crabs, blue, cooked	3 oz	100	20	0	0	0	1.0	2.0	40
Crabs, blue, steamed, flaked pieces	3 oz	87	17	0	0	0	1.5	0.1	251
Crabs, Dungeness, meat	3 oz	80	18	0	0	0	1.0	1.5	270
Crabs, queen, raw	3 oz	77	16	0	0	0	1.0	0.2	587
Crabs, queen, steamed	3 oz	98	20	0	0	0	1.3	0.1	53
Crayfish, farmed, mixed species, raw	3 oz	61	13	0	0	0	0.8	0.2	82
Crayfish, farmed, mixed species, steamed	3 oz	74	15	0	0	0	1.1	0.1	49
Crayfish, wild, mixed species, raw	3 oz	65	14	0	0	0	0.8	0.2	80
Crayfish, wild, mixed species, steamed	3 oz	70	14	0	0	0	1.0	0.1	316
Escargot, raw	3 oz	77	14	2	0	0	1.2	1.9	3118
Escargot, steamed/poached	3 oz	233	41	13	0	7	0.7	6.1	3783
Jellyfish, dried, with salt	3 oz	31	5	0	0	0	1.2	0.0	183
Jellyfish, pickled	3 oz	31	5	0	0	0	1.2	0.4	391
Lobster, cooked	3 oz	80	17	1	0	0	0.5	1.0	300
Lobster, Northern, raw	3 oz	77	16	0	0	0	0.8	0.1	323
Lobster, Northern, steamed	3 oz	83	17	1	0	0	0.5	0.2	150
Mussels, blue, raw	3 oz	73	10	3	0	0	1.9	0.4	243
Mussels, blue, steamed	3 oz	146	20	6	0	0	3.8	0.2	196
Mussels, smoked, with oil, canned, drained	3 oz	166	18	4	0	0	8.8	0.3	48

SEAFOOD continued

Item	Serving Size	Calories	Protein	Carb	Fiber	Sugar	Total Fat	Sat Fat	Sodium
Octopus, raw	3 oz	70	13	2	0	0	0.9	0.4	391
Octopus, steamed	3 oz	139	25	4	0	0	1.8	0.4	391
Oysters, Eastern, canned, drained	3 oz	59	6	3	0	0	2.1	0.6	139
Oysters, Eastern, canned, with liquid	3 oz	59	6	3	0	0	2.1	0.5	207
Oysters, Eastern, wild, raw	3 oz	58	6	3	0	0	2.1	0.7	179
Oysters, Pacific, steamed	3 oz	139	16	8	0	0	3.9	0.2	190
Prawns, mixed species, steamed	3 oz	84	18	0	0	0	0.9	3.5	1275
Roe, black/red, granular	3 oz	214	21	3	0	0	15.2	1.6	99
Scallops, cooked	3 oz	140	27	5	0	0	1.0	0.0	310
Scallops, mixed species, raw	3 oz	75	14	2	0	0	0.6	0.1	137
Sea lion, Steller, fat, Alaskan	3 oz	723	1	0	0	0	79.9	0.3	196
Sea lion, Steller, liver, Alaskan	3 oz	116	19	0	0	0	4.3	2.5	68
Shrimp, cooked	3 oz	100	21	0	0	0	1.5	0.0	360
Shrimp, mixed species, canned, drained	3 oz	85	17	0	0	0	1.2	0.2	660
Shrimp, mixed species, raw	3 oz	90	17	1	0	0	1.5	0.3	126
Shrimp, mixed species, steamed	3 oz	84	18	0	0	0	0.9	0.3	60
Snails, raw	3 oz	77	14	2	0	0	1.2	1.6	260
Snails, steamed/poached	3 oz	233	41	13	0	7	0.7	0.9	76
Squid, mixed species, raw	3 oz	78	13	3	0	0	1.2	0.0	175

SNACKS

Item	Serving Size	Calories	Protein	Carb	Fiber	Sugar	Total Fat	Sat Fat	Sodium
Bagel chips	1 oz	128	3	19	1	2	4.3	1.9	66
Bagel chips, cinnamon raisin	1 oz	130	2	17	1	7	6.0	2.5	80
Bagel chips, everything	1 oz	130	3	15	1	1	7.0	2.5	300
Bagel chips, garlic	1 oz	130	3	16	1	1	6.0	2.5	200
Bagel chips, jalapeño cheddar	1 oz	130	3	17	1	1	6.0	2.5	370

SNACKS continued

Item	Serving Size	Calories	Protein	Carb	Fiber	Sugar	Total Fat	Sat Fat	Sodium
Bagel chips, multigrain, natural	1 oz	130	4	17	2	2	6.0	2.5	180
Bagel chips, plain	1 oz	140	3	17	1	1	6.0	3.0	70
Bagel chips, ranch	1 oz	130	3	17	1	1	6.0	2.5	320
Bagel chips, sea salt	1 oz	130	3	16	1	1	6.0	2.5	310
Bagel chips, sesame	1 oz	140	3	15	1	1	7.0	2.5	290
Bagel chips, Simply Naked	1 oz	130	3	20	1	2	3.5	0.5	270
Bagel chips, toasted garlic	1 oz	130	3	20	2	2	3.5	0.5	260
Bagel chips, whole wheat	1 oz	130	4	19	2	2	4.0	0.5	260
Bagel chips, whole wheat, natural	1 oz	120	4	16	2	1	6.0	2.5	180
Baguette, with cheese dip, snack	1 oz	75	3	5	0	2	4.5	2.5	290
Baked snacks, cheddar	1 oz	130	2	21	1	1	4.5	1.0	240
Baked snacks, original	1 oz	140	2	22	1	2	4.5	1.0	200
Baked snacks, ranch	1 oz	140	2	21	1	1	5.0	1.0	170
Baked snacks, sour cream & onion	1 oz	140	2	21	1	0	5.0	1.5	190
Bread chips, rosemary & olive oil	1 oz	140	4	19	0	2	5.0	1.0	300
Bread crisps, bruschetta	1 oz	110	3	17	2	1	3.0	0.5	330
Breadsticks, with cheese dip, snack	1 oz	110	3	14	0	4	4.5	1.0	340
Bugles, nacho cheese	1 oz	160	1	18	0	1	9.0	7.0	330
Bugles, original	1 oz	160	1	18	1	1	9.0	8.0	310
Cheese twists	1 oz	160	2	15	1	1	10.5	1.6	258
Corn & potato snack, Flamin' Hot Fries, Frito-Lay	1 oz	150	2	17	1	1	8.0	1.5	270
Corn chips, BBQ	1 oz	150	2	16	1	1	10.0	1.5	280
Corn chips, blue, baked	1 oz	110	3	22	2	0	2.0	0.0	160
Corn chips, blue, whole grain	1 oz	140	2	18	2	0	7.0	0.5	60
Corn chips, chili cheese	1 oz	160	2	15	1	1	10.0	1.5	260
Corn chips, honey BBQ, Flavor Twists	1 oz	160	2	16	1	1	10.0	1.5	210
Corn chips, onion flavor, extruded	1 oz	141	2	18	1	1	6.4	1.2	278
Corn chips, plain, extruded	1 oz	147	2	18	2	0	8.1	1.0	175

SNACKS continued

Item	Serving Size	Calories	Protein	Carb	Fiber	Sugar	Total Fat	Sat Fat	Sodium
Corn chips, Scoops	1 oz	160	2	16	1	0	10.0	1.5	110
Corn chips, shrimp, artificially flavored	1 oz	140	1	19	1	0	8.0	1.5	220
Corn chips, unsalted, extruded	1 oz	158	2	16	1	0	9.5	1.2	4
Corn chips, unsalted, extruded, crushed	1 oz	158	2	16	1	0	9.5	1.2	4
Corn chips, Wild 'n' Mild Ranch, Fritos	1 oz	160	2	15	1	1	11.0	1.5	210
Corn Nuts, chili picante flavor	1 oz	130	2	19	2	0	4.5	0.5	290
Corn Nuts, nacho cheese flavor	1 oz	130	3	19	2	0	5.0	1.0	240
Corn Nuts, original	1 oz	126	2	20	2	0	4.4	0.7	156
Corn Nuts, ranch flavor	1 oz	130	3	19	2	0	5.0	1.0	240
Corn snack, Fruity Booty, Pirate's Booty	1 oz	130	2	19	0	0	5.0	0.5	0
Corn snack, spicy	1 oz	130	2	21	1	0	4.0	0.5	310
Corn snack, sunflower butter	1 oz	130	4	16	2	2	7.0	1.0	140
Corn snack, super veggie	1 oz	150	2	18	0	0	7.0	1.0	140
Corn snack, Veggie Booty, Pitrate's Booty	1 oz	140	2	17	0	0	6.0	0.5	130
Corn snack, with caramel	1 oz	120	1	23	1	12	2.0	0.0	90
Fruit crisps, apple cinnamon grove, baked	1 oz	130	1	21	2	6	4.5	1.0	35
Fruit crisps, peach mango paradise, baked	1 oz	130	1	21	1	7	4.5	1.0	35
Fruit crisps, wild berry patch, baked	1 oz	130	1	21	1	6	4.5	1.0	40
Fruit Leather, apple	1/2 oz	45	0	12	0.86	11.14	0	0	5
Fruit Leather, Chunky Cherry, Stretch Island	1/2 oz	45	0	12	1	11	0	0	0
Fruit Leather, grape, Stretch Island	1/2 oz	45	0	12	1	11	0	0	5
Fruit Leather, Great Grape, Stretch Island	1/2 oz	45	0	12	1	11	0	0	0
Fruit Leather, Mucho Mango, Stretch Island	1/2 oz	45	0	11	1	9	0	0	0

SNACKS continued

Item	Serving Size	Calories	Protein	Carb	Fiber	Sugar	Total Fat	Sat Fat	Sodium
Fruit Leather, Rare Raspberry, Stretch Island	1/2 oz	45	0	12	0.9	11.1	0	0	0
Fruit Leather, Strawberry, Stretch Island	1/2 oz	45	0	11	1	8	0	0	0
Fruit Leather, Tangy Apricot, Stretch Island	1/2 oz	45	0	11	1	7	0	0	0
Fruit Leather, Wild Apple, Stretch Island	1/2 oz	45	0	12	1	9	0	0	0
Fruit Snacks, Batman, Fruit Roll-Up	1 oz	80	0	21	0	14	0	0	20
Fruit Snacks, Finding Nemo, Kellogg's	1 oz	80	0	21	0	14	0	0	20
Fruit Snacks, Princess, Kellogg's	1 oz	80	0	21	0	14	0	0	20
Fruit Snacks, Rainbow Rush, Kellogg's	1 oz	80	1	17	0	10	1	0	80
Fruit Snacks, Right Bites, Kellogg's	1 oz	100	0	24	0	16	0	0	25
Fruit Snacks, Strawberry Fusion, Kellogg's	1 oz	80	1	17	0	10	1	0	80
Fruit Snacks, Triple Berry Twist, Kellogg's	1 oz	80	1	17	0	10	0.5	0	55
Fruit Snacks, Wild Berry Mania, Kellogg's	1 oz	80	1	17	0	10	1	0	80
Fruit Snacks, Wild Strawberry, Kellogg's	1 oz	80	1	17	0	10	0.5	0	55
Granola bites, chocolate	1 pouch	90	2	14	2	6	3.5	2.0	30
Granola bites, cinnamon	1 pouch	90	1	14	2	7	3.5	2.0	30
Granola bites, peanut butter	1 pouch	90	2	14	2	6	3.5	2.5	40
Multigrain snack, cinnamon sugar	1/2 oz	60	1	12	1	3	1.0	0.0	90
Multigrain snack, cinnamon toast	1/2 oz	50	1	12	1	3	1.0	0.0	85
Multigrain snack, French onion	1 oz	141	2	19	2	3	6.3	0.7	132
Multigrain snack, garden salsa	1 oz	140	2	19	2	2	6.0	0.9	160

SNACKS continued

Item	Serving Size	Calories	Protein	Carb	Fiber	Sugar	Total Fat	Sat Fat	Sodium
Multigrain snack, harvest cheddar	1 oz	139	2	18	2	2	6.3	0.8	153
Multigrain snack, harvest cheddar bites, 100-calorie pack	1	100	2	13	1	1	4.0	0.4	110
Multigrain snack, honey graham	1/2 oz	60	1	12	1	3	1.0	0.0	90
Pita chips, cinnamon sugar	1 oz	140	3	20	2	6	5.0	0.5	115
Pita chips, garlic & herb	1 oz	130	3	19	0	1	4.5	0.0	350
Pita chips, multigrain	1 oz	140	3	19	2	1	6.0	0.5	240
Pita chips, original	1 oz	130	2	19	0	1	4.5	0.0	310
Pita chips, parmesan garlic & herb	1 oz	140	4	19	2	1	5.0	0.5	200
Pita chips, pesto & sundried tomato	1 oz	130	3	19	2	1	5.0	0.5	250
Pita chips, salted	1 oz	130	3	19	1	1	4.3	0.4	242
Pita chips, Simply Naked	1 oz	130	3	19	2	1	5.0	0.5	270
Pita chips, Texarkana hot, Stacy's	1 oz	130	3	19	2	1	5.0	0.5	260
Pita chips, whole wheat	1 oz	130	4	17	2	0	5.0	0.0	310
Plantain chips	1 oz	150	1	17	2	0	9.0	1.0	35
Popcorn, air-popped	1 oz	110	4	22	4	0	1.3	0.2	2
Popcorn, butter	1 oz	190	3	14	4	0	13.0	1.0	140
Popcorn, butter flavor, microwaved	1 oz	149	2	16	3	0	8.5	2.0	219
Popcorn, butter flavor, with palm oil, microwaved	1 oz	150	2	16	3	0	8.5	1.8	219
Popcorn, caramel coated, original	1 oz	120	2	23	1	15	2.0	0.0	70
Popcorn, caramel coated, with peanuts	1 oz	113	2	23	1	13	2.2	0.3	84
Popcorn, caramel coated, without peanuts	1 oz	122	1	22	1	15	3.6	1.0	58
Popcorn, caramel corn	1 oz	130	1	24	1	16	3.5	1.5	50
Popcorn, caramel corn, fat-free	1 oz	112	1	27	2	16	0.0	0.0	150
Popcorn, caramel corn, with peanuts	1 oz	140	1	24	1	16	4.0	1.5	50
Popcorn, kettle korn	1 oz	80	1	10	1	4	4.5	0.5	30

SNACKS continued

Item	Serving Size	Calories	Protein	Carb	Fiber	Sugar	Total Fat	Sat Fat	Sodium
Popcorn, low fat, low sodium, microwaved	1 oz	122	4	21	4	0	2.7	0.4	139
Popcorn, low fat, microwaved	1 oz	120	4	20	4	0	2.7	0.4	251
Popcorn, low salt	1 oz	140	4	18	6	0	6.0	0.5	20
Popcorn, oil popped, microwaved	1 oz	165	2	13	2	0	12.3	1.9	300
Popcorn, sugar syrup/ caramel, fat-free	1 oz	108	1	26	1	18	0.4	0.1	81
Popcorn, unpopped	1 oz	106	3	21	4	0	1.2	0.2	2
Popcorn, white cheddar	1 oz	110	4	15	3	0	8.0	1.5	240
Pork Skins, chile limon, fried	1/2 oz	70	9	0	0	0	4.5	1.5	320
Pork Skins, cracklins, hot 'n' spicy, tender style, fried	1/2 oz	80	7	0	0	0	5.0	2.0	330
Pork Skins, cracklins, traditional, tender style, fried	1/2 oz	90	7	0	0	0	6.0	2.0	550
Pork Skins, fried, regular cracklins	1/2 oz	90	7	0	0	0	6.0	2.0	550
Pork Skins, hot 'n' spicy, fried	1/2 oz	80	7	0	0	0	5.0	2.0	470
Pork Skins, traditional, fried	1/2 oz	80	7	0	0	0	5.0	2.5	310
Potato Chip Crisps, 100-Calorie pack	1	100	1	13	1	0	6.0	1.5	110
Potato Chip Crisps, barbecue	1 oz	150	2	15	1	1	11.0	2.5	200
Potato Chip Crisps, chili cheese	1 oz	160	1	15	1	1	11.0	3.0	230
Potato Chip Crisps, Fiery Hot, Pringles	1 oz	160	2	15	1	1	10.0	1.5	135
Potato Chip Crisps, jalapeño	1 oz	160	1	14	0	0	11.0	3.0	190
Potato Chip Crisps, Pizzalicious, Pringles	1 oz	160	1	14	1	0	11.0	3.0	200
Potato Chip Crisps, Prints, Pringles	1 oz	160	1	15	1	0	11.0	3.0	170
Potato Chip Crisps, ranch	1 oz	160	1	13	1	1	11.0	3.0	190

SNACKS continued

Item	Serving Size	Calories	Protein	Carb	Fiber	Sugar	Total Fat	Sat Fat	Sodium
Potato Chip Crisps, salt & vinegar	1 oz	160	1	15	1	1	11.0	3.0	200
Potato Chip Crisps, sour cream & onion, fat-free	1 oz	70	2	15	2	0	0.0	0.0	190
Potato Chip Crisps, sour cream & onion, reduced fat	1 oz	140	2	18	1	1	7.0	2.0	140
Potato Chip Crisps, spicy Cajun	1 oz	160	1	14	1	1	11.0	3.0	200
Potato Chip Crisps, sweet mesquite BBQ	1 oz	150	2	15	1	1	10.0	2.5	200
Potato Chip Crisps, white cheddar	1 oz	160	2	15	0	0	10.0	3.0	180
Potato chips	1 oz	150	2	14	1	0	10.0	1.5	190
Potato chips, aged white cheddar, baked	1 oz	120	3	20	2	1	3.0	0.5	170
Potato chips, alder smoked	1 oz	140	2	15	1	1	8.0	2.0	200
Potato chips, Antique 1895, Robert's American Gourmet	1 oz	150	2	16	1	0	8.0	1.0	100
Potato chips, au gratin	1 oz	150	2	14	1	1	10.0	1.0	200
Potato chips, backyard BBQ	1 oz	150	2	15	2	1	9.0	1.0	170
Potato chips, baked	1 oz	133	1	20	1	1	5.2	0.7	260
Potato chips, BBQ	1 oz	130	3	19	2	1	5.0	0.5	90
Potato chips, BBQ, country	1 oz	140	2	16	1	1	9.0	2.5	290
Potato chips, BBQ, honey, reduced fat	1 oz	140	2	20	1	1	6.0	0.0	250
Potato chips, BBQ, mesquite, fat-free, Wow!	1 oz	75	2	17	1	1	0.0	0.0	250
Potato chips, BBQ, mesquite, kettle	1 oz	140	2	17	1	1	8.0	1.5	390
Potato chips, Blues	1 oz	140	3	17	1	1	6.0	1.0	110
Potato chips, Buffalo bleu	1 oz	150	2	16	2	1	9.0	1.0	150
Potato chips, cheddar	1 oz	150	1	15	1	1	10.0	2.5	190
Potato chips, cheddar & sour cream, baked	1 oz	120	2	21	2	3	3.5	1.0	210
Potato chips, cheddar & sour cream, light	1 oz	75	3	16	1	1	0.0	0.0	230
Potato chips, cheddar & sour cream, reduced fat	1 oz	140	2	17	1	0	7.0	0.5	240

SNACKS continued

Item	Serving Size	Calories	Protein	Carb	Fiber	Sugar	Total Fat	Sat Fat	Sodium
Potato chips, cheddar beer	1 oz	150	2	16	1	1	9.0	1.0	200
Potato chips, cheese & jalapeño, reduced fat	1 oz	150	2	17	1	1	8.0	1.5	350
Potato chips, chile limon	1 oz	150	2	14	1	0	10.0	3.0	210
Potato chips, chipotle chili BBQ	1 oz	150	2	16	2	1	9.0	1.0	150
Potato chips, cooked with olive oil, Red Bliss	1 oz	140	1	18	2	0	7.0	1.0	110
Potato chips, classic	1 oz	150	2	15	1	0	10.0	1.0	180
Potato chips, classic BBQ	1 oz	150	2	15	2	1	9.0	1.0	170
Potato chips, classic, with sea salt	1 oz	150	2	15	1	0	9.0	1.0	180
Potato chips, Coney Island, Snyder's of Hanover	1 oz	140	2	18	1	0	7.0	1.0	180
Potato chips, cracked peppercorn	1 oz	140	2	18	1	0	8.0	1.0	220
Potato chips, crème fraîche & dill flavor, Blues	1 oz	140	1	17	1	1	6.0		110
Potato chips, Death Valley chipotle, Kettle Chips	1 oz	150	2	16	2	0	9.0	1.0	170
Potato chips, dill & sour cream	1 oz	150	3	16	1	1	9.0	1.0	170
Potato chips, dill pickle	1 oz	160	2	13	1	1	10.0	1.0	360
Potato chips, from white potato skins	1 oz	158	2	14	1	2	10.9	2.7	186
Potato chips, fat-free	1 oz	107	3	24	2	1	0.2	0.0	182
Potato chips, fat free, from dried potatoes, with Olestra	1 oz	72	1	16	2	0	0.3	0.1	122
Potato chips, fat-free, with Olestra	1 oz	78	2	18	2	0	0.2	0.1	157
Potato chips, flamin' hot, Lay's	1 oz	160	2	15	1	1	10.0	1.0	330
Potato chips, garlic parmesan	1 oz	140	2	16	1	2	8.0	1.0	160
Potato chips, habanero	1 oz	140	2	17	2	1	7.0	1.0	260
Potato chips, hickory BBQ	1 oz	150	2	16	1	1	9.0	1.0	210
Potato chips, hickory honey BBQ, baked	1 oz	120	3	21	2	1	3.0	0.5	160

SNACKS continued

Item	Serving Size	Calories	Protein	Carb	Fiber	Sugar	Total Fat	Sat Fat	Sodium
Potato chips, honey dijon	1 oz	150	2	16	1	2	9.0	1.0	160
Potato chips, hot 'n' spicy BBQ	1 oz	150	1	15	1	2	9.0	2.5	190
Potato chips, island jerk	1 oz	150	2	16	2	1	9.0	1.0	150
Potato chips, Italian rosemary & herb	1 oz	160	2	15	1	1	10.0	1.0	200
Potato chips, jalapeño	1 oz	140	2	15	1	0	9.0	1.5	130
Potato chips, KC Masterpiece BBQ, Lay's	1 oz	150	2	16	1	1	10.0	2.5	190
Potato chips, KC Masterpiece BBQ, Lay's, baked	1 oz	120	2	22	2	2	3.0	0.0	210
Potato chips, KC Masterpiece BBQ, Lay's, hot 'n' spicy	1 oz	150	2	15	1	2	10.0	1.0	200
Potato chips, ketchup	1 oz	140	2	15	1	1	9.0	1.5	220
Potato chips, lightly salted	1 oz	150	2	15	1	0	10.0	1.0	90
Potato chips, lightly salted, baked	1 oz	120	3	21	2	0	3.0	0.5	115
Potato chips, lightly salted, baked, 100-Calorie pack	1	100	3	21	2	0	3.0	0.5	115
Potato chips, lightly salted, kettle	1 oz	140	2	17	1	0	8.0	1.5	80
Potato chips, lime & cracked black pepper, Sensations, Lay's	1 oz	150	2	17	1	1	9.0	1.0	300
Potato chips, limon	1 oz	150	2	15	1	0	10.0	1.0	370
Potato chips, Maui onion	1 oz	150	2	16	1	1	9.0	2.4	200
Potato chips, mesquite BBQ	1 oz	140	1	15	1	2	8.0	2.0	370
Potato chips, New York cheddar, with herbs	1 oz	150	3	16	1	1	9.0	1.0	150
Potato chips, olive oil & fine herb, Red Bliss	1 oz	140	2	18	3	1	7.0	1.0	70
Potato chips, olive oil, dried tomato & vinegar, Red Bliss	1 oz	140	2	18	3	1	7.0	1.0	85
Potato chips, olive oil, garlic, & parmesan, Red Bliss	1 oz	140	2	16	2	2	7.0	1.0	115
Potato chips, original	1 oz	140	2	15	1	0	9.0	1.5	70
Potato chips, original, baked	1 oz	120	2	21	2	2	3.0	0.0	200

SNACKS continued

Item	Serving Size	Calories	Protein	Carb	Fiber	Sugar	Total Fat	Sat Fat	Sodium
Potato chips, original, light	1 oz	70	2	17	1	0	0.0	0.0	190
Potato chips, original, with Olestra	1 oz	75	2	17	1	0	0.0	0.0	200
Potato chips, Parmesan & garlic	1 oz	140	2	15	1	0	8.0	1.0	180
Potato chips, Potpourri	1 oz	140	2	17	4	2	7.0	1.0	110
Potato chips, reduced fat	1 oz	140	2	18	1	0	7.0	1.0	180
Potato chips, reduced fat, lightly salted	1 oz	130	2	17	1	0	6.0	0.0	110
Potato chips, reduced fat, unsalted	1 oz	138	2	19	2	0	5.9	1.2	2
Potato chips, ripple	1 oz	150	2	15	1	0	10.0	1.0	180
Potato chips, ripple, reduced fat	1 oz	140	2	17	1	0	6.7	0.5	110
Potato chips, salt & fresh ground pepper	1 oz	150	2	16	2	0	9.0	1.0	180
Potato chips, salt & pepper	1 oz	130	2	19	1	1	5.0	0.5	120
Potato chips, salt & vinegar, reduced fat	1 oz	130	2	17	1	0	6.0	0.0	240
Potato chips, sea salt & black pepper	1 oz	150	2	16	2	0	9.0	1.0	200
Potato chips, sea salt & vinegar	1 oz	140	2	17	1	1	7.0	1.0	260
Potato chips, sea salted, reduced fat, natural	1 oz	140	2	17	1	0	7.0	0.5	160
Potato chips, sour cream & onion, baked	1 oz	120	2	21	2	3	3.0	0.0	210
Potato chips, sour cream onion & chive	1 oz	150	2	16	1	1	9.0	1.0	115
Potato chips, spicy Thai	1 oz	150	2	16	1	2	9.0	1.0	180
Potato chips, Tuscan three-cheese	1 oz	150	2	16	1	1	9.0	1.0	150
Potato chips, unsalted	1 oz	150	2	15	1	0	10.0	1.0	20
Potato chips, wasabi	1 oz	140	2	15	1	1	9.0	1.5	220
Potato chips, yogurt & green onion, reduced fat	1 oz	130	2	17	1	0	6.0	0.0	140
Potato chips, yogurt green onion	1 oz	150	3	16	1	0	9.0	1.0	170

SNACKS continued

Item	Serving Size	Calories	Protein	Carb	Fiber	Sugar	Total Fat	Sat Fat	Sodium
Potato chips, zesty dill pickle	1 oz	140	2	15	1	1	8.0	1.5	280
Potato crisps	1 oz	160	1	16	1	0	10.0	1.5	230
Potato crisps, original, fat-free	1 oz	70	2	15	2	0	0.0	0.0	160
Pretzels, bagel shaped, fat-free	1 oz	110	3	22	1	1	0.0	0.0	260
Pretzels, hard	1 oz	108	3	23	1	1	0.7	0.1	385
Pretzels, hard, unsalted, with enriched flour	1 oz	108	3	22	1	1	1.0	0.2	82
Pretzels, soft	1 oz	96	2	20	0	0	0.9	0.2	398
Pretzels, soft, unsalted	1 oz	96	2	20	0	0	0.9	0.2	196
Pretzels, sticks, cheddar, baked	1 oz	140	0	10	1	1	7.0	1.0	230
Pretzels, sticks, classic style	1 oz	100	2	23	1	1	0.0	0.0	460
Pretzels, sticks, honey mustard & onion	1 oz	140	2	19	1	2	6.0	1.0	120
Pretzels, tiny twists, cheddar	1 oz	110	3	22	1	1	1.0	0.0	370
Puffs, cheddar cheese	1 oz	180	3	13	2	3	13.0	3.0	270
Puffs, cheddar jalapeño, crunchy	1 oz	170	2	15	1	0	11.0	1.5	250
Puffs, cheese	1 oz	160	2	19	0	1	8.0	4.0	250
Puffs, cheese, crunchy, Cheetos	1 oz	160	2	15	1	1	10.0	2.0	290
Puffs, cheese, crunchy, baked, Cheetos	1 oz	130	2	19	0	1	5.0	1.0	240
Puffs, cheese, crunchy, twisted, Cheetos	1 oz	150	2	17	1	1	8.0	1.5	270
Puffs, cheese, flamin' hot limon, crunchy, Cheetos	1 oz	160	1	15	1	0	11.0	2.0	190
Puffs, cheese, flamin' hot, crunchy, Cheetos	1 oz	170	2	15	1	0	11.0	1.5	250
Puffs, cheese, flamin' hot, crunchy, baked, Cheetos	1 oz	130	3	19	1	1	5.0	0.5	240
Puffs, cheese, flamin' hot, jumbo, Cheetos	1 oz	150	1	14	1	0	10.0	1.5	300
Puffs, cheese, jalapeño	1 oz	160	2	19	0	1	8.0	4.0	250
Puffs, cheese, jumbo	1 oz	160	2	13	0	1	10.0	2.0	350

SNACKS continued

Item	Serving Size	Calories	Protein	Carb	Fiber	Sugar	Total Fat	Sat Fat	Sodium
Puffs, cheese, original	1 oz	150	2	16	0	0	10.0	1.5	130
Puffs, cheese, original, baked	1 oz	160	2	13	0	1	11.0	2.0	190
Puffs, cheese, twisted	1 oz	160	2	13	0	1	10.0	1.5	350
Puffs, cheese, white cheddar, natural	1 oz	150	2	16	1	1	9.0	1.5	290
Puffs, corn, butter	1 oz	140	2	23	1	1	4.5	0.5	270
Puffs, corn, cheddar cheese	1 oz	130	2	18	1	0	5.0	1.0	150
Puffs, corn, cheese, with twists	1 oz	160	2	15	1	1	10.5	1.6	258
Puffs, corn, cheese, with twists, low fat	1 oz	122	2	21	3	2	3.4	0.6	364
Puffs, corn, cheese, with twists, unenriched	1 oz	158	2	15	1	1	10.1	1.6	254
Puffs, corn, white cheddar	1 oz	140	3	22	1	1	4.5	0.5	340
Puffs, corn, white cheddar, Smart Puffs, Robert's American Gourmet	1 oz	130	2	17	2	1	6.0	1.0	150
Puffs, white cheddar cheese	1 oz	180	3	13	2	3	13.0	3.0	270
Puffs, white cheddar cheese, baked	1 oz	160	2	13	0	1	11.0	2.0	190
Rice cake, apple cinnamon	1/2 oz	50	1	11	0	3	0.0	0.0	0
Rice cake, brown	1 oz	107	2	24	1	0	0.7	0.2	82
Rice cake, brown rice & buckwheat, unsalted	1 oz	108	3	23	1	0	1.0	0.2	1
Rice cake, brown rice & corn	1 oz	109	2	23	1	0	0.9	0.2	82
Rice cake, brown rice & multigrain	1 oz	110	2	23	1	0	1.0	0.2	71
Rice cake, brown rice & multigrain, unsalted	1 oz	110	2	23	1	0	1.0	0.2	1
Rice cake, brown rice, plain	1 oz	110	2	23	1	0	0.8	0.2	92
Rice cake, brown rice, plain, unsalted	1 oz	110	2	23	1	0	0.8	0.2	7
Rice cake, caramel corn	1/2 oz	60	1	13	0	4	0.0	0.0	150
Rice cake, cheddar cheese	1/2 oz	70	1	11	0	0	2.5	0.0	230
Rice cake, chocolate	1/2 oz	60	1	13	0	4	1.0	0.0	45

SNACKS continued

Item	Serving Size	Calories	Protein	Carb	Fiber	Sugar	Total Fat	Sat Fat	Sodium
Rice cake, chocolate crunch	1/2 oz	60	1	12	0	4	1.0	0.0	35
Rice cake, Cracker Jack butter toffee	1/2 oz	60	1	13	0	4	0.5	0.0	70
Rice cake, double sesame	1/2 oz	50	1	10	0	1	0.0	0.0	85
Rice cake, garlic sesame	1/2 oz	50	1	10	0	0	0.0	0.0	85
Rice cake, kettle corn	1/2 oz	60	1	13	0	4	0.5	0.0	120
Rice cake, maple brown sugar	1/2 oz	50	1	12	1	3	1.0	0.0	85
Rice cake, multigrain	1 oz	102	2	23	2	0	0.6	0.1	35
Rice cake, nacho cheese	1/2 oz	70	1	11	0	1	2.5	0.0	200
Rice cake, peanut butter chocolate chip	1/2 oz	60	1	12	0	4	1.0	0.0	70
Rice cake, salted	1 oz	109	2	24	1	0	0.7	0.2	82
Rice cake, sesame	1 oz	99	2	23	2	0	0.7	0.2	95
Rice cake, sesame tamari	1 oz	107	2	22	2	0	0.9	0.2	172
Rice cake, sweet, honey nut	1 oz	106	2	24	1	2	0.7	0.2	3
Rice cake, tamari sesame	1 oz	99	2	22	2	0	0.9	0.2	172
Rice cake, teriyaki sesame	1/2 oz	50	1	10	0	1	0.0	0.0	45
Rice cake, toasted sesame	1 oz	107	2	23	2	0	0.7	0.2	95
Rice chips, original	1 oz	120	4	22	2	0	3.0	0.0	146
Rice chips, pico de gallo	1 oz	140	2	18	1	0	7.0	0.5	230
Rice chips, Santa Fe BBQ	1 oz	140	2	18	1	0	7.0	0.5	110
Rice chips, sea salt	1 oz	140	2	18	1	0	7.0	0.5	110
Rice chips, sesame seaweed	1 oz	140	2	18	1	0	7.0	0.5	90
Rice chips, with balsamic vinegar & sea salt	1 oz	110	2	22	2	0	2.5	0.0	250
Rice chips, with pesto & Parmesan	1 oz	110	2	22	2	0	2.5	0.0	250
Rye chips, roasted garlic	1 oz	160	2	16	1	1	10.0	2.0	340
Snack mix, bagel chips	1 oz	110	3	16	1	1	4.5	2.0	450
Snack mix, bold party blend	1 oz	140	3	20	1	2	6.0	1.0	390
Snack mix, camper's	1 oz	130	3	16	2	11	3.0	1.5	50
Snack mix, caramel crunch, sweet 'n' salty	1 oz	130	2	23	1	5	3.5	0.5	250

SNACKS continued

Item	Serving Size	Calories	Protein	Carb	Fiber	Sugar	Total Fat	Sat Fat	Sodium
Snack mix, cheddar	1 oz	130	2	22	1	2	4.0	1.0	330
Snack mix, cheddar, baked	1 oz	130	2	19	1	3	4.5	1.0	230
Snack mix, cheddar	1 pouch	100	2	18	1	2	2.5	0.5	320
Snack mix, Cheerios, cheddar	1 oz	120	3	21	1	2	3.0	0.5	310
Snack mix, Cheerios, original	1 oz	110	3	20	1	2	3.0	0.5	300
Snack mix, cheese fix, Munchies	1 oz	140	2	18	1	1	7.0	1.0	250
Snack mix, Chex	1 oz	120	3	21	1	1	2.8	0.4	341
Snack mix, chocolate carame	1 pouch	100	1	17	0	6	3.5	1.0	190
Snack mix, cinnamon crunch	1 oz	130	2	20	2	6	5.0	1.0	80
Snack mix, corn, wheat-free, Chaos	1 oz	140	2	18	2	1	6.0	1.0	100
Snack mix, dark chocolate	1 oz	140	2	23	1	8	4.5	2.0	170
Snack mix, flamin' hot	1 oz	140	2	18	1	1	7.0	1.0	200
Snack mix, honey graham	1 oz	130	2	20	2	6	5.0	1.0	120
Snack mix, honey nut, sweet 'n' salty	1 oz	130	2	22	1	5	4.0	0.5	280
Snack mix, hot 'n' spicy	1 oz	130	2	20	1	2	4.0	1.0	420
Snack mix, Italian cheese blend	1 oz	140	3	20	1	2	5.0	1.0	320
Snack mix, nut chocolate, freeze dried	1 pouch	480	13	25	3	17	30.0	10.0	105
Snack mix, Oriental, rice-based	1 oz	143	5	15	4	1	7.3	1.1	117
Snack mix, original recipe	1 oz	150	3	20	1	1	6.0	1.0	310
Snack mix, original recipe, reduced fat	1 oz	130	3	20	1	1	4.0	1.0	320
Snack mix, peanut lovers	1 oz	140	3	19	1	2	5.0	1.0	340
Snack mix, pretzel, deli-style mustard	1 oz	130	3	24	1	1	2.0	0.0	220
Snack mix, sesame nut	1 oz	160	5	9	2	0	13.0	2.0	240
Snack mix, soy	1 oz	120	12	8	3	0	4.5	0.0	230
Snack mix, soy, BBQ flavor	1 oz	120	12	8	3	1	4.5	0.0	310
Snack mix, soy, sour cream	1 oz	120	12	8	3	0	4.5	0.0	310

SNACKS continued

Item	Serving Size	Calories	Protein	Carb	Fiber	Sugar	Total Fat	Sat Fat	Sodium
Snack mix, special Italian recipe	1 oz	150	3	20	1	1	6.0	1.0	290
Snack mix, strawberry yogurt	1 pouch	100	1	18	0	5	2.5	1.0	170
Snack mix, totally ranch	1 oz	140	2	19	1	1	6.0	1.0	260
Snack mix, traditional	1 oz	130	2	19	1	3	5.0	1.0	220
Snack sticks, sesame, wheat-based, salted	1 oz	153	3	13	1	0	10.4	1.8	422
Soy chips, salted	1 oz	109	8	15	1	1	2.1	0.3	239
Soy crisps, BBQ	1 oz	110	6	15	2	4	4.0	0.0	400
Soy crisps, creamy ranch	1 oz	100	7	14	2	1	2.0	0.0	330
Soy crisps, onion garlic	1 oz	100	7	14	2	1	2.0	0.0	280
Soy crisps, salted	1 oz	109	8	15	1	1	2.1	0.3	239
Soy crisps, simply cheese	1 oz	130	7	13	3	2	6.0	1.0	230
Soy crisps, sticky bun	1 oz	130	6	15	3	3	5.0	0.5	180
Soy crisps, sweet BBQ	1 oz	120	6	16	3	2	4.5	0.5	390
Soy crisps, white cheddar	1 oz	120	7	14	2	3	4.5	0.5	270
Soy munchies, caramel	1/2 oz	40	2	8	1	4	0.0	0.0	10
Soy munchies, ranch	1/2 oz	60	3	8	1	1	2.0	0.0	150
Soy munchies, white cheddar	1/2 oz	60	3	6	1	1	2.5	0.5	240
Sweet potato chips	1 oz	141	1	18	1	2	7.0	0.6	10
Sweet potato chips, jalapeño flavor	1 oz	140	1	18	1	4	7.0	1.0	65
Sweet potato chips, mesquite BBQ	1 oz	140	1	18	1	4	7.0	1.5	65
Sweet potato chips, spiced	1 oz	140	1	16	3	2	7.0	1.0	105
Sweet potato chips, unsalted	1 oz	140	1	18	1	2	7.0	1.0	10
Taro chips	1 oz	141	1	19	2	1	7.1	1.8	97
Taro chips, spiced	1 oz	130	1	20	2	2	5.0	0.5	170
Taro, sweet potato, yuca, & batata chips	1 oz	140	1	18	3	1	7.0	1.0	70
Tortilla chips, black bean	1 oz	140	3	18	4	0	7.0	0.5	70
Tortilla chips, black bean, with organic corn	1 oz	140	3	18	2	0	7.0	1.0	170
Tortilla chips, black bean chili	1 oz	140	3	17	4	0	7.0	0.5	130

SNACKS continued

Item	Serving Size	Calories	Protein	Carb	Fiber	Sugar	Total Fat	Sat Fat	Sodium
Tortilla chips, black pepper jack	1 oz	150	2	18	1	1	8.0	1.0	190
Tortilla chips, blazin' buffalo & ranch	1 oz	140	2	18	1	1	7.0	1.0	250
Tortilla chips, blue corn	1 oz	110	3	22	2	0	2.0	0.0	140
Tortilla chips, blue corn, Blue Chips	1 oz	140	2	18	2	0	7.0	0.5	60
Tortilla chips, blue corn, hot & spicy	1 oz	140	2	18	1	1	7.0	1.0	140
Tortilla chips, blue corn, Red Hot Blues	1 oz	140	2	18	2	0	7.0	0.5	150
Tortilla chips, blue corn, unsalted, Blue Chips	1 oz	140	2	18	2	0	7.0	0.5	10
Tortilla chips, blue corn, with sesame seeds	1 oz	150	2	16	2	0	9.0	1.5	65
Tortilla chips, blue corn, with sesame seeds, Sesame Blues	1 oz	150	3	16	2	0	8.0	1.0	90
Tortilla chips, blue corn, with soy beans, Little Soy Blues, Garden of Eatin'	1 oz	140	3	17	2	0	7.0	0.5	70
Tortilla chips, blue corn, with sunflower seeds, Sunny Blues, Garden of Eatin'	1 oz	150	2	17	2	0	8.0	0.5	70
Tortilla chips, blue corn, with organic corn	1 oz	140	2	19	1	0	6.0	0.5	80
Tortilla chips, chili & lime	1 oz	110	2	22	2	2	2.0	0.0	200
Tortilla chips, chili lime, with organic corn	1 oz	140	3	18	2	0	7.0	1.0	140
Tortilla chips, cool ranch	1 oz	140	2	18	1	1	7.0	1.0	170
Tortilla chips, fiery habanero	1 oz	130	2	16	1	1	7.0	1.0	240
Tortilla chips, flour	1 oz	140	2	19	1	2	7.0	1.5	95
Tortilla chips, gold, bite-size	1 oz	140	2	19	1	0	7.0	1.0	110
Tortilla chips, light, baked	1 oz	132	2	21	2	0	4.3	0.8	284
Tortilla chips, light, baked, crushed	1 oz	132	2	21	2	0	4.3	0.8	284

SNACKS continued

Item	Serving Size	Calories	Protein	Carb	Fiber	Sugar	Total Fat	Sat Fat	Sodium
Tortilla chips, light, restaurant style	1 oz	90	2	20	1	0	1.0	0.0	105
Tortilla chips, low fat, baked	1 oz	118	3	23	2	0	1.6	0.2	119
Tortilla chips, low fat, unsalted	1 oz	118	3	23	2	0	1.6	0.2	4
Tortilla chips, mucho nacho	1 oz	110	2	22	2	2	2.0	0.0	200
Tortilla chips, multigrain	1 oz	150	2	18	2	1	8.0	1.0	135
Tortilla chips, multigrain, with organic corn & grains	1 oz	140	3	18	2	0	7.0	1.0	100
Tortilla chips, nacho cheese	1 oz	146	2	18	1	1	7.4	1.1	174
Tortilla chips, nacho cheese flavor, low fat, with Olestra	1 oz	90	2	18	2	1	1.0	0.3	171
Tortilla chips, nacho cheese, baked	1 oz	120	2	21	2	1	3.5	0.5	220
Tortilla chips, nacho cheese, light	1 oz	100	2	19	2	1	2.0	0.5	200
Tortilla chips, original, bite-size, baked	1 oz	110	3	24	2	0	1.0	0.0	200
Tortilla chips, picante ranch	1 oz	110	3	22	2	0	2.0	0.0	200
Tortilla chips, ranchero	1 oz	140	2	18	1	1	7.0	1.0	290
Tortilla chips, red chile & lime	1 oz	150	2	17	2	0	8.0	1.0	130
Tortilla chips, red corn	1 oz	110	3	22	2	0	2.0	0.0	140
Tortilla chips, red corn, Red Chips	1 oz	140	2	18	1	0	7.0	1.0	70
Tortilla chips, red corn, Salsa Reds	1 oz	140	2	18	3	0	7.0	1.0	170
Tortilla chips, salsa	1 oz	140	3	17	1	1	7.0	1.0	170
Tortilla chips, salsa verde	1 oz	140	2	19	1	1	7.0	1.0	210
Tortilla chips, Scoops	1 oz	140	2	18	1	0	7.0	1.0	120
Tortilla chips, Scoops, baked	1 oz	120	2	22	2	0	3.0	0.5	150
Tortilla chips, smokin' cheddar BBQ	1 oz	150	2	18	1	1	7.0	1.0	200
Tortilla chips, Southwestern ranch	1 oz	150	2	18	2	1	8.0	1.5	130
Tortilla chips, spicy black bean	1 oz	110	3	22	2	0	2.0	0.0	200
Tortilla chips, spicy nacho	1 oz	140	2	18	1	1	7.0	1.0	210

SNACKS continued

Item	Serving Size	Calories	Protein	Carb	Fiber	Sugar	Total Fat	Sat Fat	Sodium
Tortilla chips, sweet white corn	1 oz	110	3	22	2	0	2.0	0.0	140
Tortilla chips, taco	1 oz	140	2	18	1	1	7.0	1.0	170
Tortilla chips, toasted corn	1 oz	140	2	18	1	0	7.0	1.0	120
Tortilla chips, white corn	1 oz	139	2	19	2	0	6.6	0.8	119
Tortilla chips, white corn rounds	1 oz	140	2	19	2	0	6.0	0.5	60
Tortilla chips, white corn strips	1 oz	140	2	19	2	0	6.0	0.5	60
Tortilla chips, white corn, chili & lime	1 oz	140	2	18	2	1	7.0	1.0	125
Tortilla chips, white corn, lightly salted	1 oz	140	2	20	1	0	6.0	1.0	120
Tortilla chips, white corn, pico de gallo flavor	1 oz	140	2	18	3	0	7.0	0.5	150
Tortilla chips, white corn, restaurant style	1 oz	130	2	19	1	0	6.0	1.0	110
Tortilla chips, white corn, tamari flavor	1 oz	140	2	18	3	0	7.0	0.0	160
Tortilla chips, white corn, unsalted	1 oz	143	2	19	2	0	6.6	0.7	4
Tortilla chips, white corn nacho cheese, natural	1 oz	150	2	17	1	1	8.0	1.0	190
Tortilla chips, white corn, bite-size	1 oz	140	2	17	1	0	8.0	1.0	110
Tortilla chips, white corn, hint of lime	1 oz	140	2	19	1	1	6.0	1.0	160
Tortilla chips, white corn, restaurant style	1 oz	140	2	19	1	0	7.0	1.0	120
Tortilla chips, yellow corn	1 oz	139	2	19	1	0	6.1	0.7	80
Tortilla chips, yellow corn rounds	1 oz	140	2	18	2	0	7.0	0.5	60
Tortilla chips, yellow corn strips	1 oz	140	2	18	2	0	7.0	0.5	60
Tortilla chips, yellow corn, salsa flavor	1 oz	140	2	20	1	0	6.0	1.0	80
Tortilla chips, yellow corn, unsalted	1 oz	110	3	22	2	0	1.0	0.0	26
Tortilla chips, yellow corn, with organic corn	1 oz	140	2	19	1	0	6.0	0.5	100

SNACKS continued

Item	Serving Size	Calories	Protein	Carb	Fiber	Sugar	Total Fat	Sat Fat	Sodium
Vegetable chips, garden, prepared from recipe	1 oz	134	2	17	1	1	6.6	0.5	274
Vegetable chips, original	1 oz	147	1	16	3	3	8.5	0.5	70
Veggie crisps, farmland cheddar, baked	1 oz	130	2	19	2	3	5.0	1.0	190
Veggie crisps, garlic & herb field, baked	1 oz	130	2	19	2	3	5.0	0.0	190
Veggie crisps, tangy tomato ranch, baked	1 oz	130	2	19	2	3	5.0	1.0	210

SOUPS, SAUCES, AND GRAVIES

Item	Serving Size	Calories	Protein	Carb	Fiber	Sugar	Total Fat	Sat Fat	Sodium
Bouillon, beef	1 cup	17	3	0	0	0	0.5	0.3	799
Bouillon or broth, beef, low sodium	1 cup	39	5	1	0	1	1.5	0.4	74
Broth, beef	1 cup	17	3	0	0	0	0.5	0.3	799
Broth, chicken, condensed	1 cup	76	11	2	0	1	2.5	0.8	1534
Broth, chicken, low sodium	1 cup	39	5	3	0	0	1.5	0.4	74
Broth, chicken, prepared from canned with water	1 cup	39	5	1	0	1	1.4	0.4	779
Broth, chicken, reduced sodium	1 cup	17	3	1	0	1	0.0	0.0	566
Broth, fish	1 cup	39	5	1	0	0	1.5	0.3	779
Broth, stewed kidney beans	1 cup	115	4	7	0	0	7.8	2.9	5
Chili, beef, condensed	1 cup	287	12	46	6	12	6.2	3.0	1931
Chili, beef, prepared from canned with water	1 cup	140	6	23	3	6	3.0	1.5	951
Chili, con carne, with beans	1 cup	296	17	28	10	5	12.9	4.3	1039
Chili, with beans	1 cup	274	14	29	11	3	13.5	5.8	1279
Chili, without beans	1 cup	289	18	15	4	3	17.4	5.5	953
Chowder, fish	1 cup	195	24	12	1	4	5.4	2.4	180
Chowder, seafood	1 cup	195	24	12	1	4	5.4	2.4	180
Clam chowder, Manhattan style, chunky	1 cup	137	7	19	3	4	3.5	2.2	1022

SOUPS, SAUCES, AND GRAVIES continued

Item	Serving Size	Calories	Protein	Carb	Fiber	Sugar	Total Fat	Sat Fat	Sodium
Clam chowder, Manhattan style, condensed	1 cup	149	4	24	3	7	4.3	0.8	1120
Clam chowder, Manhattan style, prepared from canned with water	1 cup	74	2	12	1	3	2.1	0.4	554
Clam chowder, New England, condensed	1 cup	176	8	25	2	1	5.0	2.4	1713
Clam chowder, New England, prepared from canned with milk	1 cup	149	8	18	1	7	4.9	2.7	884
Clam chowder, New England, prepared from canned with water	1 cup	86	4	12	1	0	2.5	1.2	843
Gravy, beef	2 tbsp	18	1	2	0	0	0.8	0.4	190
Gravy, beef, instant	2 tbsp	125	3	21	1	8	3.2	1.7	1769
Gravy, brown, instant	2 tbsp	129	3	20	1	3	4.0	2.0	1718
Gravy, chicken	2 tbsp	27	1	2	0	0	1.9	0.5	196
Gravy, meat, low sodium, prepared	2 tbsp	18	1	2	0	0	0.8	0.3	6
Gravy, mushroom, dry	2 tbsp	112	3	22	2	1	1.4	0.8	2237
Gravy, pork, dry	2 tbsp	125	3	22	1	8	2.9	1.5	1821
Gravy, poultry, low sodium, prepared	2 tbsp	18	1	2	0	0	0.8	0.3	6
Gravy, sausage, country style	2 tbsp	40	1	2	0	1	3.5	0.9	156
Gravy, turkey	2 tbsp	17	1	2	0	0	0.7	0.2	196
Gravy, turkey, instant	2 tbsp	139	4	20	1	3	5.0	1.7	1391
Sauce, adobo fresco	2 tbsp	92	1	6	0	1	7.1	1.0	5832
Sauce, Alfredo, dry mix	2 tbsp	182	5	12	1	2	12.4	4.5	881
Sauce, barbecue	2 tbsp	51	0	12	0	9	0.1	0.0	380
Sauce, barbecue, low sodium	2 tbsp	51	0	12	0	9	0.1	0.0	45
Sauce, cheese	2 tbsp	59	2	2	0	0	4.5	2.0	282
Sauce, cheese, dry mix	2 tbsp	149	3	21	0	3	6.2	2.9	1089
Sauce, cheese, low fat	2 tbsp	45	3	2	0	1	2.6	1.0	171
Sauce, cheese, prepared from recipe	2 tbsp	67	4	2	0	0	5.1	2.7	168
Sauce, chili, hot, from immature green peppers	2 tbsp	7	0	2	1	1	0.0	0.0	9

SOUPS, SAUCES, AND GRAVIES continued

Item	Serving Size	Calories	Protein	Carb	Fiber	Sugar	Total Fat	Sat Fat	Sodium
Sauce, chili, hot, from mature red peppers	2 tbsp	7	0	1	0	1	0.2	0.0	9
Sauce, clam, white	2 tbsp	85	6	1	0	1	6.1	0.8	27
Sauce, fish	2 tbsp	12	2	1	0	1	0.0	0.0	2625
Sauce, hoisin	2 tbsp	75	1	15	1	9	1.2	0.2	549
Sauce, hollandaise with butter fat, prepared from dehydrated mix with water	2 tbsp	31	1	2	0	1	2.6	1.5	205
Sauce, oyster	2 tbsp	17	0	4	0	0	0.1	0.0	929
Sauce, pepper	2 tbsp	4	0	1	0	0	0.1	0.0	899
Sauce, pizza	2 tbsp	18	1	3	1	1	0.4	0.2	63
Sauce, plum, tangy, low sodium, fruit-sweetened	1/2 oz	20	0	5	1	5	0.0	0.0	10
Sauce, spaghetti, low sodium	2 tbsp	30	1	5	1	3	0.9	0.2	10
Sauce, spaghetti/marinara	2 tbsp	30	1	5	1	3	0.9	0.2	139
Sauce, stir fry, Chinese five spice	1/2 fl oz	25	1	5	0	5	0.0	0.0	310
Sauce, stir fry, garlic teriyaki	1/2 fl oz	20	0	4	0	3	0.0	0.0	210
Sauce, stir fry, sizzling General Gao	1/2 fl oz	20	0	5	0	5	0.0	0.0	190
Sauce, stir fry, spicy Korean BBQ	1/2 fl oz	20	0	3	0	3	0.5	0.0	260
Sauce, stir fry, Thai basil BBQ	1/2 fl oz	15	0	2	0	2	0.5	0.0	135
Sauce, stir fry, wasabi ginger	1/2 fl oz	35	0	6	0	5	0.0	0.0	140
Sauce, sweet & sour, prepared from recipe	2 tbsp	27	1	6	0	4	0.2	0.0	118
Sauce, teriyaki	2 tbsp	30	2	5	0	5	0.0	0.0	1303
Sauce, teriyaki, reduced sodium	2 tbsp	30	2	5	0	5	0.0	0.0	605
Sauce, tomato chili	2 tbsp	35	1	7	2	4	0.1	0.0	455
Sauce, tomato chili, low sodium	2 tbsp	35	1	10	0	3	0.1	0.0	7
Sauce, white, medium, prepared from recipe	2 tbsp	50	1	3	0	1	3.6	1.0	120

SOUPS, SAUCES, AND GRAVIES continued

Item	Serving Size	Calories	Protein	Carb	Fiber	Sugar	Total Fat	Sat Fat	Sodium
Sauce, white, thick, prepared from recipe	2 tbsp	63	1	4	0	1	4.7	1.2	127
Sauce, white, thin, prepared from recipe	2 tbsp	36	1	3	0	2	2.3	0.7	112
Sauce, white, thin, prepared from recipe with butter	2 tbsp	24	1	3	0	2	0.9	0.5	63
Soup, bean & bacon, prepared from canned with water	1 cup	154	7	20	7	4	5.3	1.4	855
Soup, bean & ham, reduced sodium, prepared with water from canned	1 cup	181	10	33	10	8	2.5	0.6	458
Soup, bean & pork, condensed	1 cup	316	14	42	14	7	10.8	2.8	1737
Soup, beef, chunky	1 cup	162	10	25	1	2	2.7	1.3	880
Soup, beef & mushroom, chunky, low sodium	1 cup	169	11	23	0	2	5.6	4.0	61
Soup, beef noodle, condensed	1 cup	164	9	18	1	5	6.0	2.2	1600
Soup, beef noodle, prepared from canned with water	1 cup	83	5	9	1	3	3.0	1.1	933
Soup, beef noodle, prepared with water	1 cup	83	5	9	1	3	3.0	1.1	933
Soup, beef Stroganoff, chunky	1 cup	240	12	22	1	4	11.3	5.7	1066
Soup, black bean, condensed	1 cup	223	12	38	17	6	3.2	0.8	2377
Soup, black bean, prepared with water	1 cup	113	6	19	8	3	1.6	0.4	1193
Soup, broccoli cheese, condensed	1 cup	213	5	19	4	5	13.0	3.9	1673
Soup, cheese, condensed	1 cup	296	10	20	2	1	20.0	12.7	1698
Soup, chicken & dumplings, condensed	1 cup	194	11	12	1	1	11.0	2.6	1514

SOUPS, SAUCES, AND GRAVIES continued

Item	Serving Size	Calories	Protein	Carb	Fiber	Sugar	Total Fat	Sat Fat	Sodium
Soup, chicken & dumplings, prepared with water	1 cup	98	6	6	0	1	5.6	1.3	875
Soup, chicken gumbo, condensed	1 cup	110	5	16	4	5	2.8	0.6	1698
Soup, chicken gumbo, prepared with water	1 cup	56	3	8	2	2	1.4	0.3	958
Soup, chicken mushroom, condensed	1 cup	267	9	19	0	3	17.9	4.7	1619
Soup, chicken noodle, chunky	1 cup	91	8	10	1	2	2.2	1.0	840
Soup, chicken noodle, condensed	1 cup	127	6	15	1	1	4.8	1.3	1318
Soup, chicken noodle, low sodium	1 cup	61	3	7	0	1	2.3	0.6	424
Soup, chicken noodle, prepared from canned with water	1 cup	61	3	7	0	1	2.3	0.6	649
Soup, chicken rice, chunky	1 cup	130	13	13	1	1	3.3	1.0	907
Soup, chicken rice, condensed	1 cup	120	7	14	1	0	3.8	0.9	1629
Soup, chicken rice, prepared from canned with water	1 cup	59	4	7	1	0	1.9	0.5	818
Soup, chicken vegetable, condensed	1 cup	149	7	17	2	3	5.7	1.7	1796
Soup, chicken vegetable, prepared from canned with water	1 cup	76	4	9	1	1	2.9	0.9	960
Soup, chicken vegetable, with potato & cheese	1 cup	159	3	13	1	2	10.9	4.0	1019
Soup, chicken, chunky	1 cup	174	12	17	1	2	6.5	1.9	867
Soup, cream of asparagus, condensed	1 cup	169	4	21	1	2	8.0	2.0	1619
Soup, cream of celery, condensed	1 cup	176	3	17	1	3	10.9	2.7	1678
Soup, cream of chicken, condensed	1 cup	221	6	18	0	1	14.1	3.9	1605

SOUPS, SAUCES, AND GRAVIES continued

Item	Serving Size	Calories	Protein	Carb	Fiber	Sugar	Total Fat	Sat Fat	Sodium
Soup, cream of chicken, reduced sodium, condensed	1 cup	142	4	23	1	1	3.2	1.2	875
Soup, cream of mushroom, condensed	1 cup	208	4	16	0	4	14.4	3.4	1580
Soup, cream of mushroom, low sodium	1 cup	130	2	11	0	4	9.1	2.5	49
Soup, cream of mushroom, prepared from canned with milk	1 cup	164	6	14	0	8	9.5	3.2	813
Soup, cream of mushroom, prepared from canned with water	1 cup	103	2	8	0	2	7.1	1.7	779
Soup, cream of mushroom, reduced sodium, condensed	1 cup	127	3	20	1	5	4.1	1.3	938
Soup, cream of onion, condensed	1 cup	216	5	25	1	9	10.3	2.9	1561
Soup, cream of potato, condensed	1 cup	145	3	22	1	4	4.6	2.4	1561
Soup, cream of shrimp, prepared from canned with water	1 cup	88	3	8	0	1	5.1	3.2	958
Soup, cream of shrimp, prepared with milk	1 cup	149	7	14	0	6	7.9	4.7	867
Soup, egg drop	1 cup	66	3	11	1	0	1.5	0.4	907
Soup, fisherman's	1 cup	195	24	12	1	4	5.4	2.4	180
Soup, gazpacho	1 cup	47	7	4	0	1	0.2	0.0	742
Soup, hot & sour	1 cup	96	6	11	1	1	3.0	0.6	921
Soup, minestrone, chunky	1 cup	130	5	21	6	5	2.9	1.5	882
Soup, minestrone, condensed	1 cup	167	9	22	2	4	5.0	1.1	1823
Soup, minestrone, reduced sodium	1 cup	123	5	22	6	5	2.0	0.3	527
Soup, mushroom, with beef stock, condensed	1 cup	167	6	18	0	6	7.9	3.0	1894
Soup, onion, condensed	1 cup	113	7	16	2	7	3.5	0.5	1793
Soup, onion, prepared with water	1 cup	56	4	8	1	3	1.7	0.2	1036

SOUPS, SAUCES, AND GRAVIES continued

Item	Serving Size	Calories	Protein	Carb	Fiber	Sugar	Total Fat	Sat Fat	Sodium
Soup, pea, green, condensed	1 cup	306	16	49	10	16	5.5	2.6	1666
Soup, pea, green, prepared from canned with water	1 cup	149	8	24	5	8	2.7	1.3	843
Soup, pea, low sodium, prepared with water	1 cup	152	8	24	5	8	2.7	1.3	25
Soup, pepper pot, prepared with water	1 cup	100	6	9	0	0	4.5	2.0	956
Soup, Scotch broth, prepared from canned with water	1 cup	81	5	9	1	1	2.6	1.1	1017
Soup, Scotch broth, prepared with water	1 cup	81	5	9	1	1	2.6	1.1	1017
Soup, split pea, reduced sodium	1 cup	174	9	29	5	12	2.3	0.7	407
Soup, split pea, with ham, chunky	1 cup	189	11	27	4	5	4.1	1.6	985
Soup, tomato beef, with noodle, prepared with water	1 cup	137	4	21	1	2	4.2	1.6	899
Soup, tomato rice, condensed	1 cup	228	4	42	3	14	5.2	1.0	1556
Soup, tomato rice, prepared with water	1 cup	115	2	21	2	7	2.6	0.5	782
Soup, tomato, condensed	1 cup	147	4	33	3	20	1.4	0.4	1350
Soup, tomato, low sodium, prepared with water	1 cup	74	2	16	1	10	0.7	0.2	59
Soup, tomato, prepared with milk	1 cup	135	6	22	1	16	3.2	1.7	711
Soup, tomato, reduced sodium, condensed	1 cup	159	4	33	3	20	1.4	0.4	54
Soup, turkey noodle, condensed	1 cup	135	8	17	1	1	3.9	1.1	1593
Soup, turkey vegetable, condensed	1 cup	147	6	17	1	3	6.1	1.8	1811
Soup, vegetable, chunky	1 cup	125	4	19	1	4	3.8	0.6	880

SOUPS, SAUCES, AND GRAVIES continued

Item	Serving Size	Calories	Protein	Carb	Fiber	Sugar	Total Fat	Sat Fat	Sodium
Soup, vegetable, low sodium, condensed	1 cup	159	5	30	5	11	2.2	0.4	943
Soup, vegetable, low sodium, prepared with water	1 cup	81	3	15	3	5	1.1	0.2	475
Soup, vegetable, vegetarian, condensed	1 cup	145	4	24	1	8	3.9	0.6	1646
Soup, vegetable, vegetarian, prepared with water	1 cup	69	2	12	1	4	1.9	0.3	828
Soup, vegetable, with beef broth, condensed	1 cup	162	6	26	3	4	3.8	0.9	1619
Soup, vegetable, with beef broth, prepared with water	1 cup	81	3	13	2	2	1.9	0.4	813
Soup, vegetable beef, condensed	1 cup	154	11	20	4	2	3.7	1.7	1546
Soup, vegetable beef, prepared with water	1 cup	76	5	10	2	1	1.9	0.8	777
Soup, vegetable chicken, low sodium	1 cup	169	12	21	1	3	4.9	1.5	86
Soup, wonton	1 cup	78	5	13	0	1	0.6	0.1	995
Stew, acorn, Apache	1 cup	233	17	23	2	1	8.5	3.1	319
Stew, beef	1 cup	243	11	19	2	4	13.5	5.4	951
Stew, hominy, with mutton, Navajo	1 cup	203	16	23	5	0	5.0	1.8	110
Stew, mutton, corn squash, Navajo	1 cup	252	21	18	4	1	10.6	4.3	120
Stew, steamed corn, Navajo	1 cup	274	22	26	6	1	9.2	3.9	255
Stew, vegetarian	1 cup	301	42	17	3	3	7.4	1.2	980
Stock, beef, prepared from recipe	1 cup	32	5	3	0	1	0.2	0.1	485
Stock, chicken, prepared from recipe	1 cup	88	6	9	0	4	2.9	0.8	350
Stock, fish, prepared from recipe	1 cup	42	6	0	0	0	2.0	0.5	382

SOY FOODS

Item	Serving Size	Calories	Protein	Carb	Fiber	Sugar	Total Fat	Sat Fat	Sodium
Cheese substitute, cheddar, soy	1 oz	35	4	1	0	0	2.0	0.0	290
Cheese substitute, jalapeño jack, soy	1 oz	35	4	0	1	0	2.0	0.0	280
Cheese, Chedarella, semisoft	1 oz	110	7	0	0	0	9.0	6.0	190
Cheese, Co-Jack, semisoft	1 oz	110	7	0	0	0	9.0	6.0	190
Cottage cheese substitute, soy	1/2 cup	166	14	8	0	2	8.9	1.3	22
Miso	1 tbsp	34	2	4	1	1	1.0	0.2	634
Miso, paste, dark red	1 tbsp	31	2	3	0	2	1.0	0.0	839
Miso, paste, light yellow	1 tbsp	31	2	3	0	2	1.0	0.0	839
Miso, paste, mellow barley	1 tbsp	28	3	3	0	0	0.0	0.0	280
Miso, paste, mellow brown	1 tbsp	28	3	6	3	3	0.0	0.0	616
Miso, paste, mellow red	1 tbsp	28	0	6	3	3	0.0	0.0	588
Miso, paste, mellow white, dried	1 tbsp	59	2	11	2	6	0.8	0.0	888
Salad dressing, vinaigrette, miso ginger	2 tbsp	100	0	1	0	1	10.0	1.5	250
Snack mix, soy	1 oz	120	12	8	3	0	5	0	230
Snack mix, soy, BBQ flavor	1 oz	120	12	8	3	1	5	0	310
Snack mix, soy, sour cream	1 oz	120	12	8	3	0	5	0	310
Soup, miso, red, instant, packet	10 g	35	2	3	0	0	1.5	0.0	750
Soup, miso, sesame, in a cup, dry	1 oz	100	4	19	0	1	1.0	0.0	690
Soup, miso, white, instant, packet	10 g	35	2	3	0	0	1.5	0.0	780
Soup, miso, with tofu, in a cup, dry	1 oz	110	5	21	0	1	1.0	0.0	690
Soy chips, salted	1 oz	109	8	15	1	1	2	0	239
Soy crisps, BBQ	1 oz	110	6	15	2	4	4	0	400
Soy crisps, BBQ flavor	1 oz	110	8	17	2	2	2	0	160
Soy crisps, creamy ranch	1 oz	100	7	14	2	1	2	0	330
Soy crisps, onion garlic	1 oz	100	7	14	2	1	2	0	280
Soy crisps, salted	1 oz	109	8	15	1	1	2	0	239
Soy crisps, simply cheese	1 oz	130	7	13	3	2	6	1	230
Soy crisps, sticky bun	1 oz	130	6	15	3	3	5	1	180

SOY FOODS continued

Item	Serving Size	Calories	Protein	Carb	Fiber	Sugar	Total Fat	Sat Fat	Sodium
Soy crisps, sweet BBQ	1 oz	120	6	16	3	2	5	1	390
Soy crisps, white cheddar	1 oz	120	7	14	2	3	5	1	270
Soy munchies, caramel	1/2 oz	40	2	8	1	4	0	0	10
Soy munchies, ranch	1/2 oz	60	3	8	1	1	2	0	150
Soy munchies, white cheddar	1/2 oz	60	3	6	1	1	3	1	240
Tempeh, five grain	3 oz	190	11	20	6	0	6.0	1.0	10
Tempeh, garden vegetable	4 oz	142	18	9	7	0	4.0	1.0	125
Tempeh, quinoa sesame	4 oz	190	21	20	7	0	3.0	1.0	3
Tempeh, soy	3 oz	160	13	20	7	0	3.5	0.5	10
Tempeh, spicy veggie	3 oz	145	13	20	7	0	3.5	0.5	25
Tempeh, three grain	4 oz	190	12	25	6	2	4.0	1.5	17
Tempeh, wild rice	4 oz	190	12	25	7	1	4.0	1.0	20
Tofu, Chinese spice, firm	3 oz	90	8	3	1	1	5.0	1.0	220
Tofu, extra firm	3 oz	83	9	2	1	0	4.4	0.6	3
Tofu, extra firm, light	3 oz	65	8	3	1	0	2.2	0.0	33
Tofu, extra firm, prep with nigari	3 oz	77	8	2	0	0	5.0	0.5	7
Tofu, firm	3 oz	76	8	2	0	0	4.4	0.5	0
Tofu, firm, light	3 oz	46	7	1	1	0	1.4	0.2	29
Tofu, firm, prepared with nigari & calcium sulfate	3 oz	60	7	1	1	1	3.5	0.7	10
Tofu, fried	3 oz	230	15	9	3	2	17.2	2.5	14
Tofu, garlic & onion, firm	3 oz	98	9	3	1	1	5.4	1.1	272
Tofu, Oriental spice	3 oz	90	8	3	1	1	5.0	1.0	220
Tofu, regular, with calcium sulfate	3 oz	65	7	2	0	0	4.1	0.6	6
Tofu, silken	3 oz	42	4	1	0	0	1.9	0.0	0
Tofu, silken, light	3 oz	37	5	1	0	0	0.9	0.0	42
Tofu, soft	3 oz	65	7	1	0	0	3.3	0.0	0
Tofu, super firm, cubed	3 oz	104	11	3	2	1	5.4	1.1	5
Tofu, zesty garlic & onion	3 oz	90	8	3	1	1	5.0	1.0	250
Vegetarian meat, bacon bits	3 oz	405	27	24	9	0	22.0	3.5	1505
Vegetarian meat, bacon, strips	3 oz	264	9	5	2	0	25.1	3.9	1245

SOY FOODS continued

Item	Serving Size	Calories	Protein	Carb	Fiber	Sugar	Total Fat	Sat Fat	Sodium
Vegetarian meat, beef, fillet	3 oz	247	20	8	5	1	15.3	2.4	417
Vegetarian meat, beef, loaf, slice	3 oz	167	18	7	4	1	7.7	1.2	468
Vegetarian meat, beef, meatballs	3 oz	167	18	7	4	1	7.7	1.2	468
Vegetarian meat, beef, meatballs, Soy Veg-T-Balls, Veggieland	3 oz	113	11	9	5	3	3.0	0.0	285
Vegetarian meat, beef, patty	3 oz	167	18	7	4	1	7.7	1.2	468
Vegetarian meat, burger, BBQ grilled tempeh	3 oz	131	11	12	0	3	3.8	1.6	196
Vegetarian meat, burger, lemon grilled tempeh	3 oz	153	12	12	0	2	6.0	2.2	305
Vegetarian meat, burger, soy veggie, original	3 oz	112	11	10	6	3	3.0	0.0	281
Vegetarian meat, burger, soy, black bean & salsa	3 oz	120	11	12	2	0	2.7	0.9	395
Vegetarian meat, burger, tamari grilled tempeh	3 oz	131	12	10	0	2	5.4	2.2	283
Vegetarian meat, chicken	3 oz	190	20	3	3	0	10.8	1.5	603
Vegetarian meat, chicken, breaded, fried	3 oz	199	18	7	4	0	10.9	1.0	340
Vegetarian meat, chicken, breaded, fried, diced	3 oz	199	18	7	4	0	10.9	1.0	340
Vegetarian meat, chicken, soy fillet	3 oz	90	15	8	4	2	2.0	0.0	170
Vegetarian meat, fish sticks	3 oz	247	20	8	5	1	15.3	2.4	417
Vegetarian meat, hot dog	3 oz	198	17	7	3	0	11.7	1.7	400
Vegetarian meat, lunchmeat, slices	3 oz	161	15	4	0	2	9.4	1.1	604
Vegetarian meat, sandwich spread	3 oz	127	7	8	3	4	7.7	1.2	536
Vegetarian meat, sausage	3 oz	218	16	8	2	0	15.4	2.5	755
Vegetarian meat, sausage, sweet Italian	3 oz	238	25	10	5	0	5.1	0.9	9

SPORTS BARS, Energy Bars

Item	Serving Size	Calories	Protein	Carb	Fiber	Sugar	Total Fat	Sat Fat	Sodium
Almond brownie, Balance Bar	1 bar	200	14	22	2	17	6.0	1.5	190
Apple Cinnamon Crisp, PowerBar Performance	1 bar	230	10	45	3	20	2.5	0.5	90
Apricot, Clif Bar	1 bar	222	9	43	5	21	2.3	0.4	71
Banana, Nestlé	1 bar	230	9	45	3	20	2.0	0.5	90
Caramel Nut Rush, Snickers Marathon	1 bar	415	25	51	13	29	12.5	6.3	238
Carrot cake, Clif Bar	1 bar	234	10	41	5	21	4.0	1.8	170
Chai tea, Luna	1 bar	175	10	26	2	11	3.9	2.7	144
Chai with almonds, BumbleBar	1 bar	210	7	21	4	11	12.0	1.5	55
Chewy chocolate peanut, Snickers Marathon	1 bar	396	24	47	3	33	13.1	4.7	462
Chocolate, Balance Bar	1 bar	200	14	22	1	17	6.0	3.5	230
Chocolate, PowerBar Performance	1 bar	363	14	70	6	30	3.1	1.3	146
Chocolate almond fudge, Clif Bar	1 bar	231	10	38	5	20	4.8	0.9	139
Chocolate brownie, Clif Bar	1 bar	236	10	41	6	20	4.2	1.0	149
Chocolate chip brownie	1 bar	270	28	24	1	1	8.0	5.0	140
Chocolate chip peanut crunch, Clif Bar	1 bar	241	12	39	5	19	5.4	1.1	274
Chocolate chip, Clif Bar	1 bar	238	10	42	5	21	4.0	1.0	76
Chocolate crisp, BumbleBar	1 bar	200	5	25	3	13	11.0	2.0	35
Chocolate peanut butter, Balance Gold	1 bar	340	24	44	0	36	7.0	1.5	230
Chocolate peanut crunch, PowerBar Pria	1 bar	110	5	16	1	10	3.5	2.0	85
Chocolate rage, energy bar, Max Muscle	1 bar	280	33	24	2	0	7.0	5.0	40
Chocolate raspberry fudge, Balance Bar	1 bar	200	14	22	1	18	6.0	3.5	150
Cookies & cream	1 bar	250	28	24	1	2	7.0	5.0	270

SPORTS BARS, Energy Bars continued

Item	Serving Size	Calories	Protein	Carb	Fiber	Sugar	Total Fat	Sat Fat	Sodium
Cookies & Cream, Clif Builders	1 bar	225	10	39	5	21	3.7	1.5	179
Double chocolate cookie, PowerBar Pria	1 bar	110	5	16	1	10	3.0	2.5	100
Double chocolate nut, Snickers Marathon	1 bar	343	22	52	11	23	9.0	4.9	333
French vanilla crisp, PowerBar Pria	1 bar	110	5	17	1	9	3.0	2.5	80
High fiber, oats & chocolate, chewy	1 bar	350	5	70	23	25	10.0	3.4	225
Honey nut oat, Snickers Marathon	1 bar	378	23	54	11	26	7.9	4.5	318
Honey peanut, Balance Bar	1 bar	200	14	22	1	17	6.0	3.5	220
Lemon zest, Luna	1 bar	179	9	27	2	14	4.4	3.4	112
Lushus Lemon, BumbleBar	1 bar	210	7	21	4	10	12.0	1.5	75
Bar, energy, mocha chip, Balance Bar	1 bar	200	14	22	1	20	6.0	4.0	160
Multigrain crunch, Snickers Marathon	1 bar	422	18	57	3	33	13.2	4.8	418
Nutz over Chocolate, Luna	1 bar	403	21	52	4	17	12.2	5.5	386
Oatmeal raisin, PowerBar Performance	1 bar	230	10	45	3	20	2.5	0.5	120
Optimum, Nature's Path	1 bar	190	10	33	5	20	3.0	0.0	115
Original, BumbleBar	1 bar	230	6	20	4	11	15.0	2.0	60
Original, with almonds, BumbleBar	1 bar	230	5	20	4	11	15.0	2.0	60
Original, with cashew, BumbleBar	1 bar	230	5	21	4	11	14.0	2.0	60
Original, with hazelnut, BumbleBar	1 bar	240	5	19	4	11	16.0	2.0	60
Original, with mixed nuts, BumbleBar	1 bar	230	5	21	4	11	15.0	2.0	60
Peanut butter chocolate chip, PowerBar Harvest	1 bar	240	7	45	4	16	4.5	1.0	80
Peanut butter, Clif Crunch	1 bar	240	12	38	5	18	5.1	0.8	289
Power oats spice, Muscle Drive	1 bar	280	33	27	1	4	6.0	5.0	110

SPORTS BARS, Energy Bars continued

Item	Serving Size	Calories	Protein	Carb	Fiber	Sugar	Total Fat	Sat Fat	Sodium
Protein rich	1 bar	145	7	18	1	14	5.0	1.0	75
Really vanilla, NuGo	1 bar	180	11	26	7	0	4.0	2.5	200
Spooky S'mores, Clif Kid	1 bar	178	10	26	2	13	4.3	3.0	183
Strawberry yogurt	1 bar	200	13	23	1	14	6.0	2.5	150
Strawberry Crunch, PowerBar Harvest	1 bar	240	7	45	4	18	4.0	0.5	80
Toasted Nuts 'N' Cranberry, Luna	1 bar	167	10	26	1	12	3.3	0.5	189
Vanilla Crisp, PowerBar Performance	1 bar	230	9	45	3	20	2.5	0.5	90
Vanilla Yogurt, PowerBar Performance	1 bar	290	24	38	2	22	5.0	3.5	190
Berry blast, PowerBar Fruit Smoothie	1 bar	230	10	45	3	14	2.5	0.5	90
Yogurt honey peanut, Balance Bar	1 bar	200	14	22	1	19	6.0	3.0	220
Zone Perfect, classic crunch, assorted flavors	1 bar	422	30	45	2	27	14.0	4.5	450
Soy, high protein, chocolate brownie, Max Muscle	1 bar	234	19	21	0	0	8.0	3.0	162
Soy, high protein, chocolate mint, Max Muscle	1 bar	234	19	20	0	0	8.0	3.0	162
Soy, high protein, chocolate peanut butter, Max Muscle	1 bar	234	19	20	0	0	8.0	3.0	162

SPORTS BARS, Diet Bars

Item	Serving Size	Calories	Protein	Carb	Fiber	Sugar	Total Fat	Sat Fat	Sodium
Breakfast, honey nut graham, Unilever	1 bar	180	10	22	1	13	6.0	3.5	200
Breakfast & lunch, Dutch chocolate, Unilever	1 bar	140	5	20	2	12	5.0	3.0	85
Breakfast & lunch, peanut butter, Unilever	1 bar	150	5	19	2	14	6.0	2.5	70
Chocolate chip, Unilever	1 bar	200	16	17	1	0	8.0	4.0	200
Chocolate coconut	1 bar	120	12	7	5	2	4.0	2.0	80
Chocolate fudge cake	1 bar	120	12	7	5	2	4.0	2.0	80

SPORTS BARS, Diet Bars continued

Item	Serving Size	Calories	Protein	Carb	Fiber	Sugar	Total Fat	Sat Fat	Sodium
Chocolate peanut butter, Unilever	1 bar	200	16	17	1	1	8.0	4.0	240
Cinnamon delight, Unilever	1 bar	200	16	17	0	0	8.0	4.0	200
High protein, granola, chocolate chip, Unilever	1 bar	190	15	20	2	9	6.0	3.0	200
High protein, granola, peanut, Unilever	1 bar	200	15	21	2	8	7.0	2.5	200
High protein, peanut butter, Optimum Nutrition	1 bar	250	30	11	1	2	4.5	3.0	95
Lemon Delite, yogurt covered	1 bar	120	12	7	5	2	4.0	2.0	80
Meal, blueberry crisp, Unilever	1 bar	180	8	28	3	12	4.0	2.5	150
Meal, caramel crispy peanut, Unilever	1 bar	220	8	33	2	15	6.0	4.0	250
Meal, cherry crisp, Unilever	1 bar	180	8	29	3	12	4.0	2.0	150
Meal, chocolate chip, chewy granola, Unilever	1 bar	220	8	35	2	15	6.0	3.5	290
Meal, milk chocolate peanut, Unilever	1 bar	386	16	60	5	25	8.9	5.4	253
Meal, oatmeal raisin, Unilever	1 bar	220	8	35	1	17	5.0	3.0	75
Meal, peanut butter, chewy granola, Unilever	1 bar	220	8	35	2	15	6.0	3.0	360
Meal, rich chocolate brownie, Unilever	1 bar	220	8	34	2	15	5.0	3.5	170
Meal, strawberry cheesecake, Unilever	1 bar	220	8	35	2	13	6.0	4.0	130
Meal, trail mix, chewy granola, Unilever	1 bar	210	8	34	2	15	5.0	1.0	190
Snack, apple cinnamon muffin, Unilever	1 bar	140	1	21	1	9	5.0	0.5	180
Snack, banana nut muffin, Unilever	1 bar	150	2	19	1	6	8.0	0.5	200
Snack, blueberry muffin, Unilever	1 bar	140	1	22	1	9	5.0	0.5	170

SPORTS BARS, Diet Bars continued

Item	Serving Size	Calories	Protein	Carb	Fiber	Sugar	Total Fat	Sat Fat	Sodium
Snack, caramel nut, Unilever	1 bar	120	2	19	1	1	5.0	2.5	70
Snack, chocolate chip cookie, Unilever	1 bar	120	2	19	1	9	3.5	2.0	110
Snack, chocolate chip muffin, Unilever	1 bar	140	1	20	1	9	6.0	1.0	100
Snack, chocolate mint crisp, Unilever	1 bar	120	2	19	1	7	4.0	3.0	100
Snack, chocolate peanut, Kellogg's	1 bar	110	4	15	2	16	6.0	4.0	220
Snack, chocolate peanut nougat, Unilever	1 bar	120	2	20	1	9	4.0	2.5	70
Snack, coconut almond, Unilever	1 bar	120	6	15	2	1	5.0	3.0	70
Snack, crispy peanut caramel, Unilever	1 bar	120	1	20	1	8	4.0	3.0	120
Snack, oatmeal raisin cookie, Unilever	1 bar	120	2	19	1	8	3.5	1.5	115
Snack, peanut butter cookie, Unilever	1 bar	120	2	19	1	8	3.5	1.5	105
Snack, rich chewy caramel, Unilever	1 bar	120	2	18	1	9	4.0	3.0	50

SPORTS DRINKS

Item	Serving Size	Calories	Protein	Carb	Fiber	Sugar	Total Fat	Sat Fat	Sodium
All Sport Body Quencher, fruit punch	8 fl oz	53	0	15	0	15	0.0	0.0	36
All Sport Body Quencher, lemon-lime	8 fl oz	46	0	13	0	13	0.0	0.0	36
All Sport Body Quencher, orange	8 fl oz	46	0	13	0	13	0.0	0.0	36
Alpha One, creatine drink, grape powder, Max Muscle	1 scoop	132	5	28	0	14	0.0	0.0	0
Berry, Gatorade G	8 fl oz	62	0	15	0	13	0.0	0.0	94
Berry Ice, Capri Sun Sport	8 fl oz	67	0	17	0	17	0.0	0.0	57
Clear Cherry Chill, Capri Sun Sport	8 fl oz	57	0	15	0	15	0.0	0.0	52
Cool Blue, Gatorade G	8 fl oz	62	0	15	0	13	0.0	0.0	94
Frost Glacier Freeze, Gatorade G	8 fl oz	62	0	15	0	13	0.0	0.0	94
Frost Riptide Rush, Gatorade G	8 fl oz	62	0	15	0	13	0.0	0.0	94
Fruit flavor sports drink	8 fl oz	65	0	16	0	13	0.0	0.0	72
Fruit flavor sports drink, low calorie	8 fl oz	26	0	7	0	0	0.0	0.0	84
Fruit punch, Gatorade G	8 fl oz	62	0	15	0	13	0.0	0.0	94
Fruit Punch, Powerade	8 fl oz	72	0	19	0	15	0.0	0.0	28
Gourmet Gainer Chocolate, protein formula, MaxMuscle	1 packet	295	45	22	1	2	1.5	0.5	250
Gourmet Gainer Vanilla, protein formula, MaxMuscle	1 packet	295	45	22	1	2	1.5	0.5	250
Grape, Gatorade G	8 fl oz	62	0	15	0	13	0.0	0.0	94
Grape, Powerade	8 fl oz	73	0	19	0	15	0.0	0.0	28
Ice Punch, Gatorade G	8 fl oz	62	0	15	0	13	0.0	0.0	94
Kiwi Strawberry, Propel	8 fl oz	12	0	3	0	3	0.0	0.0	31
Lemon, Propel	8 fl oz	12	0	3	0	3	0.0	0.0	31
Lemon-lime, Gatorade G	8 fl oz	62	0	15	0	13	0.0	0.0	94
Lemon-lime, Powerade	8 fl oz	77	0	19	0	15	0.1	0.0	53

SPORTS DRINKS continued

Item	Serving Size	Calories	Protein	Carb	Fiber	Sugar	Total Fat	Sat Fat	Sodium
Lemonade, Gatorade G	8 fl oz	62	0	15	0	13	0.0	0.0	94
Lightspeed Lemon-Lime, Capri Sun Sport	8 fl oz	57	0	15	0	15	0.0	0.0	52
Lime, Gatorade G	8 fl oz	62	0	15	0	13	0.0	0.0	94
Mango, Gatorade G	8 fl oz	62	0	15	0	13	0.0	0.0	94
Melon, Gatorade Fierce	8 fl oz	62	0	15	0	13	0.0	0.0	94
Monster energy drink, Monster Beverage Company	8 fl oz	101	0	27	0	27	0.0	0.0	180
Mountain Berry Blast, Powerade	8 fl oz	73	0	19	0	15	0.0	0.0	28
Orange, Gatorade G	8 fl oz	62	0	15	0	13	0.0	0.0	94
Orange, Powerade	8 fl oz	72	0	19	0	15	0.0	0.0	28
Orange Edge, Capri Sun Sport	8 fl oz	57	0	15	0	15	0.0	0.0	52
Orange Strawberry, Gatorade A.M.	8 fl oz	62	0	15	0	13	0.0	0.0	94
Red Bull	8 fl oz	108	1	26	0	24	0.2	0.0	202
Rockstar energy drink	8 fl oz	139	0	30	0	30	0.0	0.0	41
Sour Melon, Powerade	8 fl oz	110	1	29	0	29	0.2	0.0	84
Strawberry, Gatorade Fierce	8 fl oz	62	0	15	0	13	0.0	0.0	94
Strawberry Lemonade, Powerade	8 fl oz	110	1	29	0	29	0.2	0.0	84
Thunder Punch, Capri Sun Sport	8 fl oz	67	0	17	0	17	0.0	0.0	57
Tropical Mango, Gatorade A.M.	8 fl oz	62	0	15	0	13	0.0	0.0	94
White Cherry, Powerade	8 fl oz	110	1	29	0	29	0.2	0.0	84

SWEETENERS

Item	Serving Size	Calories	Protein	Carb	Fiber	Sugar	Total Fat	Sat Fat	Sodium
Agave, nectar, all natural	1 tbsp	60	0	16	0	16	0	0	0
Glitter, edible	1 tsp	8	0	3	3	0	0	0	0
Honey, amber light	1 tbsp	64	0	17	0	16	0	0	1
Honey, clover	1 tbsp	64	0	17	0	16	0	0	1
Honey, dark	1 tbsp	64	0	17	0	16	0	0	1
Honey, light	1 tbsp	64	0	17	0	16	0	0	1
Molasses	1 tbsp	61	0	16	0	12	0	0	8
Molasses, bead	1 tbsp	54	0	13	0	10	0	0	50
Molasses, crystals	1 tsp	15	0	4	0	3	0	0	0
Molasses, dark	1 tbsp	50	0	14	0	14	0	0	10
Molasses, light	1 tbsp	60	0	15	0	15	0	0	10
Sugar, brown	1 tsp	15	0	4	0	4	0	0	0
Sugar, brown, liquid	1 tbsp	55	0	14	0	14	0	0	6
Sugar, brown, packed	1 tsp	15	0	4	0	4	0	0	1
Sugar, cane, unrefined	1 tsp	16	0	4	0	4	0	0	0
Sugar, confectioners/ powdered	1 tsp	16	0	4	0	4	0	0	0
Sugar, date	1 tsp	11	0	3	0	3	0	0	0
Sugar, maple	1 tsp	14	0	4	0	3	0	0	0
Sugar, turbinado	1 tsp	15	0	4	0	4	0	0	0
Sugar, white, granulated	1 tsp	15	0	4	0	4	0	0	0
Sweetener, fructose, powder	1 tsp	15	0	4	0	4	0	0	0
Sweetener, granulated, brown	1 tsp	14	0	3	0	0	0	0	23
Sweetener, InstaSweet, tablet	1 tablet	0	0	0	0	0	0	0	0
Sweetener, pear juice, Pear Sweet	1/2 oz	42	0	11	0	10	0	0	1
Sweetener, saccharin, NectaSweet	1 tablet	0	0	0	0	0	0	0	20
Sweetener, Sucanat, granulated cane juice	1 tbsp	82	0	20	0	20	0	0	13
Sweetener, sucralose, Splenda	1 packet	0	0	1	0		0	0	0
Syrup, Almond Roca, with Splenda	1 fl oz	0	0	0	0	0	0	0	5

SWEETENERS continued

Item	Serving Size	Calories	Protein	Carb	Fiber	Sugar	Total Fat	Sat Fat	Sodium
Syrup, almond, with Splenda	1 fl oz	0	0	0	0	0	0	0	20
Syrup, black cherry, with Splenda	1 fl oz	0	0	0	0	0	0	0	15
Syrup, blueberry, fruit-sweetened	1/2 fl oz	30	0	8	1	7	0	0	3
Syrup, cane, with 15% maple	1 tbsp	58	0	15	0	14	0	0	22
Syrup, caramel, with Splenda	1 fl oz	0	0	0	0	0	0	0	20
Syrup, chocolate, with Splenda	1 fl oz	0	0	0	0	0	0	0	15
Syrup, coconut, with Splenda	1 fl oz	0	0	0	0	0	0	0	5
Syrup, coffee, with Splenda	1 fl oz	0	0	1	0	1	0	0	5
Syrup, corn, dark	1 tbsp	60	0	16	0	6	0	0	33
Syrup, corn, light	1 tbsp	59	0	16	0	6	0	0	13
Syrup, dietetic	1 tbsp	8	0	10	1	0	0	0	4
Syrup, English toffee, with Splenda	1 fl oz	0	0	0	0	0	0	0	20
Syrup, French vanilla, with Splenda	1 fl oz	0	0	1	0	1	0	0	5
Syrup, grenadine	1 tbsp	56	0	14	0	10	0	0	6
Syrup, hazelnut, with Splenda	1 fl oz	0	0	0	0	0	0	0	20
Syrup, Irish cream, with Splenda	1 fl oz	0	0	0	0	0	0	0	20
Syrup, lemon, with Splenda	1 fl oz	0	0	0	0	0	0	0	5
Syrup, lime, with Splenda	1 fl oz	0	0	0	0	0	0	0	5
Syrup, maple	1 tbsp	55	0	14	0	12	0	0	2
Syrup, marionberry, fruit-sweetened	1/2 fl oz	30	0	8	1	7	0	0	3
Syrup, Nesquik, chocolate, calcium-fortified	1 1/3 oz	100	0	25	1	23	0	0	55
Syrup, orange, with Splenda	1 fl oz	0	0	0	0	0	0	0	5

SWEETENERS continued

Item	Serving Size	Calories	Protein	Carb	Fiber	Sugar	Total Fat	Sat Fat	Sodium
Syrup, pancake	1 tbsp	49	0	13	0	5	0	0	17
Syrup, pancake, reduced calorie	1 tbsp	35	0	9	0	7	0	0	37
Syrup, pancake, with 2% maple	1 tbsp	56	0	15	0	9	0	0	13
Syrup, pancake, with butter	1 tbsp	62	0	16	0	11	0	0	21
Syrup, peach, with Splenda	1 fl oz	0	0	1	0	1	0	0	5
Syrup, peppermint, with Splenda	1 fl oz	0	0	0	0	0	0	0	5
Syrup, raspberry, fruit-sweetened	1/2 fl oz	30	0	8	1	7	0	0	3
Syrup, raspberry, with Splenda	1 fl oz	0	0	0	0	0	0	0	15
Syrup, sorghum	1 tbsp	61	0	16	0	16	0	0	2
Syrup, strawberry, with Splenda	1 fl oz	0	0	0	0	0	0	0	5
Syrup, strawberry, fruit-sweetened	1/2 ounce	30	0	8	1	7	0	0	3
Syrup, vanilla, with Splenda	1 fl oz	0	0	0	0	0	0	0	15
Syrup, vanilla bean, with Splenda	1 fl oz	0	0	0	0	0	0	0	5
Syrup, vanilla, with Splenda	1 fl oz	0	0	0	0	0	0	0	15
Syrup, watermelon, with Splenda	1 fl oz	0	0	0	0	0	0	0	5
Syrup, white chocolate, with Splenda	1 fl oz	0	0	0	0	0	0	0	5

VEGETABLES

Item	Serving Size	Calories	Protein	Carb	Fiber	Sugar	Total Fat	Sat Fat	Sodium
Artichokes, French, cooked from frozen with salt, drained	3 oz	38	3	8	4	1	0.4	0.1	246
Artichokes, French, fresh	3 oz	40	3	9	5	1	0.1	0.0	80
Artichokes, French, hearts, cooked, drained	3 oz	45	2	10	7	1	0.3	0.1	51
Artichokes, globe, cooked, drained	3 oz	45	2	10	7	1	0.3	0.1	51
Artichokes, globe, cooked from frozen with salt, drained	3 oz	38	3	8	4	1	0.4	0.1	246
Artichokes, globe, fresh	3 oz	40	3	9	5	1	0.1	0.0	80
Asparagus, cooked, drained	3 oz	19	2	3	2	1	0.2	0.0	12
Asparagus, cooked from frozen, drained	3 oz	15	3	2	1	0	0.4	0.1	3
Asparagus, fresh	3 oz	17	2	3	2	2	0.1	0.0	2
Asparagus, spear tips, fresh	3 oz	17	2	3	2	2	0.1	0.0	2
Asparagus, spears, cooked, drained	3 oz	19	2	3	2	1	0.2	0.0	12
Asparagus, spears, cooked from frozen, drained	3 oz	15	3	2	1	0	0.4	0.1	3
Bamboo shoots, fresh	3 oz	23	2	4	2	3	0.3	0.1	3
Beets, cooked with salt, drained	3 oz	37	1	8	2	7	0.2	0.0	242
Beets, fresh	3 oz	37	1	8	2	6	0.1	0.0	66
Bhindi, cooked, drained	3 oz	19	2	4	2	2	0.2	0.0	5
Bhindi, cooked from frozen, drained	3 oz	24	2	5	2	2	0.3	0.1	3
Bhindi, cooked with salt, drained	3 oz	19	2	4	2	2	0.2	0.0	205
Bhindi, fresh	3 oz	26	2	6	3	1	0.1	0.0	7
Borage, fresh	3 oz	18	2	3	1	1	0.6	0.1	68
Broccoli, cooked, drained	3 oz	30	2	6	3	1	0.3	0.1	35
Broccoli, cooked with salt, drained	3 oz	30	2	6	3	1	0.3	0.1	223
Broccoli, fresh	3 oz	29	2	6	2	1	0.3	0.0	28

VEGETABLES continued

Item	Serving Size	Calories	Protein	Carb	Fiber	Sugar	Total Fat	Sat Fat	Sodium
Broccoli, frozen	3 oz	22	2	4	3	1	0.2	0.0	20
Broccoli, gai lan, cooked	3 oz	19	1	3	2	1	0.6	0.1	6
Broccoli raab, cooked	3 oz	28	3	3	2	0	0.4	0.1	48
Broccoli raab, fresh	3 oz	19	3	2	2	0	0.4	0.0	28
Broccoli spears, cooked from frozen with salt, drained	3 oz	24	3	5	3	1	0.1	0.0	221
Broccoli spears, cooked from frozen, drained	3 oz	24	3	5	3	1	0.1	0.0	20
Broccoli spears, fresh	3 oz	29	2	6	2	1	0.3	0.0	28
Brussels sprouts, cooked, drained	3 oz	31	2	6	2	1	0.4	0.1	18
Brussels sprouts, cooked from frozen, drained	3 oz	36	3	7	3	2	0.3	0.1	13
Brussels sprouts, cooked from frozen with salt, drained	3 oz	36	3	7	3	2	0.3	0.1	220
Brussels sprouts, cooked with salt, drained	3 oz	31	2	6	2	1	0.4	0.1	218
Brussels sprouts, fresh	3 oz	37	3	8	3	2	0.3	0.1	21
Burdock root, cooked, drained	3 oz	75	2	18	2	3	0.1	0.0	3
Burdock root, fresh	3 oz	61	1	15	3	2	0.1	0.0	4
Cabbage, bok choy, cooked, drained	3 oz	10	1	2	1	1	0.1	0.0	29
Cabbage, bok choy, cooked with salt, drained	3 oz	10	1	2	1	1	0.1	0.0	230
Cabbage, bok choy, fresh	3 oz	11	1	2	1	1	0.2	0.0	55
Cabbage, Chinese chard, cooked, drained	3 oz	10	1	2	1	1	0.1	0.0	29
Cabbage, Chinese chard, fresh	3 oz	11	1	2	1	1	0.2	0.0	55
Cabbage, cooked, drained	3 oz	20	1	5	2	2	0.1	0.0	7
Cabbage, cooked with salt, drained	3 oz	20	1	5	2	2	0.1	0.0	217
Cabbage, fresh	3 oz	21	1	5	2	3	0.1	0.0	15
Cabbage, kale, borecole, cooked, drained	3 oz	24	2	5	2	1	0.3	0.0	20

VEGETABLES continued

Item	Serving Size	Calories	Protein	Carb	Fiber	Sugar	Total Fat	Sat Fat	Sodium
Cabbage, kale, cooked, drained	3 oz	24	2	5	2	1	0.3	0.0	20
Cabbage, kale, cooked from frozen, drained	3 oz	26	2	4	2	1	0.4	0.1	13
Cabbage, kale, cooked from frozen with salt, drained	3 oz	26	2	4	2	1	0.4	0.1	213
Cabbage, kale, cooked with salt, drained	3 oz	24	2	5	2	1	0.3	0.0	220
Cabbage, kohlrabi, cooked, drained	3 oz	25	2	6	1	2	0.1	0.0	18
Cabbage, kohlrabi, cooked with salt, drained	3 oz	25	2	6	1	2	0.1	0.0	218
Cabbage, kohlrabi, fresh	3 oz	23	1	5	3	2	0.1	0.0	17
Cabbage, mustard, salted	3 oz	24	1	5	3	1	0.1	0.0	609
Cabbage, napa, cooked with salt, drained	3 oz	12	1	2	1	0	0.1	0.0	208
Cabbage, pak choi, cooked, drained	3 oz	10	1	2	1	1	0.1	0.0	29
Cabbage, pak choi, cooked with salt, drained	3 oz	10	1	2	1	1	0.1	0.0	230
Cabbage, pak choi, fresh	3 oz	11	1	2	1	1	0.2	0.0	55
Cabbage, petsai, cooked with salt, drained	3 oz	12	1	2	1	0	0.1	0.0	208
Cabbage, petsai, fresh	3 oz	14	1	3	1	1	0.2	0.0	8
Cabbage, pickled, Japanese style	3 oz	26	1	5	3	1	0.1	0.0	235
Cabbage, red, cooked with salt, drained	3 oz	25	1	6	2	3	0.1	0.0	207
Cabbage, red, fresh	3 oz	26	1	6	2	3	0.1	0.0	23
Cabbage, savoy, cooked with salt, drained	3 oz	20	2	5	2	2	0.1	0.0	221
Cabbage, savoy, fresh	3 oz	23	2	5	3	2	0.1	0.0	24
Cabbage, Scotch kale, cooked with salt, drained	3 oz	24	2	5	2	1	0.3	0.0	239
Cabbage, Scotch kale, fresh	3 oz	36	2	7	1	2	0.5	0.1	60
Cabbage, wong bok, cooked with salt, drained	3 oz	12	1	2	1	0	0.1	0.0	208

VEGETABLES continued

Item	Serving Size	Calories	Protein	Carb	Fiber	Sugar	Total Fat	Sat Fat	Sodium
Cactus, nopales, cooked	3 oz	13	1	3	2	1	0.0	0.0	17
Cactus, nopales, fresh	3 oz	14	1	3	2	1	0.1	0.0	18
Cardoon, fresh	3 oz	14	1	3	1	1	0.1	0.0	145
Carrots, cooked, drained	3 oz	30	1	7	3	3	0.2	0.0	49
Carrots, cooked from frozen, drained	3 oz	31	0	7	3	3	0.6	0.1	50
Carrots, cooked from frozen with salt, drained	3 oz	31	0	7	3	3	0.6	0.1	251
Carrots, cooked with salt, drained	3 oz	30	1	7	3	3	0.2	0.0	257
Carrots, fresh	3 oz	35	1	8	2	4	0.2	0.0	59
Carrots, fresh, baby	3 oz	30	1	7	2	4	0.1	0.0	66
Carrots, frozen	3 oz	31	1	7	3	4	0.4	0.0	58
Cassava, fresh	3 oz	136	1	32	2	1	0.2	0.1	12
Cattail, narrow leaf shoots, Northern Plains	3 oz	21	1	4	4	0	0.0	0.0	93
Cauliflower, cooked, drained	3 oz	20	2	3	2	2	0.4	0.1	13
Cauliflower, cooked from frozen, drained	3 oz	16	1	3	2	1	0.2	0.0	15
Cauliflower, cooked from frozen with salt, drained	3 oz	14	1	3	2	0	0.2	0.0	216
Cauliflower, cooked with salt, drained	3 oz	20	2	3	2	2	0.4	0.1	206
Cauliflower, fresh	3 oz	21	2	4	2	2	0.2	0.1	26
Cauliflower, frozen	3 oz	20	2	4	2	2	0.2	0.0	20
Cauliflower, green, fresh	3 oz	26	3	5	3	3	0.3	0.0	20
Celeriac, fresh	3 oz	36	1	8	2	1	0.3	0.1	85
Celery, fresh	3 oz	15	1	4	2	0	0.0	0.0	77
Chickory root, fresh	3 oz	61	1	15	1	7	0.2	0.0	43
Chile peppers, banana, fresh	1 oz	8	0	2	1	1	0.1	0.0	4
Chile peppers, green, hot, fresh	1 oz	12	1	3	0	2	0.1	0.0	2
Chili peppers, jalapeño, fresh	1 oz	9	0	2	1	1	0.2	0.0	0
Chile peppers, serrano, fresh	1 oz	10	1	2	1	1	0.1	0.0	3

VEGETABLES continued

Item	Serving Size	Calories	Protein	Carb	Fiber	Sugar	Total Fat	Sat Fat	Sodium
Chili peppers, red, hot, fresh	1 oz	12	1	3	0	2	0.1	0.0	3
Corn, white, steamed, Navajo	3 oz	328	8	64	14	5	4.4	0.7	3
Corn, white, sweet, cooked from frozen with salt, drained	3 oz	80	3	19	2	2	0.6	0.1	204
Corn, white, sweet, cooked from frozen, drained	3 oz	80	3	19	2	2	0.6	0.1	3
Corn, white, sweet, kernels	3 oz	73	3	16	2	3	1.0	0.2	13
Corn, white, sweet, kernels, cooked, drained	3 oz	82	3	18	2	7	1.2	0.2	3
Corn, white, sweet, kernels, cooked from frozen, drained	3 oz	68	2	17	2	3	0.4	0.1	4
Corn, white, sweet, kernels, cooked from frozen with salt, drained	3 oz	68	2	17	2	3	0.4	0.1	208
Corn, white, sweet, cooked with salt, drained	3 oz	82	3	18	2	7	1.2	0.2	215
Corn, yellow, sweet, kernels, cooked, drained	3 oz	82	3	18	2	4	1.3	0.2	1
Corn, yellow, sweet, cooked from frozen, drained	3 oz	79	3	19	2	3	0.6	0.1	3
Corn, yellow, sweet, kernels, cooked from frozen with salt, drained	3 oz	67	2	16	2	3	0.6	0.1	208
Corn, yellow, sweet, kernels, cooked with salt, drained	3 oz	82	3	18	2	4	1.3	0.2	215
Corn, yellow, sweet, kernels, fresh	3 oz	73	3	16	2	5	1.1	0.3	13
Corn, yellow, sweet, kernels, frozen	3 oz	83	3	20	2	3	0.7	0.1	4
Cucumber, fresh	3 oz	13	1	3	1	2	0.0	0.0	0

VEGETABLES continued

Item	Serving Size	Calories	Protein	Carb	Fiber	Sugar	Total Fat	Sat Fat	Sodium
Cucumber, with skin, fresh	3 oz	13	1	3	0	1	0.1	0.0	2
Cucumber, without skin, fresh	3 oz	10	1	2	1	1	0.1	0.0	2
Dasheen, cooked	3 oz	121	0	29	4	0	0.1	0.0	13
Dasheen, cooked with salt	3 oz	121	0	29	4	0	0.1	0.0	213
Dasheen, fresh	3 oz	95	1	22	3	0	0.2	0.0	9
Eggplant, cooked with salt, drained	3 oz	28	1	7	2	3	0.2	0.0	203
Eggplant, fresh	3 oz	20	1	5	3	2	0.2	0.0	2
Garlic, cloves, fresh	1 oz	45	2	10	1	0	0.2	0.0	5
Gobo root, cooked, drained	3 oz	75	2	18	2	3	0.1	0.0	3
Gobo root, fresh	3 oz	61	1	15	3	2	0.1	0.0	4
Gourd, wax, cooked, drained	3 oz	12	0	3	1	1	0.2	0.0	91
Greens, arugula, fresh	3 oz	21	2	3	1	2	0.6	0.1	23
Greens, balsam pear, cooked, drained	3 oz	29	3	6	2	1	0.2	0.0	11
Greens, bathua leaf, cooked with salt, drained	3 oz	27	3	4	2	1	0.6	0.0	225
Greens, bathua leaf, cooked, drained	3 oz	27	3	4	2	1	0.6	0.0	25
Greens, beet, cooked, drained	3 oz	23	2	5	2	1	0.2	0.0	205
Greens, beet, cooked with salt, drained	3 oz	23	2	5	2	1	0.2	0.0	405
Greens, beet, fresh	3 oz	19	2	4	3	0	0.1	0.0	192
Greens, ben oil tree, cooked, drained	3 oz	51	4	9	2	1	0.8	0.1	8
Greens, bitter cucumber, cooked, drained	3 oz	29	3	6	2	1	0.2	0.0	11
Greens, bitter gourd, cooked, drained	3 oz	29	3	6	2	1	0.2	0.0	11
Greens, bitter melon, cooked, drained	3 oz	29	3	6	2	1	0.2	0.0	11
Greens, chicory, fresh	3 oz	20	1	4	3	1	0.3	0.1	38
Greens, collard, cooked, drained	3 oz	22	2	4	2	0	0.3	0.0	14

VEGETABLES continued

Item	Serving Size	Calories	Protein	Carb	Fiber	Sugar	Total Fat	Sat Fat	Sodium
Greens, collard, cooked from frozen, drained	3 oz	31	3	6	2	0	0.3	0.1	43
Greens, collard, cooked from frozen with salt, drained	3 oz	31	3	6	2	0	0.3	0.0	243
Greens, collard, cooked with salt, drained	3 oz	22	2	4	2	0	0.3	0.0	214
Greens, collard, fresh	3 oz	26	2	5	3	0	0.4	0.1	17
Greens, curly endive, fresh	3 oz	14	1	3	3	0	0.2	0.0	19
Greens, dandelion, cooked, drained	3 oz	28	2	5	2	0	0.5	0.1	37
Greens, dandelion, fresh	3 oz	38	2	8	3	1	0.6	0.1	65
Greens, dasheen leaf, fresh	3 oz	36	4	6	3	3	0.6	0.1	3
Greens, drumstick tree, cooked, drained	3 oz	51	4	9	2	1	0.8	0.1	8
Greens, endive, fresh	3 oz	14	1	3	3	0	0.2	0.0	19
Greens, escarole, fresh	3 oz	14	1	3	3	0	0.2	0.0	19
Greens, garden cress, cooked, drained	3 oz	20	2	3	1	3	0.5	0.0	7
Greens, garden cress, cooked with salt, drained	3 oz	20	2	3	1	3	0.5	0.0	207
Greens, garden cress, fresh	3 oz	27	2	5	1	4	0.6	0.0	12
Greens, garland chrysanthemum, cooked, drained	3 oz	17	1	4	2	2	0.1	0.0	45
Greens, goosefoot, cooked, drained	3 oz	27	3	4	2	1	0.6	0.0	25
Greens, grape leaf, fresh	3 oz	79	5	15	9	5	1.8	0.3	8
Greens, horseradish tree, cooked, drained	3 oz	51	4	9	2	1	0.8	0.1	8
Greens, jute, cooked, drained	3 oz	31	3	6	2	1	0.2	0.0	9
Greens, jute, cooked with salt, drained	3 oz	31	3	6	2	1	0.2	0.0	210
Greens, karela, cooked, drained	3 oz	29	3	6	2	1	0.2	0.0	11
Greens, lambs quarters, cooked, drained	3 oz	27	3	4	2	1	0.6	0.0	25

VEGETABLES continued

Item	Serving Size	Calories	Protein	Carb	Fiber	Sugar	Total Fat	Sat Fat	Sodium
Greens, lambs quarters, cooked with salt, drained	3 oz	27	3	4	2	1	0.6	0.0	225
Greens, moringa, cooked, drained	3 oz	51	4	9	2	1	0.8	0.1	8
Greens, mustard, cooked, drained	3 oz	13	2	2	2	0	0.2	0.0	14
Greens, mustard, cooked from frozen, drained	3 oz	16	2	3	2	0	0.2	0.0	21
Greens, mustard, cooked from frozen with salt, drained	3 oz	16	2	3	2	0	0.2	0.0	222
Greens, mustard, cooked with salt, drained	3 oz	13	2	2	2	0	0.2	0.0	214
Greens, mustard, fresh	3 oz	22	2	4	3	1	0.2	0.0	21
Greens, pokeberry shoots, cooked, drained	3 oz	17	2	3	1	1	0.3	0.1	15
Greens, pumpkin, cooked, drained	3 oz	18	2	3	2	1	0.2	0.1	7
Greens, pumpkin, cooked with salt, drained	3 oz	18	2	3	2	1	0.2	0.1	207
Greens, radicchio, fresh	3 oz	20	1	4	1	1	0.2	0.1	19
Greens, red-leaf chicory, fresh	3 oz	20	1	4	1	1	0.2	0.1	19
Greens, silverbeet, cooked, drained	3 oz	17	2	4	2	1	0.1	0.0	152
Greens, silverbeet, fresh	3 oz	16	2	3	1	1	0.2	0.0	181
Greens, sweet potato, steamed	3 oz	29	2	6	2	5	0.3	0.1	11
Greens, sweet potato, steamed with salt	3 oz	29	2	6	2	5	0.3	0.1	212
Greens, Swiss chard, cooked, drained	3 oz	17	2	4	2	1	0.1	0.0	152
Greens, Swiss chard, fresh	3 oz	16	2	3	1	1	0.2	0.0	181
Greens, taro leaf, fresh	3 oz	36	4	6	3	3	0.6	0.1	3
Greens, turnip, cooked, drained	3 oz	17	1	4	3	0	0.2	0.0	25
Greens, turnip, cooked from frozen, drained	3 oz	25	3	4	3	1	0.4	0.1	13

VEGETABLES continued

Item	Serving Size	Calories	Protein	Carb	Fiber	Sugar	Total Fat	Sat Fat	Sodium
Greens, turnip, cooked from frozen with salt, drained	3 oz	25	3	4	3	1	0.4	0.1	213
Greens, turnip, cooked with salt, drained	3 oz	17	1	4	3	0	0.2	0.0	225
Greens, turnip, fresh	3 oz	27	1	6	3	1	0.3	0.1	34
Greens, watercress, fresh	3 oz	9	2	1	0	0	0.1	0.0	35
Hash browns, plain, prepared from frozen	3 oz	185	3	24	2	1	9.8	3.8	29
Jicama, fresh	3 oz	32	1	7	4	2	0.1	0.0	3
Kale, Chinese, cooked	3 oz	19	1	3	2	1	0.6	0.1	6
Lady's fingers, cooked, drained	3 oz	19	2	4	2	2	0.2	0.0	5
Lady's fingers, cooked from frozen, drained	3 oz	24	2	5	2	2	0.3	0.1	3
Lady's fingers, cooked from frozen with salt, drained	3 oz	24	2	5	2	2	0.3	0.1	203
Lady's fingers, cooked with salt, drained	3 oz	19	2	4	2	2	0.2	0.0	205
Lady's fingers, fresh	3 oz	26	2	6	3	1	0.1	0.0	7
Lady's fingers, frozen	3 oz	26	1	6	2	3	0.2	0.1	3
Leeks, bulb & lower leaf, cooked, drained	3 oz	26	1	6	1	2	0.2	0.0	9
Leeks, bulb & lower leaf, cooked with salt, drained	3 oz	26	1	6	1	2	0.2	0.0	209
Leeks, bulb & lower leaf, fresh	3 oz	52	1	12	2	3	0.3	0.0	17
Lettuce, bibb, fresh	3 oz	11	1	2	1	1	0.2	0.0	4
Lettuce, Boston, fresh	3 oz	11	1	2	1	1	0.2	0.0	4
Lettuce, butterhead, fresh	3 oz	11	1	2	1	1	0.2	0.0	4
Lettuce, crisphead, fresh	3 oz	12	1	3	1	2	0.1	0.0	9
Lettuce, green leaf, fresh	3 oz	13	1	2	1	1	0.1	0.0	24
Lettuce, iceberg, fresh	3 oz	12	1	3	1	2	0.1	0.0	9
Lettuce, romaine, fresh	3 oz	14	1	3	2	1	0.3	0.0	7
Lotus root, cooked, drained	3 oz	56	1	14	3	0	0.1	0.0	38
Manioc, fresh	3 oz	136	1	32	2	1	0.2	0.1	12

VEGETABLES continued

Item	Serving Size	Calories	Protein	Carb	Fiber	Sugar	Total Fat	Sat Fat	Sodium
Mushrooms, brown, fresh	3 oz	19	2	4	1	1	0.1	0.0	5
Mushrooms, cooked, drained	3 oz	24	2	4	2	2	0.4	0.1	2
Mushrooms, cooked with salt, drained	3 oz	24	2	4	2	2	0.4	0.1	202
Mushrooms, crimini, fresh	3 oz	19	2	4	1	1	0.1	0.0	5
Mushrooms, enoki, fresh	3 oz	31	2	7	2	0	0.2	0.0	3
Mushrooms, fresh	3 oz	19	3	3	1	2	0.3	0.0	4
Mushrooms, golden needle, fresh	3 oz	31	2	7	2	0	0.2	0.0	3
Mushrooms, hen of the woods, fresh	3 oz	26	2	6	2	2	0.2	0.0	1
Mushrooms, Italian, fresh	3 oz	19	2	4	1	1	0.1	0.0	5
Mushrooms, maitake, fresh	3 oz	26	2	6	2	2	0.2	0.0	1
Mushrooms, morel, fresh	3 oz	26	3	4	2	0	0.5	0.1	18
Mushrooms, oyster, fresh	3 oz	28	3	5	2	1	0.3	0.0	15
Mushrooms, portobella, sliced, grilled	3 oz	25	3	4	2	2	0.5	0.1	9
Mushrooms, ram's head, fresh	3 oz	26	2	6	2	2	0.2	0.0	1
Mushrooms, sheep's head, fresh	3 oz	26	2	6	2	2	0.2	0.0	1
Mushrooms, shiitake, cooked	3 oz	48	1	12	2	0	0.2	0.0	3
Mushrooms, shiitake, cooked with salt	3 oz	48	1	12	2	0	0.2	0.1	204
Mushrooms, shitake, sliced, stir-fried	3 oz	33	3	7	3	0	0.3	0.0	4
Mushrooms, white, microwaved	3 oz	30	3	5	2	0	0.4	0.1	14
Mushrooms, white, sliced, stir-fried	3 oz	22	3	3	2	0	0.3	0.0	10
Natto, fermented soybeans	3 oz	180	15	12	5	4	9.4	1.4	6
Okra, cooked, drained	3 oz	19	2	4	2	2	0.2	0.0	5
Okra, cooked from frozen, drained	3 oz	24	2	5	2	2	0.3	0.1	3
Okra, cooked from frozen with salt, drained	3 oz	24	2	5	2	2	0.3	0.1	203

VEGETABLES continued

Item	Serving Size	Calories	Protein	Carb	Fiber	Sugar	Total Fat	Sat Fat	Sodium
Okra, cooked with salt, drained	3 oz	19	2	4	2	2	0.2	0.0	205
Okra, fresh	3 oz	26	2	6	3	1	0.1	0.0	7
Okra, frozen	3 oz	26	1	6	2	3	0.2	0.1	3
Olives, black, canned	5 oz	161	1	9	4	0	15.0	2.0	1221
Olives, black, jumbo, canned	5 oz	113	1	8	4	0	9.6	1.3	1257
Olives, green, pickled, canned	1 oz	44	0	1	1	0	4.6	0.6	654
Onion, cooked from frozen, drained	3 oz	24	1	6	2	2	0.1	0.0	10
Onion, cooked with salt, drained	3 oz	36	1	8	1	4	0.2	0.0	203
Onion, green, tops & bulb, fresh	1 oz	10	1	2	1	1	0.1	0.0	5
Onion, green, tops only, fresh	1 oz	8	0	2	0	1	0.1	0.0	5
Onion, pearl, cooked, drained	3 oz	37	1	9	1	4	0.2	0.0	3
Onion, pearl, fresh	3 oz	34	1	8	1	4	0.1	0.0	3
Onion, red, cooked, drained	3 oz	37	1	9	1	4	0.2	0.0	3
Onion, red, fresh	3 oz	34	1	8	1	4	0.1	0.0	3
Onion, scallions, tops & bulb, fresh	1 oz	10	1	2	1	1	0.1	0.0	5
Onion, Vidalia, cooked, drained	3 oz	37	1	9	1	4	0.2	0.0	3
Onion, Vidalia, fresh	3 oz	34	1	8	1	4	0.1	0.0	3
Onion, Walla Walla, cooked, drained	3 oz	37	1	9	1	4	0.2	0.0	3
Onion, Walla Walla, fresh	3 oz	34	1	8	1	4	0.1	0.0	3
Onion, white, cooked, drained	3 oz	37	1	9	1	4	0.2	0.0	3
Onion, white, fresh	3 oz	34	1	8	1	4	0.1	0.0	3
Onion, whole, cooked from frozen, drained	3 oz	24	1	6	1	2	0.0	0.0	7
Onion, whole, cooked from frozen with salt, drained	3 oz	22	1	5	1	2	0.0	0.0	207
Onion, whole, frozen	3 oz	30	1	7	1	3	0.1	0.0	9

VEGETABLES continued

Item	Serving Size	Calories	Protein	Carb	Fiber	Sugar	Total Fat	Sat Fat	Sodium
Onion, yellow, cooked, drained	3 oz	37	1	9	1	4	0.2	0.0	3
Onion, yellow, fresh	3 oz	34	1	8	1	4	0.1	0.0	3
Palm hearts, fresh	3 oz	98	2	22	1	15	0.2	0.0	12
Parsnips, cooked with salt, drained	3 oz	60	1	14	3	4	0.3	0.0	209
Parsnips, fresh	3 oz	64	1	15	4	4	0.3	0.0	9
Peppers, bell, green, sweet, cooked, drained	3 oz	24	1	6	1	3	0.2	0.0	2
Peppers, bell, green, sweet, cooked with salt, drained	3 oz	22	1	5	1	3	0.2	0.0	202
Potatoes, microwaved in skin, peeled, salted	3 oz	85	2	20	1	2	0.1	0.0	207
Potatoes, peeled, cooked	3 oz	73	1	17	2	1	0.1	0.0	4
Potatoes, peeled, cooked with salt	3 oz	73	1	17	2	1	0.1	0.0	205
Potatoes, red, with skin, baked	3 oz	76	2	17	2	1	0.1	0.0	10
Potatoes, roasted	3 oz	120	3	27	2	2	0.2	0.0	9
Potatoes, russet, with skin, baked	3 oz	82	2	18	2	1	0.1	0.0	12
Potatoes, skin, baked	3 oz	168	4	39	7	1	0.1	0.0	18
Potatoes, skin, baked with salt	3 oz	168	4	39	7	1	0.1	0.0	218
Potatoes, skin, from cooked potato	3 oz	66	2	15	3	1	0.1	0.0	12
Potatoes, skin, from cooked potato, salted	3 oz	66	2	15	3	1	0.1	0.0	213
Potatoes, skin, from microwaved potato	3 oz	112	4	25	5	1	0.1	0.0	14
Potatoes, skin, from microwaved potato, salted	3 oz	112	4	25	5	1	0.1	0.0	214
Pumpkin, cooked, drained	3 oz	17	1	4	1	1	0.1	0.0	1
Radishes, daikon, cooked with salt, drained	3 oz	14	1	3	1	2	0.2	0.1	212
Radishes, fresh	3 oz	14	1	3	1	2	0.1	0.0	33

VEGETABLES continued

Item	Serving Size	Calories	Protein	Carb	Fiber	Sugar	Total Fat	Sat Fat	Sodium
Radishes, icicle, cooked with salt, drained	3 oz	14	1	3	1	2	0.2	0.1	212
Radishes, Oriental, cooked, drained	3 oz	14	1	3	1	2	0.2	0.1	11
Radishes, wasabi, cooked with salt, drained	3 oz	14	1	3	1	2	0.2	0.1	212
Rutabaga, cooked, drained	3 oz	33	1	7	2	5	0.2	0.0	17
Rutabaga, fresh	3 oz	31	1	7	2	5	0.2	0.0	17
Salsify, cooked, drained	3 oz	58	2	13	3	2	0.1	0.0	14
Seaweed, agar, fresh	3 oz	22	0	6	0	0	0.0	0.0	8
Seaweed, carrageen, fresh	3 oz	42	1	10	1	1	0.1	0.0	57
Seaweed, Irish moss, fresh	3 oz	42	1	10	1	1	0.1	0.0	57
Seaweed, kelp, fresh	3 oz	37	1	8	1	1	0.5	0.2	198
Seaweed, laver, fresh	3 oz	30	5	4	0	0	0.2	0.1	41
Seaweed, oarweed, fresh	3 oz	37	1	8	1	1	0.5	0.2	198
Seaweed, wakame, fresh	3 oz	38	3	8	0	1	0.5	0.1	741
Spinach, cooked, drained	3 oz	20	3	3	2	0	0.2	0.0	60
Spinach, cooked from frozen, drained	3 oz	29	3	4	3	0	0.7	0.1	82
Spinach, cooked from frozen with salt	3 oz	29	3	4	3	0	0.7	0.0	274
Spinach, cooked with salt, drained	3 oz	20	3	3	2	0	0.2	0.0	260
Spinach, fresh	3 oz	20	2	3	2	0	0.3	0.1	67
Spinach, leaf, frozen	3 oz	25	3	4	2	1	0.5	0.0	63
Squash, acorn, baked with salt	3 oz	48	1	12	4	3	0.1	0.0	204
Squash, acorn, cooked with salt	3 oz	29	1	7	2	3	0.1	0.0	203
Squash, acorn, fresh	3 oz	34	1	9	1	2	0.1	0.0	3
Squash, bitter cucumber, cooked, drained	3 oz	16	1	4	2	2	0.2	0.0	5
Squash, bitter gourd, cooked, drained	3 oz	16	1	4	2	2	0.2	0.0	5
Squash, bitter melon, cooked, drained	3 oz	16	1	4	2	2	0.2	0.0	5
Squash, brionne, fresh	3 oz	16	1	4	1	1	0.1	0.0	2

VEGETABLES continued

Item	Serving Size	Calories	Protein	Carb	Fiber	Sugar	Total Fat	Sat Fat	Sodium
Squash, butternut, baked with salt	3 oz	34	1	9	3	2	0.1	0.0	204
Squash, butternut, cooked from frozen with salt	3 oz	33	1	9	3	3	0.1	0.0	202
Squash, butternut, fresh	3 oz	38	1	10	2	2	0.1	0.0	3
Squash, crookneck, cooked from frozen, drained	3 oz	21	1	5	1	2	0.2	0.0	5
Squash, crookneck, cooked from frozen with salt, drained	3 oz	21	1	5	1	2	0.2	0.0	206
Squash, crookneck, fresh	3 oz	16	1	3	1	3	0.2	0.1	2
Squash, hubbard, baked with salt	3 oz	43	2	9	2	2	0.5	0.1	207
Squash, hubbard, cooked	3 oz	26	1	5	2	2	0.3	0.1	4
Squash, mango, fresh	3 oz	16	1	4	1	1	0.1	0.0	2
Squash, scallop, cooked, drained	3 oz	14	1	3	2	1	0.1	0.0	1
Squash, scallop, cooked with salt, drained	3 oz	14	1	3	2	1	0.1	0.0	201
Squash, spaghetti, baked or cooked, drained	3 oz	23	1	5	1	2	0.2	0.1	15
Squash, spaghetti, baked with salt, drained	3 oz	23	1	5	1	2	0.2	0.1	216
Squash, straightneck, cooked, drained	3 oz	20	1	3	1	2	0.3	0.1	1
Squash, straightneck, cooked from frozen, drained	3 oz	21	1	5	1	2	0.2	0.0	5
Squash, straightneck, cooked from frozen with salt, drained	3 oz	21	1	5	1	2	0.2	0.0	206
Squash, straightneck, cooked with salt, drained	3 oz	16	1	3	1	2	0.3	0.1	201
Squash, straightneck, fresh	3 oz	16	1	3	1	3	0.2	0.1	2
Squash, summer, all types, cooked, drained	3 oz	17	1	4	1	2	0.3	0.1	1

VEGETABLES continued

Item	Serving Size	Calories	Protein	Carb	Fiber	Sugar	Total Fat	Sat Fat	Sodium
Squash, summer, all types, cooked with salt, drained	3 oz	17	1	4	1	2	0.3	0.1	201
Squash, summer, all types, fresh	3 oz	14	1	3	1	2	0.2	0.0	2
Squash, vegetable pear, fresh	3 oz	16	1	4	1	1	0.1	0.0	2
Squash, winter, all types, baked	3 oz	31	1	8	2	3	0.3	0.1	1
Squash, winter, all types, baked with salt	3 oz	33	1	7	2	3	0.5	0.1	201
Squash, winter, all types, fresh	3 oz	29	1	7	1	2	0.1	0.0	3
Squash, xoxo, fresh	3 oz	16	1	4	1	1	0.1	0.0	2
Squash, zucchini, with skin, cooked, drained	3 oz	13	1	2	1	2	0.3	0.1	3
Squash, zucchini, with skin, cooked from frozen, drained	3 oz	14	1	3	1	1	0.1	0.0	2
Squash, zucchini, with skin, cooked from frozen with salt, drained	3 oz	12	1	3	1	1	0.1	0.0	202
Squash, zucchini, with skin, cooked with salt, drained	3 oz	13	1	2	1	2	0.3	0.1	203
Squash, zucchini, with skin, fresh	3 oz	14	1	3	1	2	0.3	0.1	7
Squash, zucchini, with skin, frozen	3 oz	14	1	3	1	1	0.1	0.0	2
Sweet potatoes, dark orange, baked from frozen	3 oz	85	1	20	2	8	0.1	0.0	7
Sweet potatoes, dark orange, baked from frozen with salt	3 oz	85	1	20	2	10	0.1	0.0	207
Sweet potatoes, dark orange, baked in skin, peeled	3 oz	77	2	18	3	6	0.1	0.0	31

VEGETABLES continued

Item	Serving Size	Calories	Protein	Carb	Fiber	Sugar	Total Fat	Sat Fat	Sodium
Sweet potatoes, dark orange, baked in skin with salt	3 oz	78	2	18	3	9	0.1	0.0	209
Sweet potatoes, dark orange, cooked without skin	3 oz	65	1	15	2	5	0.1	0.0	23
Sweet potatoes, dark orange, fresh	3 oz	73	1	17	3	4	0.0	0.0	47
Sweet potatoes, dark orange, peeled, cooked with salt	3 oz	65	1	15	2	5	0.1	0.0	224
Takenoko, fresh	3 oz	23	2	4	2	3	0.3	0.1	3
Taro, cooked	3 oz	121	0	29	4	0	0.1	0.0	13
Taro, cooked with salt	3 oz	121	0	29	4	0	0.1	0.0	213
Taro, fresh	3 oz	95	1	22	3	0	0.2	0.0	9
Tomatillo, fresh	3 oz	27	1	5	2	3	0.9	0.1	1
Tomatoes, green, cooked, fried	3 oz	168	3	11	1	3	12.8	2.7	79
Tomatoes, green, fresh	3 oz	20	1	4	1	3	0.2	0.0	11
Tomatoes, Italian/plum, fresh	3 oz	15	1	3	1	2	0.2	0.0	4
Tomatoes, red, cherry, fresh	3 oz	15	1	3	1	2	0.2	0.0	4
Tomatoes, red, cooked from fresh	3 oz	15	1	3	1	2	0.1	0.0	9
Tomatoes, red, cooked with salt	3 oz	15	1	3	1	2	0.1	0.0	210
Tomatoes, red, fried	3 oz	142	2	10	1	7	10.7	2.3	65
Tomatoes, roma, fresh, year-round average, fresh	3 oz	15	1	3	1	2	0.2	0.0	4
Tung sun, fresh	3 oz	23	2	4	2	3	0.3	0.1	3
Turnips, cooked, drained	3 oz	19	1	4	2	3	0.1	0.0	14
Turnips, cooked from frozen, drained	3 oz	20	1	4	2	2	0.2	0.0	31
Turnips, cooked from frozen with salt, drained	3 oz	18	1	3	2	1	0.2	0.0	231
Turnips, cooked with salt, drained	3 oz	19	1	4	2	3	0.1	0.0	243
Turnips, fresh	3 oz	24	1	5	2	3	0.1	0.0	57

VEGETABLES continued

Item	Serving Size	Calories	Protein	Carb	Fiber	Sugar	Total Fat	Sat Fat	Sodium
Turnips, with greens, cooked from frozen, drained	3 oz	30	3	4	3	1	0.3	0.1	16
Turnips, with greens, cooked from frozen with salt, drained	3 oz	29	3	4	3	1	0.3	0.1	217
Vegetable oyster, cooked, drained	3 oz	58	2	13	3	2	0.1	0.0	14
Vegetables, cooked from frozen, drained	3 oz	55	2	11	4	3	0.1	0.0	30
Vegetables, cooked from frozen with salt, drained	3 oz	51	2	11	4	3	0.1	0.0	230
Vegetables, peas & carrots, cooked from frozen, drained	3 oz	41	3	9	3	4	0.4	0.1	58
Vegetables, peas & carrots, cooked from frozen with salt, drained	3 oz	41	3	9	3	4	0.4	0.1	258
Vegetables, peas & onions, cooked from frozen, drained	3 oz	38	2	7	2	3	0.2	0.0	31
Vegetables, peas & onions, cooked from frozen with salt, drained	3 oz	38	2	7	2	3	0.2	0.0	232
Water chestnuts, Matai, fresh	3 oz	82	1	20	3	4	0.1	0.0	12
Yams, domestic, baked from frozen	3 oz	85	1	20	2	8	0.1	0.0	7
Yams, domestic, baked from frozen with salt	3 oz	85	1	20	2	10	0.1	0.0	207
Yams, domestic, baked in skin, peeled	3 oz	77	2	18	3	6	0.1	0.0	31
Yams, domestic, baked in skin with salt	3 oz	78	2	18	3	9	0.1	0.0	209

VEGETABLES continued

Item	Serving Size	Calories	Protein	Carb	Fiber	Sugar	Total Fat	Sat Fat	Sodium
Yams, domestic, cooked without skin	3 oz	65	1	15	2	5	0.1	0.0	23
Yams, domestic, fresh	3 oz	73	1	17	3	4	0.0	0.0	47
Yams, domestic, peeled, cooked with salt	3 oz	65	1	15	2	5	0.1	0.0	224
Yams, tropical, cooked/baked	3 oz	99	1	23	3	0	0.1	0.0	7
Yams, tropical, cooked/baked with salt, drained	3 oz	97	1	23	3	0	0.1	0.0	207
Yams, tropical, fresh	3 oz	100	1	24	3	0	0.1	0.0	8
Yellow pond lily, tuber, cooked, Pacific Northwest	3 oz	29	1	6	2	0	0.3	0.0	9
Yuca, fresh	3 oz	136	1	32	2	1	0.2	0.1	12

dining out

APPLEBEE'S

Item	Serving Size	Calories	Protein	Carb	Fiber	Sugar	Total Fat	Sat Fat	Sodium
ENTRÉES									
Asiago Peppercorn Steak	as served	390	43	26	5	n/a	14.0	6.0	1520
Asian Crunch Salad	as served	490	51	57	7	n/a	9.0	1.0	3170
Bourbon Street Steak	as served	700	54	31	4	n/a	41.0	10.0	2310
Grilled Dijon Chicken & Portobellos	as served	450	54	32	6	n/a	16.0	6.0	1810
Grilled Shrimp & Island Rice	as served	380	29	59	6	n/a	4.5	1.0	2370
Sizzling Asian Shrimp	as served	710	30	117	7	n/a	15.0	3.0	3830
Sizzling Chicken with Spicy Queso Blanco	as served	550	53	37	6	n/a	22.0	8.0	2500
Sizzling Skillet Fajitas, chicken	as served	1150	72	103	10	n/a	50.0	22.0	4570
Sizzling Skillet Fajitas, shrimp	as served	1040	47	104	10	n/a	49.0	22.0	4840
Sizzling Skillet Fajitas, steak	as served	1180	72	105	10	n/a	53.0	24.0	5330
Sizzling Steak & Cheese	as served	1070	67	54	7	n/a	65.0	22.0	3430
Spicy Shrimp Diavolo	as served	500	32	79	12	n/a	10.0	3.5	1910
SALADS									
Apple Walnut Chicken Salad	as served	1000	55	53	6	n/a	65.0	16.0	1670
Asian Crunch Salad	as served	490	51	57	7	n/a	9.0	1.0	3170
California Shrimp Salad	as served	730	32	21	8	n/a	61.0	11.0	2080
Crispy Shrimp Caesar	as served	1060	33	57	7	n/a	78.0	15.0	2270
Fried Chicken Salad	as served	1060	47	49	6	n/a	75.0	21.0	2130
Grilled Chicken Caesar	as served	820	54	25	6	n/a	57.0	11.0	1640
Grilled Shrimp 'n' Spinach	as served	1050	50	68	13	n/a	72.0	11.0	2530
Grilled Steak Caesar	as served	900	54	25	6	n/a	66.0	15.0	1860
Oriental Chicken Salad	as served	1310	34	88	11	n/a	93.0	15.0	1470
Oriental Grilled Chicken Salad	as served	1240	53	87	9	n/a	77.0	12.0	2000

APPLEBEE'S continued

Item	Serving Size	Calories	Protein	Carb	Fiber	Sugar	Total Fat	Sat Fat	Sodium
Pecan-Crusted Chicken Salad	as served	1340	46	108	14	n/a	81.0	17.0	2600
Santa Fe Chicken Salad	as served	1300	60	58	11	n/a	94.0	25.0	3540
Weight Watchers® Paradise Chicken Salad	as served	340	45	35	6	n/a	4.5	1.0	2060

ARBY'S

Item	Serving Size	Calories	Protein	Carb	Fiber	Sugar	Total Fat	Sat Fat	Sodium
SANDWICHES & SUBS									
All-American Roastburger®	1	390	19	40	2	10	16.0	5.0	1720
Arby's Melt	1	320	18	38	2	6	11.0	3.5	900
Bacon & Bleu Roastburger®	1	450	24	39	2	9	21.0	7.0	1750
Bacon Cheddar Roastburger®	1	430	26	39	2	8	18.0	8.0	1810
Chicken Bacon & Swiss, Roasted	1	470	32	43	3	10	19.0	6.0	1380
Chicken Cordon Bleu, Roasted	1	490	35	40	3	8	20.0	5.0	1670
Ham & Swiss Melt	1	131	6	35	37	2	70.0	8.0	1070
Pecan Chicken Salad Sandwich	1	830	30	82	6	22	44.0	6.0	1390
Regular Beef 'n' Cheddar	1	430	23	42	2	10	19.0	6.0	1220
Regular Roast Beef	1	350	23	37	2	5	13.0	4.5	960
Reuben Sandwich	1	690	36	65	4	7	32.0	9.0	2050
Roast Beef Gyro	1	420	20	32	2	3	23.0	6.0	1030
Roast Beef Patty Melt	1	470	26	44	3	5	22.0	6.0	1790
Roast Beef & Swiss Sandwich	1	780	39	78	5	17	37.0	11.0	1700
Roast Chicken Club	1	500	31	38	2	8	23.0	7.0	1370
Roast Chicken Ranch Sandwich	1	360	26	42	3	5	10.0	1.5	1030

ARBY'S continued

Item	Serving Size	Calories	Protein	Carb	Fiber	Sugar	Total Fat	Sat Fat	Sodium
Roast Ham & Swiss Sandwich	1	710	37	79	5	19	30.0	7.0	2030
Roast Turkey & Swiss Sandwich	1	710	41	78	5	18	28.0	7.0	1790
Roast Turkey, Ranch & Bacon Sandwich	1	820	48	78	6	18	36.0	10.0	2270
Super Roast Beef	1	430	24	44	3	11	18.0	6.0	1070
Ultimate BLT Sandwich	1	850	34	78	6	18	46.0	10.0	1680
Classic Italian Toasted Sub	1	590	24	57	3	5	30.0	8.0	1870
French Dip & Swiss Toasted Sub Au Jus	1	500	29	59	2	2	17.0	7.0	2080
Philly Beef Toasted Sub	1	570	29	55	3	3	27.0	8.0	1490
Turkey Bacon Club Toasted Sub	1	570	33	56	3	4	24.0	6.0	1700

SIDES & SALADS

Item	Serving Size	Calories	Protein	Carb	Fiber	Sugar	Total Fat	Sat Fat	Sodium
Chopped Farmhouse Chicken Salad	1	460	32	29	4	5	25.0	9.0	1090
Chopped Farmhouse Salad: Turkey and Ham	1	250	23	9	3	5	14.0	7.0	900
Chopped Side Salad	1	70	4	4	1	2	5.0	3.0	100
Crispy Chicken Tenders	regular	360	23	28	2	0	17.0	2.5	730
Curly Fries	small	410	5	48	5	0	22.0	3.0	920
Homestyle Fries	small	350	4	49	4	0	15.0	2.0	720
Jalapeño Bites®	regular	300	5	32	2	2	17.0	7.0	640
Loaded Potato Bites®	regular	340	10	29	2	1	20.0	6.0	760
Mozzarella Sticks	regular	430	20	36	2	3	23.0	9.0	1480
Onion Petals	regular	330	4	38	2	7	18.0	2.5	280
Popcorn Chicken	regular	360	26	27	2	0	16.0	2.5	980
Potato Cakes	small	260	2	16	2	0	14.0	2.0	440

AUNTIE ANNIE'S

Item	Serving Size	Calories	Protein	Carb	Fiber	Sugar	Total Fat	Sat Fat	Sodium
Cinnamon sugar, soft pretzel, without butter	1	350	9	74	2	16	2.0	0.0	410
Garlic, soft pretzel, without butter	1	320	9	66	2	9	1.0	0.0	830
Glazin' Raisin, soft pretzel, without butter	1	470	11	104	3	37	0.5	0.0	460
Jalapeño, soft pretzel, without butter	1	270	8	58	2	8	1.0	0.0	780
Kidstix, soft pretzel, without butter	4	227	7	48	2	7	1.0	0.0	600
Original, soft pretzel, without butter	1	340	10	72	3	10	1.0	0.0	900
Sesame, soft pretzel, without butter	1	350	11	63	3	9	6.0	1.0	840
Wwhole wheat, soft pretzel, without butter	1	350	11	72	7	10	1.5	0.0	1100

BAJA FRESH

Item	Serving Size	Calories	Protein	Carb	Fiber	Sugar	Total Fat	Sat Fat	Sodium
BURRITOS									
Bean and cheese	1 order	840	39	96	n/a	n/a	33.0	17.0	1790
Bean and cheese with chicken	1 order	970	67	96	n/a	n/a	35.0	18.0	2230
Bean and cheese with grilled veggie	1 order	800	32	94	n/a	n/a	33.0	17.0	1880
Bean and cheese with mahimahi	1 order	960	65	96	n/a	n/a	35.0	18.0	1930
Bean and cheese with pork carnitas	1 order	1010	59	98	n/a	n/a	42.0	20.0	2370
Bean and cheese with shrimp	1 order	950	61	96	n/a	n/a	34.0	17.0	2320
Bean and cheese with steak	1 order	1030	64	97	n/a	n/a	43.0	21.0	2350
QUESADILLAS									
Chicken	1 order	1330	75	84	n/a	n/a	80.0	37.0	2590
Cheese	1 order	1200	47	84	n/a	n/a	78.0	37.0	2140
Veggie	1 order	1260	48	96	n/a	n/a	78.0	37.0	2310

BAJA FRESH continued

Item	Serving Size	Calories	Protein	Carb	Fiber	Sugar	Total Fat	Sat Fat	Sodium
SIDES									
Cheese nachos	1 order	1890	63	163	n/a	n/a	108.0	40.0	2530
Chicken nachos	1 order	2020	91	164	n/a	n/a	110.0	41.0	2980
Chips with guacamole	1 order	1340	21	141	n/a	n/a	83.0	8.0	950
Chips with Baja salsa	1 order	810	13	98	n/a	n/a	37.0	4.0	1140
Tostada salad with beans	1 order	1010	32	98	n/a	n/a	53.0	13.0	1930
Tostada salad with chicken	1 order	1140	60	98	n/a	n/a	55.0	14.0	2370
Tostada salad with steak	1 order	1230	65	98	n/a	n/a	63.0	17.0	2380
TACOS									
Americano chicken, soft	1 order	230	16	20	n/a	n/a	10.0	4.5	590
Americano mahimahi, soft	1 order	240	17	20	n/a	n/a	10.0	4.5	490
Americano pork carnitas, soft	1 order	250	13	21	n/a	n/a	12.0	5.0	640
Americano shrimp, soft	1 order	230	15	21	n/a	n/a	10.0	4.5	640
Americano steak, soft	1 order	260	15	21	n/a	n/a	13.0	6.0	640
Baja pork carnitas	1 order	220	10	29	n/a	n/a	7.0	2.0	280
Baja shrimp	1 order	200	11	28	n/a	n/a	5.0	1.0	280
Baja steak	1 order	230	11	28	n/a	n/a	8.0	2.0	260

BASKIN ROBBINS

Item	Serving Size	Calories	Protein	Carb	Fiber	Sugar	Total Fat	Sat Fat	Sodium
ICE CREAMS, SORBETS, & FROZEN YOGURTS									
Butter almond crunch reduced fat ice cream	2.5 oz	140	4	19	3	4	7.0	3.0	90
Butter pecan, old-fashioned ice cream	2.5 oz	170	3	15	1	14	11.0	6.0	60
Chocolate chip cookie dough ice cream	2.5 oz	180	3	22	0	19	9.0	6.0	80

BASKIN ROBBINS continued

Item	Serving Size	Calories	Protein	Carb	Fiber	Sugar	Total Fat	Sat Fat	Sodium
Fat-free vanilla frozen yogurt	2.5 oz	90	4	20	0	19	0.0	0.0	65
Lemon blueberry frozen yogurt	2.5 oz	120	3	21	0	19	3.5	2.5	45
Lemon sorbet	2.5 oz	80	0	21	0	20	0.0	0.0	10
Pink grapefruit sorbet	2.5 oz	80	0	21	0	20	0.0	0.0	10
Premium churned light aloha brownie ice cream	2.5 oz	150	3	26	1	21	5.0	3.0	95
Premium churned light cappuccino chip ice cream	2.5 oz	140	3	20	1	18	5.0	2.5	70
Premium churned light dulce de leche ice cream	2.5 oz	140	3	24	0	22	4.5	3.0	90
Premium churned reduced fat, no-sugar-added cabana berry banana ice cream	2.5 oz	90	3	17	2	4	3.5	2.0	45
Premium churned reduced fat, no-sugar-added caramel turtle truffle ice cream	2.5 oz	120	3	24	2	4	5.0	3.5	75
Rocky road ice cream	2.5 oz	180	3	22	0	20	10.0	5.0	75
Strawberry sorbet	2.5 oz	80	0	21	0	21	0.0	0.0	5
Vanilla pomegranate parfait frozen yogurt	2.5 oz	150	3	23	0	19	5.0	3.5	55

BLIMPIE

Item	Serving Size	Calories	Protein	Carb	Fiber	Sugar	Total Fat	Sat Fat	Sodium
SUBS & WRAPS									
Blimpie Best	6"	450	24	49	3	10	17.0	6.0	1330
BLT	6"	430	15	43	2	6	22.0	5.0	960
Chicken Caesar wrap	1	560	30	56	4	5	24.0	8.0	1480
Chicken Cheddar Bacon Ranch	6"	600	36	48	3	8	29.0	10.0	1570
Chicken Teriyaki	6"	450	33	52	2	13	12.0	5.0	1280
Club	6"	410	23	49	3	9	13.0	4.0	1050
Cuban	6"	410	29	43	1	6	11.0	4.5	1630

BLIMPIE continued

Item	Serving Size	Calories	Protein	Carb	Fiber	Sugar	Total Fat	Sat Fat	Sodium
French Dip	6"	410	30	46	1	3	11.0	5.0	1650
Ham, Salami and Provolone	6"	470	24	49	3	9	20.0	7.0	1270
Ham and American Cheese Kids' sub	3"	260	14	32	2	6	8.0	4.5	900
Ham and Swiss	6"	420	23	49	3	10	14.0	4.5	1020
Hot Pastrami	6"	430	30	42	1	5	16.0	7.0	1350
Meatball	6"	580	27	50	4	6	31.0	13.0	1960
Philly Steak and Onion	6"	600	25	46	1	7	35.0	11.0	1410
Reuben	6"	530	34	52	3	7	20.0	6.0	1740
Roast Beef and Provolone	6"	430	28	46	3	7	14.0	5.0	980
Special Vegetarian (Doritos Sub)	6"	590	16	66	4	10	30.0	9.0	1170
Southwestern wrap	1	530	23	61	4	10	22.0	6.0	1770
Tuna	6"	470	24	43	2	5	21.0	3.0	770
Tuna Kids' sub	3"	280	14	30	2	4	11.0	1.5	460
Turkey and Avocado	6"	360	21	51	4	8	7.0	1.0	1340
Turkey and Cranberry	6"	350	20	58	3	14	4.0	0.5	1220
Turkey and Provolone	6"	410	24	49	3	8	13.0	4.0	1310
Turkey Kids' sub	3"	190	10	31	2	5	2.5	0.0	600
Veggie and Cheese	6"	460	19	50	3	9	21.0	9.0	1420
Veggie Supreme	6"	550	26	50	3	9	27.0	13.0	1500
VegiMax	6"	520	28	56	5	8	20.0	6.0	1270

BOSTON MARKET

Item	Serving Size	Calories	Protein	Carb	Fiber	Sugar	Total Fat	Sat Fat	Sodium

DESSERTS

Item	Serving Size	Calories	Protein	Carb	Fiber	Sugar	Total Fat	Sat Fat	Sodium
Apple cinnamon pie	1 slice	550	4	66	3	16	31.0	13.0	690
Brownie	1 order	580	9	88	6	65	23.0	5.0	350
Chocolate cake	1 slice	650	4	86	2	68	32.0	8.0	320
Chocolate chip cookie	1 order	390	4	51	2	28	19.0	10.0	340
Hot apples with cinnamon	1 order	250	0	56	3	49	4.5	0.5	45

BOSTON MARKET continued

Item	Serving Size	Calories	Protein	Carb	Fiber	Sugar	Total Fat	Sat Fat	Sodium
ENTRÉES & SANDWICHES									
Chicken, dark meat, without skin, rotisserie garlic	1/4 chicken	190	22	1	0	1	10.0	3.0	440
Chicken and queso sandwich	1	550	38	62	3	5	21.0	7.0	1590
Chicken Carver sandwich, with cheese and sauce	1	640	38	61	4	13	29.0	7.0	980
Chicken with skin, rotisserie garlic	1/2 chicken	590	70	4	0	4	33.0	10.0	1010
Chicken pot pie	as served	750	26	57	2	4	46.0	14.0	1530
Country chicken, crispy baked	as served	420	26	31	5	1	22.0	5.0	880
Lean pork ham, honey-glazed	as served	210	24	10	0	10	8.0	3.0	1460
Marinated grilled chicken sandwich	1	670	42	45	2	5	36.0	6.0	810
Meatloaf, double sauce Angus	as served	310	22	16	1	9	19.0	8.0	650
Meatloaf Carver sandwich, with cheese	1	730	39	85	5	18	29.0	12.0	1590
Turkey, breast, without skin, low fat, rotisserie	as served	170	36	3	0	3	1.0	0.0	850
Turkey Carver sandwich, with cheese and sauce	1	630	40	64	4	14	26.0	7.0	1350
SIDES									
Asian grilled chicken salad, with dressing and noodles	1	570	39	56	8	44	19.0	3.5	1810
Caesar salad, entrée-size	1	470	14	17	3	3	40.0	9.0	1070
Caesar salad, side	1	300	5	13	1	2	26.0	4.5	960
Chicken gravy	as served	15	0	2	0	0	0.5	0.0	180
Cornbread	1 piece	200	3	33	1	13	6.0	1.5	390
Creamed spinach	as served	260	9	11	2	2	20.0	13.0	740
Macaroni & cheese	as served	280	13	33	1	8	11.0	7.0	1100
Mashed potatoes with gravy, homestyle	as served	230	4	32	3	4	9.0	5.0	780

BOSTON MARKET continued

Item	Serving Size	Calories	Protein	Carb	Fiber	Sugar	Total Fat	Sat Fat	Sodium
Potato salad, homestyle	as served	200	3	22	2	5	12.0	2.0	440
Rice pilaf with vegetables	as served	140	2	24	1	2	4.0	0.5	520
Sesame broccoli	as served	80	3	13	2	10	2.5	0.0	390
Squash, butternut	as served	150	2	25	6	12	6.0	4.0	560
Steamed vegetables	as served	30	2	6	2	2	0.0	0.0	135
Stuffing, savory	as served	190	4	27	2	5	8.0	1.5	620
Tomato bisque soup	as served	380	6	25	4	11	29.0	13.0	1660
Tortilla soup, with toppings	as served	170	8	18	2	2	8.0	2.5	1060

BRUEGGER'S

Item	Serving Size	Calories	Protein	Carb	Fiber	Sugar	Total Fat	Sat Fat	Sodium
BAGELS, BREADS, & WRAPS									
Asiago Parmesan, bagel	1	330	14	61	4	7	4.0	1.0	730
Bagel bowl	1	720	30	136	8	22	9.0	3.0	152
Baked apple, bagel	1	320	10	67	5	18	2.0	0.0	510
Blueberry, bagel	1	14	500	62	3	310	2.0	0.0	500
Chocolate chip, bagel	1	330	10	65	3	18	3.5	2.0	470
Ciabatta	1	250	9	48	2	2	2.5	0.0	730
Cinnamon raisin, bagel	1	310	11	65	4	10	2.0	0.0	480
Cinnamon sugar, bagel	1	320	14	63	4	13	2.0	0.0	420
Cranberry orange, bagel	1	310	10	64	4	16	2.0	0.0	480
Egg, bagel	1	310	11	63	4	10	2.5	0.0	530
Everything, bagel	1	310	12	62	4	7	2.5	0.0	710
Fortified multigrain, bagel	1	340	12	66	6	10	2.5	0.0	500
Garlic, bagel	1	300	12	61	4	7	2.0	0.0	520
Hearty white, slice	2	260	10	54	2	2	1.0	0.0	620
Honey grain, bagel	1	310	11	61	4	10	2.5	0.0	490
Honey wheat, slice	2	280	12	54	2	6	3.0	0.0	520
Jalapeño, bagel	1	310	12	62	4	7	2.0	0.0	530
Onion, bagel	1	300	12	61	4	8	2.0	0.0	530
Plain, bagel	1	300	12	60	4	7	2.0	0.0	530

BRUEGGER'S continued

Item	Serving Size	Calories	Protein	Carb	Fiber	Sugar	Total Fat	Sat Fat	Sodium
Poppy, bagel	1	310	12	61	4	7	2.5	0.0	610
Pumpernickel, bagel	1	300	11	62	4	10	2.0	0.0	560
Rosemary olive oil, bagel	1	330	11	59	4	8	6.0	0.5	510
Rye, bagel	1	330	11	59	5	8	2.0	0.0	560
Salt, bagel	1	300	12	61	4	7	2.0	0.0	1540
Sesame, bagel	1	310	12	60	4	7	3.0	0.0	610
Sourdough, bagel	1	290	11	56	4	7	2.0	0.0	540
Square asiago Parmesan, bagel	1	360	15	68	4	11	4.5	1.5	76
Square everything, bagel	1	350	12	64	4	8	2.0	0.0	740
Square plain, bagel	1	330	12	67	4	11	2.5	0.0	640
Square sesame, bagel	1	370	14	70	4	11	3.5	0.0	690
Sundried tomato, bagel	1	280	10	57	4	10	2.0	0.0	550
White wrap	1	180	6	32	3	1	1.5	1.0	420
Whole wheat, bagel	1	300	13	56	5	10	3.5	0.0	670

SWEETS

Item	Serving Size	Calories	Protein	Carb	Fiber	Sugar	Total Fat	Sat Fat	Sodium
Banana nut muffin	1	450	5	50	2	24	26.0	4.0	379
Blueberry muffin	1	430	5	53	1	30	22.0	3.5	310
Cappuccino muffin	1	490	6	60	1	34	26.0	5.0	340
Chocolate chip cookie	1	390	5	52	2	32	17.0	8.0	150
Chocolate chunk brownies	1	310	4	38	2	26	18.0	9.0	25
Double chocolate cookie	1	390	5	51	3	33	19.0	9.0	160
Everything cookie	1	380	5	49	2	29	18.0	9.0	260
Marshmallow chew	1	280	2	55	0	29	6.0	3.0	330
Seven layer bar	1	650	10	58	5	42	43.0	23.0	280
Toffee almond bar	1	400	4	53	1	34	19.0	8.0	340

BURGER KING

Item	Serving Size	Calories	Protein	Carb	Fiber	Sugar	Total Fat	Sat Fat	Sodium
BREAKFASTS									
Bacon, egg, cheese, with biscuit, sandwich	1	520	20	38	1	4	46.0	16.0	1360
Egg, with biscuit, sandwich	1	390	11	37	1	4	22.0	5.0	1020
Egg and cheese, with croissant, sandwich	1	340	14	26	1	5	19.0	8.0	840
Egg, cheese, and sausage, with croissant, sandwich	1	460	19	27	1	5	31.0	11.0	1000
Sausage, with biscuit, sandwich	1	510	13	35	1	3	35.0	15.0	1090
Sausage and cheese, with croissant, sandwich	1	380	14	26	1	3	24.0	10.0	780
BURGERS & SANDWICHES									
BK Big Fish., sandwich	1	710	24	67	4	4	38.0	5.0	1370
BK Broiler, chicken sandwich	1	550	30	52	3	5	25.0	5.0	1110
Cheeseburger	1	286	15	24	3	5	14.8	6.8	602
Cheeseburger, double with bacon	1	610	38	32	2	5	37.0	15.0	1380
Chicken Tenders sandwich	1	450	14	37	2	4	27.0	7.0	1100
Hamburger	1	275	14	27	2	5	12.0	5.1	455
Hamburger, double	1	480	31	30	2	5	26.0	8.0	550
Whopper, chicken sandwich	1	216	12	19	2	3	11.0	2.2	433
SIDES									
Chicken Tenders	4 pieces	289	17	17	2	0	16.7	4.2	721
Chocolate milk shake	medium	440	13	80	4	68	8.0	5.0	270
French fries	small	331	4	40	3	1	17.4	4.4	455
French toast sticks	3 pieces	349	6	41	1	10	18.0	2.0	280
Hash browns	small	369	3	35	3	0	24.4	5.9	511
Onion rings	small	180	2	22	2	3	9.0	3.0	490
Strawberry milk shake, added syrup	medium	500	12	95	2	81	8.0	5.0	350
Vanilla milk shake	medium	520	12	84	2	69	16.0	12.0	420

CARL'S JUNIOR

Item	Serving Size	Calories	Protein	Carb	Fiber	Sugar	Total Fat	Sat Fat	Sodium
BREAKFASTS									
Bacon strips	2	50	3	0	0	0	4.0	1.5	140
Bran raisin muffin	1	370	7	61	6	35	13.0	2.0	410
Burrito, breakfast	1	480	27	26	2	2	30.0	13.0	750
French toast, without syrup	1 order	370	6	42	1	11	20.0	2.5	430
Hash browns	1 order	330	3	32	3	0	21.0	4.5	470
Pork patty sausage	1 order	200	8	2	1	1	19.0	17.0	480
BURGERS & SANDWICHES									
Cheeseburger, Western Bacon	1	650	32	63	2	16	30.0	12.0	1430
Cheeseburger, double Western Bacon	1	900	51	64	2	16	49.0	21.0	1770
Chicken sandwich, BBQ flavor, charbroiled	1	280	25	37	2	9	3.0	1.0	830
Chicken sandwich, club, charbroiled	1	460	32	33	2	6	22.0	7.0	1110
Chicken sandwich, crispy, bacon, Swiss cheese	1	720	32	66	3	10	36.0	10.0	1610
Chicken sandwich, crispy, ranch	1	620	25	65	3	10	29.0	6.0	1220
Chicken sandwich, Santa Fe, charbroiled	1	510	28	32	2	6	31.0	7.0	1240
Fish sandwich, Carl's Catch	1	510	18	50	1	7	27.0	7.0	1030
Hamburger, Big	1	460	24	54	3	14	17.0	8.0	1090
Hamburger, Carl's Famous Star	1	580	25	49	2	10	32.0	9.0	910
Hamburger, Kids	1	230	9	24	1	5	19.0	3.5	550
Steak sandwich, sirloin, charbroiled	1	580	33	50	2	7	26.0	5.0	1110
Baked potato with bacon and cheese	1	630	20	76	6	7	29.0	7.0	1700
SIDES									
Breadstick	1 stick	35	1	7	1	0	0.5	0.0	60
Chicken Stars	6 pieces	280	12	15	0	0	19.0	4.5	330

CARL'S JUNIOR continued

Item	Serving Size	Calories	Protein	Carb	Fiber	Sugar	Total Fat	Sat Fat	Sodium
Chocolate cake	1 slice	300	3	49	4	27	10.0	3.0	350
Crisscut French fries	1 order	410	5	43	4	0	24.0	5.0	950
French fries, regular	1 order	290	5	37	3	0	14.0	3.0	170
Onion rings	1 order	430	7	53	3	5	21.0	4.0	478
Salad with charbroiled chicken	1	200	25	12	3	5	7.0	3.5	440
Strawberry swirl cheesecake	1 slice	290	6	30	0	20	17.0	9.0	230

CHEESECAKE FACTORY

Item	Serving Size	Calories	Protein	Carb	Fiber	Sugar	Total Fat	Sat Fat	Sodium
DESSERTS									
Black-Out cake	as served	1289	n/a	178	n/a	n/a	n/a	26.0	900
Carrot cake	as served	1549	n/a	183	n/a	n/a	n/a	24.0	490
Chocolate Tower Truffle Cake™	as served	1679	n/a	206	n/a	n/a	n/a	49.0	970
Chris' Outrageous Chocolate Cake™	as served	1507	n/a	183	n/a	n/a	n/a	44.0	580
Factory Mud Pie	as served	2065	n/a	251	n/a	n/a	n/a	55.0	950
Fresh strawberry shortcake	as served	878	n/a	105	n/a	n/a	n/a	27.0	904
Goblet of fresh strawberries	as served	108	n/a	15	n/a	n/a	n/a	2.0	0
Godiva® chocolate brownie sundae	as served	1018	n/a	103	n/a	n/a	n/a	35.0	206
Hot fudge sundae	as served	1534	n/a	162	n/a	n/a	n/a	52.0	416
Lemoncello Cream Torte™	as served	1034	n/a	114	n/a	n/a	n/a	30.0	490
Linda's Fudge Cake	as served	1369	n/a	280	n/a	n/a	n/a	17.0	1080
Tiramisu	as served	932	n/a	74	n/a	n/a	n/a	33.0	301
Warm apple crisp	as served	1305	n/a	193	n/a	n/a	n/a	28.0	176

CHEESECAKE FACTORY continued

Item	Serving Size	Calories	Protein	Carb	Fiber	Sugar	Total Fat	Sat Fat	Sodium
ENTRÉES									
Beef ribs	as served	2306	n/a	110	n/a	n/a	n/a	74.0	1613
Farfalle with chicken and roasted garlic	as served	2193	n/a	164	n/a	n/a	n/a	58.0	1833
Filet mignon	as served	992	n/a	24	n/a	n/a	n/a	26.0	1705
Grilled skirt steak	as served	894	n/a	29	n/a	n/a	n/a	14.0	1285
Pan-seared albacore	as served	1649	n/a	135	n/a	n/a	n/a	21.0	1879
Pan-seared pork tenderloin	as served	1698	n/a	82	n/a	n/a	n/a	54.0	1891
Pasta bolognese	as served	1641	n/a	176	n/a	n/a	n/a	15.0	1497
Pasta carbonara	as served	2134	n/a	144	n/a	n/a	n/a	81.0	1246
Rigatoni with marinara	as served	1211	n/a	173	n/a	n/a	n/a	3.0	749
Shrimp scampi	as served	1195	n/a	92	n/a	n/a	n/a	37.0	676
Shrimp with angel hair	as served	845	n/a	106	n/a	n/a	n/a	2.0	1586
Wasabi-crusted ahi tuna	as served	1750	n/a	113	n/a	n/a	n/a	58.0	1302
SALADS									
BLT salad	as served	465	n/a	15	n/a	n/a	n/a	14.0	1405
Boston house salad	as served	305	n/a	11	n/a	n/a	n/a	10.0	713
Caesar salad with chicken	as served	976	n/a	16	n/a	n/a	n/a	10.0	923
Endive, pecan, & blue cheese salad	as served	333	n/a	16	n/a	n/a	n/a	6.0	464
Factory-chopped salad	as served	518	n/a	28	n/a	n/a	n/a	10.0	995
French country salad	as served	389	n/a	27	n/a	n/a	n/a	6.0	668
Tomato and mozzarella salad	as served	490	n/a	22	n/a	n/a	n/a	17.0	1057
Tossed green salad	as served	189	n/a	21	n/a	n/a	n/a	4.0	173
Vegetable chopped salad with chicken	as served	390	n/a	30	n/a	n/a	n/a	6.0	576

CHICK-FIL-A

Item	Serving Size	Calories	Protein	Carb	Fiber	Sugar	Total Fat	Sat Fat	Sodium
DESSERTS									
Cheesecake	1 slice	340	6	30	2	25	21.0	12.0	270
Fudge nut brownie	1	330	4	45	2	29	15.0	3.5	210
Ice cream, Icedream	small	230	5	39	0	39	6.0	3.5	100
Lemon pie	1 slice	320	7	51	3	39	10.0	3.5	220
SANDWICHES AND WRAPS									
Charbroiled chicken wrap	1	390	31	53	3	6	7.0	3.0	1120
Chicken breast fillet, chargrilled	1	100	20	1	0	1	1.5	0.0	690
Chicken caesar wrap	1	460	38	51	3	5	11.0	6.0	1540
Chicken deluxe sandwich	1	420	28	39	2	5	16.0	3.5	1300
Chicken salad sandwich on whole wheat	1	350	20	32	5	6	15.0	3.0	880
Chicken sandwich	1	410	28	38	1	5	16.0	3.5	1300
Spicy chicken wrap	1	390	31	51	3	5	7.0	3.5	1150
SIDES & SALADS									
Chicken Caesar salad, chargrilled	1	240	31	6	2	3	10.0	6.0	1170
Chicken nuggets	8 pieces	260	26	12	1	3	12.0	2.5	1090
Chick-N-Strips salad	1	340	30	19	3	5	16.0	5.0	680
Chick-N-Strips, breaded and fried	4 pieces	250	25	12	0	2	11.0	2.5	570
French fries, waffle-style	small	280	3	37	5	0	14.0	5.0	105
Garden salad with chargrilled chicken	1	180	23	8	3	4	6.0	3.0	730
Hearty chicken breast soup	1 cup	100	9	13	1	2	1.5	0.0	940
Salad	1	80	5	6	2	3	5.0	2.5	110

CHILI'S

Item	Serving Size	Calories	Protein	Carb	Fiber	Sugar	Total Fat	Sat Fat	Sodium
ENTRÉES									
Cajun pasta with grilled chicken	as served	1350	70	37	104	n/a	71.0	7.0	3100
Chicken platter	as served	563	38	83	4	5	9.0	3.0	3284
Chicken salad with dressing	as served	272	29	27	6	20	5.0	1.0	1475
Chili's classic sirloin without sides	as served	450	26	11	19	n/a	34.0	2.0	1730
Classic bacon burger	as served	1520	64	115	9	0	88.0	26.0	3630
Crispy chicken tacos with corn tortillas	as served	1120	48	13	115	n/a	59.0	13.0	2820
Crispy shrimp tacos with corn tortillas	as served	830	28	5	111	n/a	34.0	21.0	2620
Flame-grilled rib eye without sides	as served	900	68	32	18	n/a	50.0	2.0	1980
Grilled BBQ chicken salad with dressing	as served	1060	76	50	12	4	63.0	19.0	2190
Grilled salmon with garlic and herbs	as served	620	29	11	44	n/a	48.0	5.0	1700
Memphis dry rub ribs 1/2 rack, without sides	as served	620	44	14	24	n/a	29.0	3.0	2820
Original ribs, 1/2 rack, without sides	as served	560	41	13	17	n/a	28.0	1.0	2050
Pasta with veggies and chicken	as served	786	53	106	6	6	15.0	5.0	1195
Pulled pork tacos with corn tortillas	as served	800	22	8	99	n/a	52.0	12.0	2870
Shiner Bock® BBQ ribs, 1/2 rack, without sides	as served	610	41	14	29	n/a	29.0	0.0	1940
Smoked chicken tacos with corn tortillas	as served	700	15	6	98	n/a	45.0	12.0	3060
SIDES & SALADS									
Asian salad with grilled chicken	small	540	33	5	40	n/a	29.0	8.0	2110
Asian salad with salmon	small	650	42	9	40	n/a	32.0	8.0	2310
Asian salad with steak	small	610	39	7	41	n/a	33.0	8.0	2760

CHILI'S continued

Item	Serving Size	Calories	Protein	Carb	Fiber	Sugar	Total Fat	Sat Fat	Sodium
Buffalo chicken salad	as served	1150	84	17	52	n/a	45.0	7.0	4410
Caribbean salad with grilled chicken	small	560	24	4	64	n/a	24.0	7.0	470
Carribean salad with grilled shrimp	small	550	28	5	64	n/a	11.0	6.0	760
Chicken caesar salad	as served	710	42	8	25	n/a	58.0	6.0	1010
Guiltless Grill Asian salad	as served	360	22	3	22	n/a	26.0	7.0	930
Guiltless Grill Caribbean salad	as served	520	24	4	52	n/a	23.0	7.0	630
Buffalo wings, boneless, with blue cheese	1 order	1060	38	44	2	2	81.0	14.0	3330
Loaded beef nachos	1/8 order	144	8	5	1	0	10.3	4.8	418

CHIPOTLE

Item	Serving Size	Calories	Protein	Carb	Fiber	Sugar	Total Fat	Sat Fat	Sodium
COMPONENTS									
Black beans	4 oz	120	7	23	11	<1	1.0	0.0	250
Carnitas	4 oz	190	27	1	0	0	8.0	2.5	540
Cheese	1 oz	100	8	0	0	0	8.5	5.0	180
Chicken	4 oz	190	32	1	0	1	6.5	2.0	370
Chips	4 oz	570	8	73	8	4	27.0	3.5	420
Cilantro–lime rice	3 oz	130	2	23	0	0	3.0	0.5	150
Corn salsa	3.5 oz	80	3	15	3	4	1.5	0.0	410
Crispy taco shell	1 each	60	<1	9	1	<1	2.0	0.5	10
Fajita vegetables	2.5 oz	20	1	4	1	2	0.5	0.0	170
Flour burrito tortilla	1 piece	290	7	44	2	0	9.0	3.0	670
Flour taco tortilla	1 piece	90	2	13	<1	0	2.5	1.0	200
Green tomatillo salsa	1/4 cup	15	1	3	1	2	0.0	0.0	230
Guacamole	3.5 oz	150	2	8	6	1	13.0	2.0	190
Pinto beans	4 oz	120	7	22	10	<1	1.0	0.0	330
Red tomatillo salsa	1/4 cup	40	2	8	4	4	1.0	0.0	510
Sour cream	2 oz	120	2	2	0	2	10.0	7.0	30
Steak	4 oz	190	30	2	0	1	6.5	2.0	320
Tomato salsa	3.5 oz	20	1	4	<1	3	0.0	0.0	470

COLDSTONE CREAMERY

Item	Serving Size	Calories	Protein	Carb	Fiber	Sugar	Total Fat	Sat Fat	Sodium
ICE CREAMS									
Butter pecan	5 oz.*	320	5	32	0	28	19.0	12.0	105
Chocolate peanut butter	5 oz.*	410	10	36	3	31	28.0	13.0	200
Cookie batter	5 oz.*	380	5	44	0	34	20.0	11.0	240
French vanilla	5 oz.*	340	5	37	0	33	19.0	14.0	80
Ghirardelli chocolate	5 oz.*	330	7	37	4	27	20.0	12.0	75
Mint	5 oz.*	330	5	36	0	31	19.0	12.0	75
Mocha	5 oz.*	320	6	33	1	29	20.0	12.0	95
Pecan praline	5 oz.*	330	5	37	0	31	19.0	12.0	90
Pistachio	5 oz.*	330	5	34	0	29	20.0	12.0	85
Sinless cake batter	5 oz.*	190	7	43	0	14	1.0	0.0	190
Sinless Sans Fat™ sweet cream	5 oz.*	140	6	34	<1	9	0.0	0.0	110
Strawberry cheesecake	5 oz.*	320	5	39	0	32	21.0	12.0	50
Strawberry	5 oz.*	320	5	35	0	30	18.0	12.0	75
Vanilla bean	5 oz.*	330	5	32	0	28	19.0	12.0	75
SHAKES & SMOOTHIES									
2 to Mango™ smoothie	5 oz.*	220	0	55	1	43	0.0	0.00	25
Berry Trinity™ smoothie	5 oz.*	110	2	28	6	15	1.0	0.00	25
Citrus Sunsation™ smoothie	5 oz.*	190	0	48	1	42	0.0	0.00	40
Man-Go Bananas™ smoothie	5 oz.*	240	1	59	2	42	0.0	0.00	20
Sinless Cake 'n Shake	16 fl oz	670	1	15	780	140	7.0	2.0	0
Sinless Milk and Cookies shake	16 fl oz	510	1	0	400	109	4.5	1.0	0
Sinless Oh Fudge shake	16 fl oz	490	0	0	360	110	2.0	2.0	0
Sinless Very Vanilla shake	16 fl oz	500	0	5	330	113	1.0	0.5	0
Strawberry Bananza™ smoothie	5 oz.*	140	2	37	4	24	1.0	0.0	30
SORBETS & FROZEN YOGURTS									
Lemon sorbet	5 oz.*	150	0	40	0	34	0.0	0.0	15
Raspberry sorbet	5 oz.*	160	0	42	0	36	0.0	0.0	15
Tart and tangy berry yogurt	5 oz.*	150	3	36	0	27	0.0	0.0	65

*A 5 oz. serving for Coldstone Creamery is the equivalent of the Like It™ serving size.

COLDSTONE CREAMERY continued

Item	Serving Size	Calories	Protein	Carb	Fiber	Sugar	Total Fat	Sat Fat	Sodium
Tart and tangy yogurt	5 oz.*	140	3	33	0	24	0.0	0.0	70
Watermelon sorbet	5 oz.*	160	0	41	0	35	0.0	0.0	15

*A 5 oz. serving for Coldstone Creamery is the equivalent of the Like It™ serving size.

DAIRY QUEEN

Item	Serving Size	Calories	Protein	Carb	Fiber	Sugar	Total Fat	Sat Fat	Sodium
Frozen dessert, banana split	1 order	510	8	96	3	82	12.0	8.0	180
Frozen dessert, strawberry shortcake	1 order	430	7	70	1	57	14.0	9.0	360
Frozen dessert, sundae, chocolate	small	280	5	49	0	42	7.0	4.5	140
Frozen dessert, sundae, strawberry	small	240	5	40	0	35	7.0	4.5	110
Ice cream cone, chocolate	small	240	6	37	0	25	8.0	5.0	115
Ice cream cone, dipped	small	340	6	42	1	31	17.0	9.0	130
Ice cream cone, vanilla	small	230	6	38	0	27	7.0	4.5	115
Ice cream sandwich	1	200	4	31	1	18	6.0	3.0	140
Ice cream, soft serve, chocolate	1 order	150	4	22	0	17	5.0	3.5	75
Ice cream, soft serve, vanilla	1 order	140	3	22	0	19	4.5	3.0	70

DENNY'S

Item	Serving Size	Calories	Protein	Carb	Fiber	Sugar	Total Fat	Sat Fat	Sodium
BREAKFASTS									
All-American Slam	as served	820	42	5	1	1	69.0	26.0	1520
Bacon avocado burrito	as served	1010	29	91	8	6	59.0	15.0	2210
Belgian Waffle Slam	as served	820	30	32	2	2	64.0	27.0	1270
Country fried steak & eggs	as served	660	39	29	3	0	42.0	15.0	1620
French toast slam	as served	940	47	68	4	14	53.0	17.0	1820
Grand Slamwich without hash browns	as served	1320	52	71	3	9	90.0	42.0	3070

DENNY'S continued

Item	Serving Size	Calories	Protein	Carb	Fiber	Sugar	Total Fat	Sat Fat	Sodium
Ham & cheddar omelette	as served	590	40	4	0	1	44.0	17.0	1330
Lumberjack Slam	as served	850	45	60	3	11	46.0	15.0	2770
Moons Over My Hammy	as served	780	46	50	2	3	42.0	16.0	2580
Prime Rib Premium Sizzlin' Breakfast Skillet	as served	850	41	77	6	14	40.0	15.0	2110
Southwestern Sizzlin' Skillet	as served	990	35	71	6	10	61.0	21.0	2140
Southwestern steak burrito	as served	910	33	76	5	4	52.0	14.0	1970
T-bone steak & eggs	as served	780	110	4	0	1	36.0	19.0	1210
Two-egg breakfast	as served	200	13	1	0	0	15.0	5.0	330
Ultimate omelette	as served	670	36	8	2	3	54.0	18.0	740
Veggie-cheese omelette	as served	500	29	10	2	4	37.0	12.0	940

BREAKFAST BUILDERS

Item	Serving Size	Calories	Protein	Carb	Fiber	Sugar	Total Fat	Sat Fat	Sodium
Bacon strips	2 slices	90	7	1	0	1	7.0	3.0	350
Buttermilk biscuit	1	105	2	13	0	0	6.0	2.0	285
Buttermilk pancakes	2 pieces	340	2	68	2	12	4.0	0.5	1180
Chicken sausage patty	1 1/2 oz	110	7	0	0	1	9.0	3.0	460
Egg whites	4 oz	50	11	1	0	0	0.0	0.0	180
English muffin	1 piece	180	4	25	1	1	3.0	1.0	300
Granola with 8 oz of milk	as served	690	20	131	9	53	12.0	3.0	430
Grits	12 oz	260	5	47	1	0	5.0	1.0	840
Hash browns	as served	210	2	26	2	1	12.0	2.5	650
Hearty wheat pancakes	2 pieces	310	10	64	8	2	1.5	0.5	950
Low fat yogurt	6 oz	160	6	30	0	25	1.5	1.0	100
Oatmeal with 8 oz of milk	16 oz	270	14	37	4	20	7.0	4.0	290
Sausage links	2 links	182	5	2	1	0	18.0	6.0	330
Scrambled eggs	4 oz	250	13	1	0	0	21.0	5.0	380
Seasonal fruit	4 oz	70	1	18	3	17	0.0	0.0	7
Toast	2 slices	260	6	32	1	4	14.0	2.0	110
Turkey bacon	2 slices	76	8	0	0	0	4.0	0.5	304

DOMINO'S PIZZA

Item	Serving Size	Calories	Protein	Carb	Fiber	Sugar	Total Fat	Sat Fat	Sodium
PIZZAS									
America's Favorite Feast, 12"	1/4 pizza	508	22	57	4	5	22.0	9.2	1340
Bacon Cheeseburger Feast, 12"	1/4 pizza	549	25	55	3	5	25.9	11.6	1274
Barbecue Feast, bacon, 12"	1/4 pizza	506	22	62	3	9	19.7	9.1	1206
Cheese, 12"	1/4 pizza	375	15	55	3	5	11.1	4.8	776
Deluxe Feast, 12"	1/4 pizza	465	20	57	4	5	18.0	8.0	1063
ExtravaganZZa, Feast, 12"	1/4 pizza	576	27	59	4	5	26.9	11.6	1511
Hawaiian Feast, 12"	1/4 pizza	450	21	58	3	7	15.6	7.2	1102
Pepperoni Feast, 12"	1/4 pizza	534	24	56	3	5	24.7	10.9	1349
Ultimate Deep Dish, cheese 12"	1/4 pizza	450	16	54	6	5	24.0	7.0	1050
Ultimate Deep Dish, pepperoni 12"	1/4 pizza	530	20	54	6	5	31.0	9.0	1330
Veggie Feast, 12"	1/4 pizza	439	19	57	4	5	15.8	7.1	987
SIDES									
Breadsticks, cheesy	1	142	4	18	1	1	6.2	2.0	183
Breadsticks, cinnamon sugar, CinnaStix	1	122	2	15	1	3	6.1	1.2	110
Dipping sauce, garlic	1 pack	440	0	5	1	0	50.0	10.0	390
Dipping sauce, sweet icing	1 pack	250	0	57	0	55	3.0	2.5	0
Fried chicken, buffalo wings	1 wing	50	6	2	0	1	2.4	0.7	175

DUNKIN' DONUTS

Item	Serving Size	Calories	Protein	Carb	Fiber	Sugar	Total Fat	Sat Fat	Sodium
Cookie, chocolate chunk	1	540	7	80	3	48	23.0	13.0	550
Cookie, oatmeal raisin	1	480	8	83	5	51	14.0	7.0	310
Cookie, peanut butter cup	1	590	11	73	3	49	29.0	13.0	530

DUNKIN DONUTS continued

Item	Serving Size	Calories	Protein	Carb	Fiber	Sugar	Total Fat	Sat Fat	Sodium
Doughnut, Bavarian cream	1	210	3	30	1	9	9.0	2.0	270
Doughnut, Boston cream	1	240	3	36	1	14	9.0	2.0	280
Doughnut, chocolate frosted	1	200	3	29	1	10	9.0	2.0	260
Doughnut, chocolate glazed	1	290	3	33	1	14	16.0	3.5	370
Doughnut, chocolate cream filled	1	270	3	35	1	16	13.0	3.0	260
Doughnut, glazed	1	180	3	25	1	6	8.0	1.5	250
Doughnut, jelly filled	1	210	3	32	1	14	8.0	1.5	280
Doughnut, maple frosted	1	210	3	30	1	12	9.0	2.0	260
Doughnut, sugar	1	170	3	22	1	4	8.0	1.5	250
Eclair pastry	1	270	3	39	1	17	11.0	2.5	290
Fritter, apple	1	300	4	41	1	12	14.0	3.0	360
Fritter, glazed	1	260	4	31	1	7	14.0	3.0	330

HARDEE'S

Item	Serving Size	Calories	Protein	Carb	Fiber	Sugar	Total Fat	Sat Fat	Sodium

BURGERS & SANDWICHES

Item	Serving Size	Calories	Protein	Carb	Fiber	Sugar	Total Fat	Sat Fat	Sodium
1/3 lb original Thickburger®	1	860	35	52	4	10	58.0	17.0	1630
1/3 Low carb Thickburger®	1	420	30	5	2	3	32.0	12.0	1010
Charbroiled chicken club sandwich	1	630	32	54	4	16	32.0	8.0	1730
Cheeseburger	1	313	16	26	1	5	14.0	4.0	780
Hamburger	1	267	14	26	1	5	10.0	3.0	560
Jumbo chili dog	1	400	16	25	1	6	26.0	9.0	1170
Little Thickburger®	1	570	24	35	3	7	39.0	12.0	1140
Regular roast beef sandwich	1	310	17	28	1	3	15.0	5.0	840
Six Dollar Thickburger®	1	930	46	57	4	15	59.0	21.0	1960

HARDEE'S continued

Item	Serving Size	Calories	Protein	Carb	Fiber	Sugar	Total Fat	Sat Fat	Sodium
SIDES									
Beer-battered onion rings	1 order	410	3	45	3	5	24.0	4.5	470
Crispy Curls™	small	340	4	43	4	0	17.0	4.0	840
Natural-cut French fries	small	320	4	45	3	0	14.0	3.0	710
Side salad without dressing	1	120	7	7	2	4	7.0	5.0	160

IHOP

Item	Serving Size	Calories	Protein	Carb	Fiber	Sugar	Total Fat	Sat Fat	Sodium
Belgian waffle	1	390	8	48	1	0	19.0	12.0	850
Breakfast sampler	1	757	43	36	0	0	47.0	0.0	2422
French toast combo, stuffed	1 order	1476	29	173	11	95	76.0	42.0	1327
Garden Scramble, without pancakes	1 order	267	18	15	0	0	15.0	0.0	0
Hash browns	1 order	225	2	20	2	0	14.0	2.0	424
Omelette, spinach and mushroom	1	679	45	14	3	1	74.0	26.4	1098
Pancakes, buttermilk	1 pancake	110	3	17	0	0	3.0	1.0	450
Pancakes, Harvest Grain 'N Nut	1 pancake	180	5	20	2	0	9.0	1.5	410
Rooty Tooty Fresh and Fruity	1 order	865	28	84	2	20	45.0	14.0	1577
Syrup	2 fl oz	230	0	58	0	58	0.0	0.0	230

IN-N-OUT BURGER

Item	Serving Size	Calories	Protein	Carb	Fiber	Sugar	Total Fat	Sat Fat	Sodium
Cheeseburger wth onion	1	480	22	39	3	10	27.0	10.0	1000
Chocolate shake	15 oz	690	9	83	0	62	36.0	24.0	350
Double-Double burger with onion	1	670	37	39	3	10	41.0	18.0	1440
French fries	1	400	7	54	2	0	18.0	5.0	245
Hamburger with onion	1	390	16	39	3	10	19.0	5.0	650
Strawberry shake	15 oz	690	9	91	0	75	33.0	22.0	280
Vanilla shake	15 oz	680	9	78	0	57	37.0	25.0	390

JACK IN THE BOX

Item	Serving Size	Calories	Protein	Carb	Fiber	Sugar	Total Fat	Sat Fat	Sodium
BURGERS									
Cheeseburger	1	350	18	31	1	7	17.0	8.0	790
Cheeseburger, bacon ultimate	1	1090	46	53	2	12	77.0	30.0	2040
Cheeseburger, deluxe	1	460	21	33	2	7	28.0	11.0	930
Cheeseburger, double bacon	1	840	34	51	2	9	56.0	19.0	1610
Cheeseburger, Jumbo Jack	1	690	25	54	3	12	42.0	16.0	1310
Cheeseburger, junior bacon	1	430	20	30	1	6	25.0	9.0	820
Cheeseburger, ultimate	1	1010	40	53	2	12	71.0	28.0	1580
Hamburger	1	310	16	30	1	6	14.0	6.0	600
Hamburger, with ciabatta	1	720	25	67	3	5	42.0	13.0	1280
SIDES									
Chicken strips	2 pieces	500	35	36	3	1	25.0	6.0	1260
Egg rolls	3 pieces	400	14	44	6	4	19.0	6.0	920
Fish and chips	medium	680	18	60	4	0	41.0	10.0	1100
French fries, curly	small	550	8	60	6	1	31.0	6.0	1200
French fries, natural cut	1 kids size	530	8	69	5	1	25.0	6.0	870
Stuffed jalapeños	3 pieces	530	15	51	4	5	30.0	13.0	1600

JAMBA JUICE

Item	Serving Size	Calories	Protein	Carb	Fiber	Sugar	Total Fat	Sat Fat	Sodium
BREADS									
Bread, Grin and Carrot	1 slice	250	5	36	1	20	10.0	1.0	250
Bread, honey berry bran	1 slice	320	6	48	6	28	12.0	2.0	360
JUICES									
Orange banana, power	1 power size	510	7	123	6	113	2.0	0.0	10
Orange, power	1 power size	450	7	103	2	101	2.0	0.0	10

JAMBA JUICE continued

Item	Serving Size	Calories	Protein	Carb	Fiber	Sugar	Total Fat	Sat Fat	Sodium
Pineapple orange banana blend, Vibrant C, power	1 power size	470	5	113	6	104	1.0	0.0	30
Wheatgrass	1 oz	5	1	1	0	1	0.0	0.0	0

SMOOTHIES

Item	Serving Size	Calories	Protein	Carb	Fiber	Sugar	Total Fat	Sat Fat	Sodium
Aloha Pineapple	16 fl oz	320	6	75	3	67	1.0	0.0	80
Banana Berry	16 fl oz	270	2	66	3	57	1.5	0.0	35
Berry Lime Sublime	16 fl oz	270	2	63	5	47	1.0	0.0	45
Bounce Back Blast	16 fl oz	300	6	65	3	51	1.0	0.0	95
Caribbean Passion	16 fl oz	270	2	62	3	54	1.0	0.0	40
Chocolate Moo'd	16 fl oz	540	12	112	2	100	6.0	3.5	270
Coldbuster	16 fl oz	280	3	65	3	60	1.5	0.0	15
Mango-A-Go-Go	16 fl oz	300	2	71	2	62	1.0	0.5	40
PowerBoost	16 fl oz	280	4	67	6	56	1.0	0.0	30
Razzmatazz	16 fl oz	300	2	72	3	56	1.0	0.0	45
Strawberries Wild	16 oz	280	3	67	3	58	0.0	0.0	95

JASON'S DELI

Item	Serving Size	Calories	Protein	Carb	Fiber	Sugar	Total Fat	Sat Fat	Sodium
Amy's Turkey-O, sandwich	1	648	33	72	8	11	27.0	11.0	2063
Bird to the Wise with mayo, sandwich	1	1491	71	49	0	7	113.0	49.0	2053
Bird to the Wise without mayo, sandwich	1	1391	71	49	0	7	102.0	47.0	1978
BLT, sandwich	1	800	30	68	10	10	49.0	14.0	1850
California Club, sandwich	1	826	39	42	2	7	57.0	27.0	1548
Chicago Club, sandwich	1	776	46	46	7	2	50.0	15.0	2785
Club Royale, sandwich	1	846	53	44	2	11	51.0	27.0	2188
Deli Club, sandwich	1	882	58	80	9	10	44.0	16.0	2280
Philly Chick Wrap, sandwich	1	610	47	53	6	8	25.0	10.0	1499
Ranchero Wrap, sandwich	1	890	61	53	13	6	50.0	18.0	3879
Reuben the Great, sandwich	1	860	75	56	7	2	35.0	15.0	4186
Santa Fe Chicken, sandwich	1	757	57	52	7	9	38.0	14.0	1909

JASON'S DELI continued

Item	Serving Size	Calories	Protein	Carb	Fiber	Sugar	Total Fat	Sat Fat	Sodium
The New York Yankee, sandwich	1	1189	92	47	2	0	69.0	32.0	2270
Tuna Melt, sandwich	1	960	55	47	7	7	62.0	18.0	1310

JIMMY JOHN'S

Item	Serving Size	Calories	Protein	Carb	Fiber	Sugar	Total Fat	Sat Fat	Sodium
Big John®, sandwich	1	533	26	49	1	n/a	24.0	4.0	1014
Double provolone Slim, sandwich	1	545	29	65	0	n/a	16.0	9.0	991
Ham and cheese Slim, sandwich	1	508	31	66	0	n/a	9.6	5.0	1244
JJBLT®, sandwich	1	634	25	49	1	n/a	35.0	9.0	1329
Pepe®, sandwich	1	617	28	50	1	n/a	31.0	8.0	1262
Roast beef Slim, sandwich	1	424	29	64	0	n/a	2.8	1.0	966
Salami, capicola, cheese Slim, sandwich	1	599	33	66	0	n/a	19.8	8.8	1450
Totally Tuna®, sandwich	1	548	33	54	3	n/a	31.0	4.0	1592
Tuna salad Slim, sandwich	1	722	35	68	1	n/a	30.5	4.0	1746
Turkey breast Slim, sandwich	1	401	27	65	0	n/a	0.6	0.0	1075
Turkey Tom®, sandwich	1	515	24	50	1	n/a	22.0	3.0	1094
Vegetarian, sandwich	1	578	19	53	2	n/a	30.0	7.6	873
Vito®, sandwich	1	600	30	52	1	n/a	28.0	9.0	1377

KFC

Item	Serving Size	Calories	Protein	Carb	Fiber	Sugar	Total Fat	Sat Fat	Sodium
MAINS									
Chicken sandwich, honey barbecue flavor with sauce	1	300	21	41	4	16	6.0	1.5	640
Chicken sandwich, original recipe with sauce	1	450	29	22	0	0	27.0	6.0	1010
Chicken sandwich, tenders with sauce	1	390	31	24	1	0	19.0	4.0	810

KFC continued

Item	Serving Size	Calories	Protein	Carb	Fiber	Sugar	Total Fat	Sat Fat	Sodium
Chicken sandwich, Triple Crunch Zinger with sauce	1	680	35	42	1	3	41.0	8.0	1650
Chicken sandwich, Twister	1	670	27	55	3	7	38.0	7.0	1650
Chicken, breast, extra crispy, fried	1	510	39	16	0	1	33.0	7.0	1010
Chicken thigh, original recipe, fried	1	220	18	5	0	0	15.0	4.0	620
Chicken, popcorn, fried	1 order	400	21	22	3	0	26.0	4.5	1160

SIDES

Item	Serving Size	Calories	Protein	Carb	Fiber	Sugar	Total Fat	Sat Fat	Sodium
Baked beans	1 order	230	8	46	7	22	1.0	1.0	720
Corn on the cob	1 piece	150	5	26	7	10	3.0	1.0	10
Macaroni & cheese	1 order	180	6	20	2	4	9.0	3.0	880
Mashed potatoes, with gravy	1 order	130	2	18	1	1	4.5	2.0	580
Snap beans, green	1 order	20	1	3	1	1	0.0	0.0	290

LITTLE CAESAR'S

Item	Serving Size	Calories	Protein	Carb	Fiber	Sugar	Total Fat	Sat Fat	Sodium

PIZZAS

Item	Serving Size	Calories	Protein	Carb	Fiber	Sugar	Total Fat	Sat Fat	Sodium
3 Meat Treat®	1/8 pizza	350	17	30	1	3	18.0	8.0	730
Deep-dish cheese	1/8 pizza	320	14	38	1	3	13.0	5.0	490
Deep-dish pepperoni	1/8 pizza	360	16	38	1	4	16.0	6.0	610
Hula Hawaiian	1/8 pizza	270	15	33	1	6	9.0	4.5	600
Just cheese	1/8 pizza	240	12	30	1	3	9.0	4.5	410
Meat and vegetable	1/8 pizza	350	17	30	1	3	18.0	8.0	730
Pepperoni	1/8 pizza	280	14	30	1	3	11.0	5.0	520
Thin crust, cheese	1/8 pizza	148	8	11	1	1	8.0	4.0	218
Ultimate Supreme	1/8 pizza	310	15	31	2	3	14.0	6.0	640
Vegetarian	1/8 pizza	270	13	32	2	4	10.0	4.5	530

LITTLE CAESAR'S continued

Item	Serving Size	Calories	Protein	Carb	Fiber	Sugar	Total Fat	Sat Fat	Sodium
SIDES									
Italian cheese bread	1 piece	130	6	13	0	1	7.0	2.5	230
Oven-roasted wings	1 wing	50	4	0	0	0	3.5	1.0	150
Pepperoni cheese bread	1 piece	150	7	13	0	1	8.0	3.0	280

LONG JOHN SILVER'S

Item	Serving Size	Calories	Protein	Carb	Fiber	Sugar	Total Fat	Sat Fat	Sodium
DOLLAR-STRETCHER MENU									
Chicken & fries	1 piece & 3 oz.	370	11	42	4	0	18.0	4.5	820
Fish & fries	1 piece & 3 oz.	490	14	50	4	0	26.0	6.0	1140
Fish sandwich	1	470	18	49	3	4	23.0	5.0	1180
Four battered shrimp	4 pieces	170	7	10	0	0	12.0	3.0	640
Popcorn shrimp	1 snack box	270	9	23	1	1	16.0	4.0	570
Six hushpuppies	6 pieces	360	9	56	4	5	19.0	4.5	1210
Small golden fries	3 oz.	230	3	33	3	0	10.0	2.5	350
Three shrimp & fries	3 pieces & 3 oz.	360	8	41	3	1	19.0	5.0	830
Zesty chicken sandwich	1	380	14	39	3	2	19.0	4.0	880
Baja chicken taco	1	370	11	31	3	2	23.0	5.0	890
Baja fish taco	1	360	9	30	3	2	23.0	4.5	810
FISH & SEAFOOD									
Clam strips, battered	1 snack box	320	9	29	2	1	19.0	4.5	1190
Fish, battered	1 piece	260	12	17	0	0	16.0	4.0	790
Langostino lobster bites, battered	1 snack box	230	13	24	2	0	9.0	3.0	520
Langostino lobster-stuffed crab cake	1 cake	170	6	16	1	0	9.0	2.0	390
Pacific salmon, grilled	2 fillets	150	24	2	0	1	5.0	1.0	440
Shrimp, battered	3 pieces	130	5	8	0	0	9.0	2.5	480
Shrimp, popcorn	1 snack box	270	9	23	1	1	16.0	4.0	570
Shrimp, scampi	8 pieces	200	17	3	0	1	13.0	2.5	650
Tilapia, grilled	1 fillet	110	22	1	0	1	2.5	1.0	250
Whitefish, crispy-breaded	1 piece	190	9	17	1	0	10.0	2.5	540

MCDONALD'S

Item	Serving Size	Calories	Protein	Carb	Fiber	Sugar	Total Fat	Sat Fat	Sodium
BREAKFASTS									
Bacon, egg, cheese, with biscuit, sandwich	1 biscuit	420	15	37	2	3	23.0	12.0	1160
Burrito, breakfast, sausage	1 burrito	300	12	26	1	2	16.0	7.0	830
Meal, hotcakes and sausage, without syrup and margarine	1 order	520	15	61	3	14	24.0	7.0	930
Muffin, apple bran, low fat	1	300	6	61	3	32	3.0	0.0	380
Pancakes, plain	3 pancakes	340	9	58	2	14	9.0	2.0	590
Parfait, fruit and yogurt with granola	7 oz	160	4	31	1	21	2.0	1.0	85
BURGERS									
Cheeseburger	1	300	15	33	2	6	12.0	6.0	750
Cheeseburger, Big Mac	1	540	25	45	3	9	29.0	10.0	1040
Cheeseburger, Big N' Tasty	1	510	27	38	3	8	28.0	11.0	960
Cheeseburger, double	1	440	25	34	2	7	23.0	11.0	1150
Cheeseburger, Quarter Pounder	1	510	29	40	3	9	26.0	12.0	1190
Cheeseburger, Quarter Pounder, double	1	740	48	40	3	9	42.0	19.0	1380
Hamburger	1	252	12	31	1	7	9.3	2.9	507
Hamburger, Big N' Tasty	1	460	24	37	3	8	24.0	8.0	720
Hamburger, Quarter Pounder	1	410	24	37	2	8	19.0	7.0	730
DESSERTS									
Apple pie	1 slice	250	2	32	4	13	13.0	7.0	170
Cookie, chocolate chip, package	1	160	2	21	1	15	8.0	3.5	90

MCDONALD'S continued

Item	Serving Size	Calories	Protein	Carb	Fiber	Sugar	Total Fat	Sat Fat	Sodium
Cookie, McDonaldland, package	2 oz	260	4	43	1	14	8.0	2.5	300
Danish, apple	1	340	5	47	2	21	15.0	5.0	290
Frozen dessert, McFlurry, Oreo, regular	12 oz	580	20	89	3	73	19.0	10.0	320
Frozen dessert, sundae, hot fudge	1	330	8	54	2	48	10.0	7.0	180
Frozen dessert, sundae, strawberry	1	280	6	49	1	45	6.0	4.0	95
Ice cream cone, vanilla, low fat	1	150	4	24	0	18	3.5	2.0	60
Sweet roll, cinnamon	1	398	7	53	2	25	18.1	2.5	378

SALADS & SIDES

Item	Serving Size	Calories	Protein	Carb	Fiber	Sugar	Total Fat	Sat Fat	Sodium
Chicken, McNuggets	10 pieces	460	24	27	0	0	29.0	5.0	1000
Chicken strips, breast, premium, breaded, fried, Selects	3 pieces	400	23	23	0	0	24.0	3.5	1010
Hash browns	1 order	150	1	15	2	0	9.0	1.5	310
Salad, Caesar, with chicken, crispy	1	330	26	20	3	6	17.0	4.5	840
Salad, California cobb, without chicken	1	160	11	7	3	4	11.0	4.5	450
Salad, California cobb, with grilled chicken	1	380	35	12	4	5	11.0	5.0	1110
Salad, chef, shaker	1	150	17	5	2	2	8.0	4.0	740
Salad, garden, shaker	1	100	7	4	2	1	6.0	3.5	115
Side salad	1	20	1	4	2	2	0.2	0.0	12

SANDWICHES

Item	Serving Size	Calories	Protein	Carb	Fiber	Sugar	Total Fat	Sat Fat	Sodium
Sandwich, chicken, classic, premium crispy	1	530	28	32	3	12	20.0	3.5	1150
Sandwich, Filet-O-Fish	1	380	15	38	2	5	18.0	3.5	640
Sandwich, McChicken	1	360	14	40	2	5	16.0	3.0	830

MRS. FIELDS

Item	Serving Size	Calories	Protein	Carb	Fiber	Sugar	Total Fat	Sat Fat	Sodium
Butter cookie	1	200	2	29	<1	15	8.0	3.5	180
Cut Out cookie	1	400	2	56	0	32	19.0	7.0	230
Debra's special cookie	1	200	3	28	1	16	9.0	3.0	160
Peanut butter cookie	1	210	4	24	1	12	12.0	4.0	190
Semi-sweet chocolate cookie	1	210	2	29	1	19	10.0	5.0	170
Semi-sweet chocolate with walnuts cookie	1	220	2	29	2	18	11.0	4.5	140
Triple chocolate cookie	1	210	2	28	2	18	11.0	5.0	140
White chunk macadamia cookie	1	230	3	27	1	18	12.0	5.0	150

OLIVE GARDEN

Item	Serving Size	Calories	Protein	Carb	Fiber	Sugar	Total Fat	Sat Fat	Sodium
APPETIZERS									
Alfredo dipping sauce	1 order	380	n/a	9	1	n/a	35.0	22.0	510
Breadstick (with garlic-butter spread)	1 order	150	n/a	28	2	n/a	2.0	0.0	400
Bruschetta	1 order	610	n/a	100	10	n/a	13.0	2.5	1760
Calamari	1 order	890	n/a	64	2	n/a	54.0	5.0	2340
Caprese flatbread	1 order	600	n/a	46	5	n/a	36.0	11.0	1520
Grilled chicken flatbread	1 order	760	n/a	47	5	n/a	44.0	15.0	1500
Hot artichoke-spinach dip	1 order	650	n/a	68	6	n/a	31.0	15.0	1430
Lasagna fritta	1 order	1030	n/a	82	9	n/a	63.0	21.0	1590
Marinara dipping sauce	1 order	70	n/a	10	3	n/a	2.5	0.0	540
Mussels di Napoli	1 order	180	n/a	13	0	n/a	8.0	4.0	1770
Sicilian scampi	1 order	500	n/a	43	7	n/a	22.0	10.0	1850
Smoked mozzarella fonduta	1 order	940	n/a	72	7	n/a	48.0	28.0	1940
Stuffed mushrooms	1 order	280	n/a	15	3	n/a	19.0	5.0	720
ENTRÉES									
Braised beef & tortelloni	1 order	1020	n/a	82	10	n/a	53.0	22.0	2060

OLIVE GARDEN continued

Item	Serving Size	Calories	Protein	Carb	Fiber	Sugar	Total Fat	Sat Fat	Sodium
Capellini di mare	1 order	650	n/a	82	7	n/a	18.0	5.0	1830
Capellini pomodoro	1 order	840	n/a	141	19	n/a	17.0	3.0	1250
Cheese ravioli with marinara sauce	1 order	660	n/a	84	7	n/a	22.0	11.0	1440
Cheese ravioli with meat sauce	1 order	790	n/a	88	12	n/a	28.0	14.0	1510
Chianti-braised short ribs	1 order	1060	n/a	71	17	n/a	58.0	26.0	2970
Chicken Alfredo	1 order	1440	n/a	103	5	n/a	82.0	48.0	2070
Chicken Marsala	1 order	770	n/a	59	16	n/a	37.0	5.0	1800
Chicken Parmigiana	1 order	1090	n/a	79	27	n/a	49.0	18.0	3380
Chicken scampi	1 order	1070	n/a	88	8	n/a	53.0	20.0	2220
Chicken & shrimp carbonara	1 order	1440	n/a	80	9	n/a	88.0	38.0	3000
Eggplant Parmigiana	1 order	850	n/a	98	19	n/a	35.0	10.0	1900
Fettuccine Alfredo	1 order	1220	n/a	99	5	n/a	75.0	47.0	1350
Five-cheese ziti al forno	1 order	1050	n/a	112	9	n/a	48.0	26.0	2370
Garlic-herb chicken con broccoli	1 order	960	n/a	90	12	n/a	41.0	18.0	2180
Grilled shrimp caprese	1 order	900	n/a	82	0	n/a	40.0	17.0	3490
Herb-grilled salmon	1 order	510	n/a	5	2	n/a	26.0	6.0	760
Lasagna classico	1 order	850	n/a	39	19	n/a	47.0	25.0	2830
Lasagna rollata al forno	1 order	1170	n/a	90	11	n/a	68.0	39.0	2510
Mixed grill	1 order	830	n/a	72	10	n/a	28.0	5.0	1840
Parmesan-crusted bistecca	1 order	690	n/a	40	7	n/a	35.0	19.0	1480
Parmesan-crusted tilapia	1 order	590	n/a	42	6	n/a	25.0	10.0	910
Pork Milanese	1 order	1510	n/a	118	11	n/a	87.0	37.0	3100
Ravioli di portobello	1 order	670	n/a	74	15	n/a	30.0	17.0	1400
Seafood Alfredo	1 order	1020	n/a	88	9	n/a	52.0	31.0	2430
Seafood brodetto	1 order	480	n/a	35	7	n/a	16.0	3.0	2250
Seafood Portofino	1 order	800	n/a	85	16	n/a	33.0	14.0	1880
Shrimp & crab tortelli romana	1 order	840	n/a	67	4	n/a	42.0	24.0	1710
Shrimp primavera	1 order	730	n/a	110	14	n/a	12.0	2.0	1620
Spaghetti & Italian sausage	1 order	1270	n/a	97	15	n/a	67.0	24.0	3090

OLIVE GARDEN continued

Item	Serving Size	Calories	Protein	Carb	Fiber	Sugar	Total Fat	Sat Fat	Sodium
Spaghetti & meatballs	1 order	1110	n/a	103	9	n/a	50.0	20.0	2180
Spaghetti with meat sauce	1 order	710	n/a	94	9	n/a	22.0	8.0	1340
Steak gorgonzola-Alfredo	1 order	1310	n/a	82	9	n/a	73.0	41.0	2190
Steak Toscano	1 order	810	n/a	62	11	n/a	35.0	8.0	1690
Stuffed chicken Marsala	1 order	800	n/a	40	6	n/a	36.0	16.0	2830
Tour of Italy	1 order	1450	n/a	97	10	n/a	74.0	33.0	3830
Venetian apricot chicken	1 order	380	n/a	32	8	n/a	4.0	1.5	1420

SOUPS & SALADS

Item	Serving Size	Calories	Protein	Carb	Fiber	Sugar	Total Fat	Sat Fat	Sodium
Chicken & gnocchi	1 order	250	n/a	29	2	n/a	8.0	3.0	1180
Garden-fresh salad	1/2 order	120	n/a	17	3	n/a	3.5	0.5	550
Garden-fresh salad	1 order	350	n/a	22	3	n/a	26.0	4.5	1930
Grilled chicken Caesar	1 order	850	n/a	14	4	n/a	64.0	13.0	1880
Minestrone	1 order	100	n/a	18	3	n/a	1.0	0.0	1020
Pasta e fagioli	1 order	130	n/a	17	6	n/a	2.5	1.0	680
Zuppa toscana	1 order	170	n/a	24	2	n/a	4.0	2.0	960

ON THE BORDER

Item	Serving Size	Calories	Protein	Carb	Fiber	Sugar	Total Fat	Sat Fat	Sodium
APPETIZERS									
Border sampler	1 order	2010	101	105	15	n/a	135.0	50.0	4490
Chicken flautas with original queso	1 order	1070	51	69	10	n/a	66.0	17.0	1910
Chips and salsa	1 order	430	5	52	5	n/a	22.0	4.0	440
Empanadas, chicken with original queso	1 order	1220	41	79	4	n/a	83.0	29.0	1310
Empanadas with ground beef with original queso	1 order	1250	39	79	5	n/a	88.0	30.0	1370
Fajita quesadillas with chicken	1 order	1240	62	59	5	n/a	85.0	32.0	2740
Fajita quesadillas with steak	1 order	1230	50	59	7	n/a	90.0	36.0	1930
Firecracker-stuffed jalapeños with original queso	1 order	1950	67	123	3	n/a	134.0	36.0	6540
Grande fajita nachos with chicken	1 order	1540	112	88	17	n/a	85.0	38.0	5180
Grande fajita nachos with steak	1 order	1530	87	87	21	n/a	95.0	48.0	3560
Shaken margarita shrimp cocktail with cocktail sauce	1 order	640	36	62	10	n/a	36.0	7.0	2890
Ultimate loaded queso without chips	1 order	780	45	36	11	n/a	52.0	27.0	2750
MAINS									
Cheese stuffed chile relleno with ranchero sauce	1 order	680	31	28	6	n/a	57.0	5.0	1190
Chicken flautas with chile con queso	1 order	330	17	19	2	n/a	21.0	7.0	790
Chicken tortilla soup	1 order	330	17	26	4	n/a	18.0	7.0	960
Crispy taco with chicken	1 order	260	18	19	3	n/a	12.0	4.0	530
Crispy taco with ground beef	1 order	320	18	19	4	n/a	19.0	7.0	600
Enchiladas, cheese and onion with chile con carne	1 order	360	17	20	2	n/a	24.0	12.0	930

ON THE BORDER continued

Item	Serving Size	Calories	Protein	Carb	Fiber	Sugar	Total Fat	Sat Fat	Sodium
Empanadas, chicken with chile con queso	1 order	540	20	33	1	n/a	37.0	14.0	780
Enchiladas, chicken with sour cream sauce	1 order	210	12	18	1	n/a	11.0	5.0	490
Enchiladas, ground beef with chile con carne	1 order	260	14	19	2	n/a	15.0	6.0	650
Empanadas, ground beef with chile con queso	1 order	550	19	33	2	n/a	39.0	15.0	810
House salad without dressing	1 order	200	6	20	4	n/a	12.0	4.0	260
Pork tamale with chile con carne	1 order	290	13	14	3	n/a	20.0	7.0	960
Soft taco with chicken	1 order	240	19	24	2	n/a	11.0	4.0	830
Soft taco with ground beef	1 order	310	19	24	3	n/a	18.0	8.0	900

SIDES

Item	Serving Size	Calories	Protein	Carb	Fiber	Sugar	Total Fat	Sat Fat	Sodium
Black beans with cheese	1 order	130	8	20	6	n/a	3.0	1.0	630
Grilled vegetables	1 order	70	2	16	3	n/a	0.0	0.0	20
Guacamole	1 order	50	1	3	3	n/a	5.0	1.0	90
House vegetables	1 order	180	2	13	3	n/a	14.0	3.0	190
Mexican rice	1 order	290	6	54	0	n/a	5.0	1.0	620
Pico de gallo	1 order	10	0	1	0	n/a	1.0	0.0	55
Refried beans with cheese	1 order	230	10	24	7	n/a	10.0	4.0	730

SOUPS & SALADS

Item	Serving Size	Calories	Protein	Carb	Fiber	Sugar	Total Fat	Sat Fat	Sodium
Chicken tortilla soup	side	330	17	26	4	n/a	18.0	7.0	960
Chicken tortilla soup	regular	510	25	50	6	n/a	25.0	8.0	1950
Citrus chipotle chicken salad with mango citrus vinaigrette	1 order	290	25	42	11	n/a	4.0	2.0	840
Grande taco salad with chicken with dressing	1 order	1290	53	83	12	n/a	85.0	28.0	2110
Grande taco Salad with ground beef with dressing	1 order	1380	53	83	14	n/a	95.0	33.0	2200

ON THE BORDER continued

Item	Serving Size	Calories	Protein	Carb	Fiber	Sugar	Total Fat	Sat Fat	Sodium
House salad without dressing	1 order	200	6	20	4	n/a	12.0	4.0	260
Sizzling chicken fajita salad, without dressing	1 order	710	52	25	7	n/a	46.0	20.0	1930
Sizzling steak fajita salad, without dressing	1 order	830	56	24	8	n/a	58.0	29.0	2090

OUTBACK STEAKHOUSE

Item	Serving Size	Calories	Protein	Carb	Fiber	Sugar	Total Fat	Sat Fat	Sodium
ENTRÉES									
Alice Springs Chicken® without sides	as served	1297	84	30	2	n/a	93.0	40.0	2292
Atlantic salmon	as served	582	39	2	1	0	45.0	17.0	708
Baby back ribs without sides	full rack	2013	109	24	1	n/a	160.0	59.0	2600
Chicken, Grilled on the barbie	as served	587	54	32	4	0	26.0	13.0	1533
Chicken and Swiss grilled sandwich	1 sandwich	750	48	50	3	0	39.0	13.0	1371
Filet with wild mushroom sauce without sides	as served	344	36	7	1	n/a	18.0	10.0	1193
Grilled chicken on the barbie without sides	as served	444	52	21	1	n/a	15.0	7.3	1256
New York strip steak	8 oz	566	27	92	13	0	36.0	14.0	1683
New Zealand rack of lamb without sides	as served	1303	61	5	1	n/a	112.0	58.0	1473
No Rules Parmesan pasta	as served	909	20	89	4	n/a	53.0	31.0	1075
Outbacker burger	1 burger	759	43	43	4	0	45.0	17.0	1250
Prime rib	8 oz	537	29	2	0	n/a	45.0	18.6	888
Ribs, 1/2 rack, with fries	as served	1403	59	66	6	0	99.0	39.0	1727
Sweet-glazed roasted pork tenderloin without sides	as served	385	37	32	1	n/a	12.0	6.0	462
Victoria's Filet® without sides	9 oz	725	50	1	0	n/a	57.0	25.5	593

OUTBACK STEAKHOUSE continued

Item	Serving Size	Calories	Protein	Carb	Fiber	Sugar	Total Fat	Sat Fat	Sodium
SIDES & SALADS									
Baked potato, dressed	1 potato	520	8	65	7	0	26.0	13.0	2456
Chicken Caesar salad	1 salad	1044	68	27	6	0	73.0	24.0	2101
Fresh seasonal vegetables	1 order	143	3	11	4	0	11.0	6.0	277
Queensland salad without dressing	as served	839	54	53	5	n/a	59.0	22.5	1322

P.F. CHANG'S

Item	Serving Size	Calories	Protein	Carb	Fiber	Sugar	Total Fat	Sat Fat	Sodium
APPETIZERS									
Chang's chicken lettuce wraps	5 oz	160	8	17	2	n/a	7.0	1.0	650
Chang's vegetarian lettuce wraps	5 oz	140	6	11	2	n/a	7.0	1.0	530
Crispy green beans	4 oz	260	2	21	2	n/a	18.0	3.0	140
Egg rolls	3 oz	174	5	22	3	n/a	8.0	1.0	673
Northern-style spare ribs	4 oz	343	31	11	0	n/a	19.0	2.0	925
Pork dumplings, steamed	2 oz	60	4	6	0	n/a	2.0	1.0	125
Salt and pepper calamari	2 oz	160	6	11	0	n/a	10.0	2.0	208
Shrimp dumplings, steamed	4 oz	45	4	6	0	n/a	0.0	0.0	180
Spring rolls	3 oz	156	4	17	2	n/a	8.0	1.0	271
Vegetable dumplings, steamed	6 oz	45	2	8	0	n/a	0.0	0.0	80
BEEF									
Asian marinated New York Strip	8 oz	370	33	17	0	n/a	20.0	9.0	933
Beef with broccoli	7 oz	290	24	21	2	n/a	12.0	3.0	1573
Hong Kong beef with snow peas	9 oz	310	24	24	3	n/a	14.0	3.0	826
Orange-peel beef	5 oz	283	12	21	1	n/a	13.0	3.0	833
Pepper steak	8 oz	297	24	19	1	n/a	13.0	3.0	1300

P.F. CHANG'S continued

Item	Serving Size	Calories	Protein	Carb	Fiber	Sugar	Total Fat	Sat Fat	Sodium
CHICKEN									
Chang's spicy chicken	6 oz	323	28	23	0	n/a	16.0	2.0	550
Chicken with black bean sauce	7 oz	300	29	14	0	n/a	16.0	2.0	1850
Crispy honey chicken	6 oz	477	16	49	0	n/a	23.0	4.0	510
Ginger chicken with broccoli	9 oz	273	28	18	2	n/a	11.0	2.0	1457
Kung pao chicken	5 oz	383	33	14	2	n/a	23.0	4.0	940
Orange-peel chicken	5 oz	333	27	20	1	n/a	15.0	3.0	770
Sesame chicken	8 oz	343	30	25	2	n/a	14.0	2.0	1020
Sweet & sour chicken	5 oz	370	12	38	0	n/a	19.0	3.0	367
SEAFOOD									
Kung pao scallops	5 oz	307	16	17	2	n/a	20.0	3.0	1126
Oolong marinated sea bass	9 oz	315	24	15	2	n/a	19.0	5.0	1550
Salmon steamed with ginger	10 oz	330	31	12	3	n/a	19.0	3.0	605
Salt and pepper prawns	6 oz	197	21	8	2	n/a	11.0	2.0	1070
Shrimp with candied walnuts	7 oz	377	16	25	1	n/a	24.0	4.0	654
Shrimp with lobster sauce	10 oz	250	23	11	1	n/a	14.0	2.0	1745
VEGETARIAN									
Buddha's feast	6 oz	55	4	11	4	n/a	0.0	0.0	40
Coconut curry vegetables	13 oz	510	22	26	5	n/a	36.0	12.0	650
Ma po tofu	10 oz	350	20	17	2	n/a	23.0	5.0	1060
Stir-fried eggplant	6 oz	270	2	14	2	n/a	22.0	3.0	760
Vegetable chow fun	7 oz	250	2	46	3	n/a	2.0	0.0	750
Vegetarian fried rice	7 oz	190	5	38	2	n/a	2.0	0.0	230

PANDA EXPRESS

Item	Serving Size	Calories	Protein	Carb	Fiber	Sugar	Total Fat	Sat Fat	Sodium
BEEF & PORK									
BBQ pork	4.6 oz	360	34	13	1	12	19.0	8.0	1310
Broccoli beef	5.4 oz	150	11	12	3	2	6.0	1.5	720
Mongolian beef	6.9 oz	230	17	17	3	6	11.0	2.5	1040
Sweet & sour pork	5.6 oz	400	13	36	2	15	23.0	4.5	360
CHICKEN									
Broccoli chicken	5.5 oz	180	13	11	3	2	9.0	2.0	630
Kung pao chicken	6.1 oz	300	19	13	2	4	19.0	3.5	880
Mushroom chicken	5.9 oz	220	17	9	2	3	13.0	3.0	780
Orange chicken	5.4 oz	400	15	42	0	18	20.0	3.5	640
Pineapple chicken breast	6 oz	220	17	20	1	14	8.0	1.5	640
String bean chicken	5.1 oz	190	12	11	2	4	10.0	2.0	720
String bean chicken breast	5.6 oz	170	15	13	2	5	7.0	1.5	720
Sweet and sour chicken	5.5 oz	400	15	46	1	23	17.0	3.0	370
Thai cashew chicken breast	6.3 oz	280	23	21	2	6	19.0	3.5	980
SHRIMP									
Crispy shrimp	6 pieces	260	9	26	1	2	13.0	2.5	810
Honey walnut shrimp	3.7 oz	370	14	27	2	9	23.0	4.0	470
Kung pao shrimp	6.4 oz	250	14	14	2	4	15.0	2.5	880
Tangy shrimp	6.4 oz	190	13	19	2	14	7.0	1.5	820
SOUPS & SIDES									
Chicken egg roll	1	200	8	16	2	2	12.0	4.0	390
Chicken potstickers	3 pieces	220	7	23	1	2	11.0	2.5	280
Chow mein	8.3 oz	400	12	61	8	10	12.0	2.0	1060
Eggplant and tofu	6.1 oz	310	7	19	3	13	24.0	3.0	680
Fortune cookie	1	32	1	7	0	5	0.0	0.0	8
Fried rice	10 oz	570	16	85	8	0	18.0	4.0	900
Hot and sour soup	10.6 oz	90	4	12	1	3	3.5	0.5	970
Mixed veggies	8.6 oz	70	4	13	5	4	0.5	0.0	530
Veggie spring rolls	2	160	4	22	4	2	7.0	1.0	540

PANERA BREAD

Item	Serving Size	Calories	Protein	Carb	Fiber	Sugar	Total Fat	Sat Fat	Sodium
BAGELS									
Asiago cheese	1	330	13	55	2	3	6.0	3.5	570
Blueberry	1	330	10	67	2	9	1.5	0.0	490
Chocolate chip	1	370	10	69	2	14	6.0	4.0	480
Cinnamon crunch	1	430	9	81	3	30	8.0	5.0	430
Cinnamon swirl and raisin	1	320	10	65	3	11	2.5	1.0	460
Everything	1	300	10	59	2	4	2.5	0.0	630
French toast	1	350	9	67	2	15	5.0	2.0	610
Jalapeño and cheddar	1	310	12	56	2	3	3.0	1.5	740
Plain	1	290	10	59	2	3	1.5	0.0	450
Sesame	1	310	10	59	2	3	3.0	0.0	450
Sweet onion poppy seed	1	400	14	72	4	7	7.0	1.0	510
Whole grain	1	370	13	70	6	5	3.5	0.0	420
Asiago cheese, demi	1	160	7	22	1	0	4.0	2.5	320
BREADS									
Ciabatta	6.25 oz	460	16	84	3	3	6.0	1.0	760
Cinnamon raisin loaf	2 oz	180	5	34	1	11	3.0	1.5	135
Focaccia	2 oz	180	5	28	1	1	4.5	0.5	320
Focaccia with Asiago cheese	2 oz	160	5	23	1	1	5.0	1.5	230
French baguette	2 oz	150	5	30	1	0	1.0	0.0	370
Honey wheat loaf	2 oz	170	5	30	2	4	3.0	1.5	240
Sesame semolina loaf	2 oz	140	4	29	1	1	0.5	0.0	350
Sourdough round loaf	2 oz	140	5	28	1	0	0.5	0.0	290
Sourdough soup bowl	8 oz	590	21	118	4	1	2.5	0.0	1210
Stone-milled rye loaf	2 oz	140	5	28	2	0	0.5	0.0	380
Three-cheese demi	2 oz	160	6	29	1	1	2.0	0.0	320
Three-Seed demi	2 oz	160	6	27	2	0	3.5	0.0	300
Tomato basil loaf	2 oz	140	5	27	1	1	0.5	0.0	330
White whole-grain loaf	2 oz	140	5	26	2	1	2.5	1.0	310
Whole-grain loaf	2 oz	140	6	27	3	2	1.0	0.0	300

PANERA BREAD continued

Item	Serving Size	Calories	Protein	Carb	Fiber	Sugar	Total Fat	Sat Fat	Sodium
BREAKFAST SANDWICHES									
Asiago cheese bagel with bacon	6.5 oz	480	23	55	2	3	18.0	9.0	800
Asiago cheese bagel with egg and cheese	8.25 oz	640	31	56	2	4	31.0	14.0	1130
Asiago cheese bagel with sausage	7.25 oz	590	32	58	3	4	25.0	11.0	1430
Bacon, egg, & cheese on ciabatta	5.75 oz	380	18	43	2	1	14.0	6.0	620
Breakfast power sandwich	7.5 oz	610	33	56	3	4	27.0	13.0	1240
Egg & cheese on ciabatta	7.5 oz	540	26	44	2	2	28.0	11.0	950
Grilled breakfast sandwiches	6.6 oz	510	28	44	2	2	24.0	10.0	1060
Jalapeño & cheddar bagel with bacon	7.25 oz	490	28	58	3	3	15.0	8.0	1270
Sausage, egg, & cheese on ciabatta	6 oz	360	23	36	4	3	14.0	6.0	860
PASTRIES, COOKIES & CAKES									
Apple crunch muffin	5 oz	450	7	80	2	49	12.0	3.0	340
Carrot walnut muffin	5 oz	500	8	72	3	37	21.0	4.5	580
Cheese pastry	3.75 oz	400	8	42	1	15	22.0	14.0	340
Cherry pastry	5 oz	500	7	77	2	45	18.0	11.0	320
Chocolate Chip Muffie	2.5 oz	280	4	40	1	24	12.0	3.5	180
Chocolate Chipper	3.25 oz	440	5	59	2	33	23.0	14.0	250
Chocolate Duet with walnuts	3.25 oz	450	6	55	3	36	24.0	13.0	150
Chocolate fudge brownie	3.5 oz	410	5	64	2	33	14.0	8.0	260
Chocolate pastry	3.5 oz	410	8	46	2	18	24.0	14.0	260
Cinnamon coffee crumb cake	4.25 oz	470	6	54	1	30	25.0	9.0	310
Macadamia nut blondie	3.5 oz	460	4	62	1	25	21.0	11.0	200
Oatmeal raisin	3.25 oz	370	5	57	2	28	14.0	8.0	310
Pecan braid	4.25 oz	470	8	52	2	23	26.0	12.0	270
Pumpkin Muffie	3 oz	290	3	45	1	26	11.0	2.0	240

PANERA BREAD continued

Item	Serving Size	Calories	Protein	Carb	Fiber	Sugar	Total Fat	Sat Fat	Sodium
Pumpkin muffin	6 oz	580	7	89	2	51	22.0	4.0	470
Shortbread	2.5 oz	350	3	36	1	11	21.0	12.0	160
Wild blueberry muffin	4.5 oz	440	6	66	2	39	17.0	3.0	330

SANDWICHES AND PANINI

Item	Serving Size	Calories	Protein	Carb	Fiber	Sugar	Total Fat	Sat Fat	Sodium
Asiago roast beef on Asiago cheese	1/2	350	24	32	1	2	13.0	7.0	630
Bacon Turkey Bravo® on tomato basil	1/2	420	26	44	2	6	14.0	5.0	1500
Chicken Caesar on three cheese	1/2	360	21	33	2	2	16.0	4.5	730
Chipotle chicken on artisan French	1/2	500	26	34	2	3	28.0	8.0	1180
Cuban chicken panini	1/2	430	23	43	2	5	19.0	5.0	950
Frontega Chicken® on focaccia	1/2	430	23	40	2	3	20.0	4.5	1080
Italian combo on ciabatta	1/2	520	31	47	2	3	23.0	9.0	1510
Mediterranean veggie on tomato basil	1/2	300	11	50	5	3	7.0	1.5	730
Napa almond chicken salad on sesame semolina	1/2	340	15	44	2	6	13.0	2.0	660
Sierra turkey on focaccia with Asiago cheese	1/2	480	19	40	2	3	27.0	6.0	990
Smoked ham and Swiss on stone-milled rye	1/2	350	23	33	3	2	14.0	5.0	1180
Smoked turkey breast on country	1/2	280	16	34	2	2	9.0	1.5	980
Smokehouse Turkey® on three-cheese	1/2	360	25	33	2	3	14.0	6.0	1230
Tomato and mozzarella on ciabatta	1/2	380	15	48	3	5	15.0	5.0	650
Tuna salad on honey wheat	1/2	380	10	32	3	6	23.0	4.5	570
Turkey artichoke on focaccia	1/2	370	20	44	3	5	13.0	3.5	1170

PANERA BREAD continued

Item	Serving Size	Calories	Protein	Carb	Fiber	Sugar	Total Fat	Sat Fat	Sodium
SOUPS & SIDES									
Baked potato	12 oz	340	7	29	0	2	22.0	11.0	1210
Baked potato with You Pick Two®	8 oz	210	5	18	0	1	14.0	7.0	760
Broccoli Cheddar soup	12 oz	290	12	24	7	0	16.0	9.0	1540
Cream of Chicken and wild rice soup	12 oz	320	10	33	0	3	17.0	7.0	1270
French onion soup	13.25 oz	240	9	24	1	7	12.0	5.0	2210
Low fat chicken noodle soup	12 oz	110	8	10	0	2	4.0	1.5	1360
Low fat chicken tortilla soup	12.75 oz	190	10	24	1	1	6.0	1.5	1110
Low fat garden vegetable with pesto soup	12 oz	160	5	28	6	8	3.5	0.0	1240
Low fat vegetarian black bean soup	12 oz	170	10	29	5	4	4.0	1.5	1590
New England clam chowder	12 oz	450	8	29	3	0	34.0	20.0	1190
Signature macaroni & cheese	15.5 oz	980	33	75	3	14	61.0	26.0	2030
Signature macaroni & cheese	7.75 oz	490	17	37	1	7	30.0	13.0	1020

PAPA JOHN'S

Item	Serving Size	Calories	Protein	Carb	Fiber	Sugar	Total Fat	Sat Fat	Sodium
PIZZAS									
BBQ chicken & bacon, 14"	1/8 pizza	350	15	44	2	7	12.0	5.0	1020
Cheese, 14"	1/8 pizza	290	11	37	2	4	10.0	4.5	720
Garden Fresh, 14"	1/8 pizza	280	11	39	2	5	9.0	4.0	700
Hawaiian BBQ chicken, 14"	1/8 pizza	290	11	37	2	4	10.0	4.5	720
Pepperoni, 14"	1/8 pizza	330	13	37	2	4	14.0	6.0	870
Sausage, 14"	1/8 pizza	330	12	37	2	4	15.0	6.0	830
Spicy Italian, 14"	1/8 pizza	380	14	38	2	4	18.0	7.0	980
Spinach Alfredo, 14"	1/8 pizza	290	10	36	1	4	11.0	6.0	640

PAPA JOHN'S continued

Item	Serving Size	Calories	Protein	Carb	Fiber	Sugar	Total Fat	Sat Fat	Sodium
The Meats, 14"	1/8 pizza	370	15	38	2	5	19.0	7.0	1050
The Works, 14"	1/8 pizza	330	13	39	2	5	14.0	6.0	930
Tuscan six-cheese, 14"	1/8 pizza	320	14	38	2	4	13.0	6.0	800

PAPA MURPHY'S

Item	Serving Size	Calories	Protein	Carb	Fiber	Sugar	Total Fat	Sat Fat	Sodium
PIZZAS									
50/50	1/8 pizza	330	16	29	<1	6	17.0	8.0	850
5-meat	1/8 pizza	370	18	39	0	7	16.0	7.0	910
All-meat	1/8 pizza	320	17	28	0	5	16.0	8.0	790
Awesome Foursome	1/8 pizza	320	116	34	<1	9	15.0	8.0	800
Barbeque chicken	1/8 pizza	310	17	35	0	11	11.0	6.0	680
Big Murphy	1/8 pizza	370	17	40	<1	7	16.0	7.0	890
Cheese	1/8 pizza	250	12	27	0	5	10.0	6.0	500
Cherry dessert pizza	1/8 pizza	240	4	44	<1	16	4.5	1.0	330
Chicago-style	1/8 pizza	370	17	40	<1	7	16.0	7.0	850
Chicken and bacon	1/8 pizza	370	20	39	0	6	15.0	7.0	820
Chicken Florentine	1/8 pizza	460	26	46	1	7	19.0	9.0	1040
Combo	1/8 pizza	450	21	46	<1	8	21.0	11.0	1030
Cowboy	1/8 pizza	320	16	29	<1	5	16.0	8.0	810
Forty-Niner	1/8 pizza	370	18	31	<1	6	19.0	9.0	880
Gourmet chicken garlic	1/8 pizza	290	17	27	0	4	13.0	6.0	560
Gourmet classic Italian	1/8 pizza	350	17	31	<1	5	18.0	8.0	790
Gourmet supreme	1/8 pizza	280	13	30	2	6	12.0	6.0	600
Gourmet vegetarian	1/8 pizza	300	14	31	1	5	14.0	7.0	700
Hawaiian	1/8 pizza	270	13	30	<1	8	10.0	6.0	600
Herb chicken Mediterranean	1/8 pizza	340	17	35	3	7	14.0	7.0	630
Italian	1/8 pizza	450	22	46	<1	8	20.0	10.0	1090
Meat sampler	1/8 pizza	280–340	15–17	31–32	<1	6	11-16	6–8	670–840
Murphy's combo	1/8 pizza	330	16	29	<1	6	17.0	8.0	850
Papa's Favorite	1/8 pizza	330	16	29	<1	6	17.0	8.0	820

PAPA MURPHY'S continued

Item	Serving Size	Calories	Protein	Carb	Fiber	Sugar	Total Fat	Sat Fat	Sodium
Papa-Roni	1/8 pizza	300	14	28	0	5	15.0	8.0	690
Pepperoni	1/8 pizza	290	13	27	0	5	14.0	7.0	640
Perfect	1/8 pizza	290-320	15	30-34	<1	6-9	11-15	6-8	670-710
Rancher	1/8 pizza	300	16	28	0	6	14.0	7.0	700
Specialty of the house	1/8 pizza	320	16	32	<1	6	15.0	7.0	800
Taco grande	1/8 pizza	310	16	30	1	5	14.0	6.0	760
Vegetarian combo	1/8 pizza	270	13	30	<1	6	11.0	6.0	610
Veggie Mediterranean	1/8 pizza	280	12	31	2	6	12.0	6.0	540

SIDES

Item	Serving Size	Calories	Protein	Carb	Fiber	Sugar	Total Fat	Sat Fat	Sodium
Apple dessert pizza	1 slice	240	4	46	<1	19	4.5	1.0	340
Caesar salad	1/2	50	4	4	2	2	2.0	1.0	120
Caesar salad dressing	1 oz	140	1	2	0	1	14.0	1.0	170
Cheesy bread, without sauce	1/8	220	7	31	0	5	7.0	3.0	480
Chicken Caesar salad	1/2	140	18	5	3	2	5.0	2.5	320
Cinnamon wheel	2 slices	250	5	42	0	13	7.0	2.0	410
Club salad	1/2 salad	140	13	6	3	2	8.0	4.0	480
Cookie dough with Hershey's chocolate chips	1 oz	120	1	17	0	10	6.0	2.0	115
Garden salad	1/2	100	6	8	3	2	6.0	3.0	260
Italian salad	1/2	140	7	7	3	1	10.0	4.0	400
Lasagna	1/8	330	17	26	2	9	18.0	9.0	760
Low-calorie Italian salad dressing	1 oz	10	0	1	0	1	0.5	0.0	280

PIZZA HUT

Item	Serving Size	Calories	Protein	Carb	Fiber	Sugar	Total Fat	Sat Fat	Sodium
Cheese	1/8 pizza	240	11	27	1	2	11.0	4.5	530
Chicken supreme	1/8 pizza	270	13	28	1	3	12.0	4.0	580
Italian sausage	1/8 pizza	270	11	28	1	3	13.0	4.5	560
Meat Lover's	1/8 pizza	330	14	27	1	2	18.0	7.0	830
Pepperoni Lover's	1/8 pizza	250	11	26	1	2	12.0	4.5	590
Sausage Lover's	1/8 pizza	330	13	29	2	2	20.0	7.0	830
Super supreme	1/8 pizza	340	14	30	2	7	18.0	6.0	760
Supreme	1/8 pizza	240	11	26	2	3	12.0	5.0	690
Veggie Lover's, medium	1/8 pizza	230	9	28	2	3	9.0	3.5	500
Veggie Lover's, small	1/8 pizza	200	9	27	2	3	7.0	3.5	540

POPEYES

Item	Serving Size	Calories	Protein	Carb	Fiber	Sugar	Total Fat	Sat Fat	Sodium
Cajun-battered French fries	1 order	660	30	60	3	9	33.0	9.0	2280
Cajun chicken, wings, fried	6 pieces	595	34	19	0	0	43.0	15.0	1274
Cajun chicken with rice	1 order	630	30	72	1	0	18.0	6.0	2229
Chicken, breast, mild, fried	1 order	265	22	9	0	0	15.5	5.4	530
Chicken deluxe sandwich, with mayo	1	480	33	54	3	5	15.0	6.0	1290
Chicken strips	2 pieces	271	19	19	1	0	13.0	5.4	922
Chicken, thigh, mild, fried	1 order	313	19	11	1	0	22.0	7.4	595
Étouffée Creole chicken, with rice	1 order	480	36	18	6	3	30.0	9.0	2610
Red beans and rice	1 order	320	10	31	17	2	19.0	6.0	710
Shrimp, popcorn, batter-fried	as served	280	12	22	1	0	16.0	6.0	1110

RED LOBSTER

Item	Serving Size	Calories	Protein	Carb	Fiber	Sugar	Total Fat	Sat Fat	Sodium
LOBSTERS & CRABS									
Chef's Signature lobster and shrimp pasta	1/2	510	n/a	43	n/a	n/a	25.0	11.0	1090
Crab linguini Alfredo	1/2	560	n/a	47	n/a	n/a	25.0	12.0	1310
Live Maine lobster	1 1/4 lb	45	n/a	0	n/a	n/a	0.0	0.0	350
North Pacific king crab legs	1 order	390	n/a	2	n/a	n/a	3.5	1.0	3520
Rock lobster tail	1	90	n/a	0	n/a	n/a	1.0	0.0	490
Rockzilla®	1 order	130	n/a	0	n/a	n/a	1.5	0.0	690
Snow crab legs	1 lb	160	n/a	0	n/a	n/a	1.0	0.0	1960
Stuffed Maine lobster	1 order	240	n/a	12	n/a	n/a	7.0	2.5	1150
SHRIMP									
Crunchy popcorn shrimp	1 order	560	n/a	51	n/a	n/a	27.0	2.5	2100
Parrot Isle jumbo coconut shrimp	1 order	980	n/a	90	n/a	n/a	55.0	12.0	1950
Shrimp linguini Alfredo	1/2	550	n/a	41	n/a	n/a	29.0	10.0	1580
Walt's Favorite Shrimp	1 order	700	n/a	52	n/a	n/a	39.0	3.5	2410
SIGNATURE COMBOS									
Admiral's Feast	1 order	1500	n/a	110	n/a	n/a	87.0	7.0	4400
Seaside Shrimp Trio	1 order	1030	n/a	68	n/a	n/a	57.0	14.0	3480
Ultimate Feast®	1 order	620	n/a	29	n/a	n/a	30.0	3.5	3370
SOUPS & SALADS									
Bayou seafood gumbo	1 cup	190	n/a	15	n/a	n/a	6.0	2.0	1130
Caesar salad with chicken	1 order	670	n/a	14	n/a	n/a	52.0	10.0	1750
Caesar salad with shrimp	1 order	620	n/a	14	n/a	n/a	51.0	10.0	1370
Creamy potato bacon soup	1 cup	220	n/a	19	n/a	n/a	15.0	9.0	790
Manhattan clam chowder	1 cup	80	n/a	12	n/a	n/a	1.0	0.0	690
New England clam chowder	1 cup	230	n/a	13	n/a	n/a	17.0	10.0	680

RED LOBSTER continued

Item	Serving Size	Calories	Protein	Carb	Fiber	Sugar	Total Fat	Sat Fat	Sodium
seafood gumbo	1 cup	230	n/a	25	n/a	n/a	8.0	2.5	1160
Spicy Shrimp Soup	1 cup	160	n/a	15	n/a	n/a	6.0	2.5	1010

RED ROBIN

Item	Serving Size	Calories	Protein	Carb	Fiber	Sugar	Total Fat	Sat Fat	Sodium
A.1.® peppercorn burger	1	1025	51	70	3	15	59.0	n/a	2032
All-American patty melt	1	1315	48	60	3	12	98.0	n/a	2064
Banzai burger	1	1033	47	68	3	25	62.0	n/a	1922
Bleu Ribbon cheeseburger	1	1042	47	69	4	21	57.0	6.0	2076
Burnin' Love burger™	1	936	45	55	3	10	60.0	n/a	2198
Chili Chili™ cheeseburger	1	923	55	59	5	10	50.0	20.0	1601
Gardenburger	1	561	10	73	6	9	23.0	4.0	1724
Gourmet cheeseburger	1	931	45	53	3	9	60.0	n/a	1818
Guacamole bacon burger	1	1046	61	54	4	10	64.0	n/a	1515
Natural burger	1	569	37	51	3	9	24.0	n/a	989
Pub burger	1	957	54	57	4	14	55.0	n/a	1310
Red Robin bacon cheeseburger	1	1030	51	51	3	8	69.0	n/a	1930
Royal Red Robin Burger®	1	1196	59	52	3	9	83.0	n/a	2113
Sauteed 'Shroom burger	1	961	59	58	6	10	56.0	n/a	1352
Teriyaki chicken sandwich	1	905	56	64	3	20	48.0	n/a	1616
Whiskey River BBQ burger	1	1114	48	72	4	16	68.0	n/a	1815

RUBY TUESDAY

Item	Serving Size	Calories	Protein	Carb	Fiber	Sugar	Total Fat	Sat Fat	Sodium
BURGERS & SANDWICHES									
Alpine Swiss burger	as served	1251	n/a	65	6	n/a	82.0	n/a	2041
Avocado turkey burger	as served	1234	n/a	62	6	n/a	81.0	n/a	2961
Bacon cheeseburger	as served	1252	n/a	61	6	n/a	86.0	n/a	2270
Bella turkey burger	as served	1126	n/a	67	4	n/a	69.0	n/a	2760
Bison bacon cheeseburger	as served	1032	n/a	61	6	n/a	61.0	n/a	2250
Brewmaster burger	as served	1244	n/a	70	6	n/a	82.0	n/a	2249
Buffalo chicken burger	as served	1127	n/a	74	5	n/a	67.0	n/a	2454
Chicken BLT	as served	1137	n/a	74	5	n/a	66.0	n/a	2204
Classic cheeseburger	as served	1192	n/a	61	6	n/a	81.0	n/a	2060
Pimento cheese burger	as served	1282	n/a	61	6	n/a	89.0	n/a	2092
Ruby's classic burger	as served	1122	n/a	60	6	n/a	75.0	n/a	1820
Smokehouse burger	as served	1461	n/a	83	7	n/a	97.0	n/a	2629
The Ultimate Chicken	as served	1222	n/a	60	6	n/a	67.0	n/a	2477
Three-cheese burger	as served	1352	n/a	61	6	n/a	94.0	n/a	2245
Turkey burger	as served	997	n/a	62	4	n/a	61.0	n/a	2538
Boston blue burger	as served	1446	n/a	80	9	n/a	96.0	n/a	2745
SIDES & SALADS									
Asian dumplings	1/4	114	n/a	11	1	n/a	5.0	n/a	295
Asian salmon spinach salad	as served	494	n/a	35	9	n/a	20.0	n/a	729
Asian sesame wings	1/4	190	n/a	5	1	n/a	10.0	n/a	709
Avocado shrimp salad	as served	516	n/a	29	14	n/a	31.0	n/a	822
Beef queso dip	1/4	378	n/a	28	3	n/a	24.0	n/a	727
Boston barbecue wings	1/4	167	n/a	6	1	n/a	7.0	n/a	676
Buffalo shrimp	1/4	126	n/a	11	1	n/a	6.0	n/a	580
Carolina chicken salad	as served	1157	n/a	48	11	n/a	70.0	n/a	2891
Cheddar fries	1/4	335	n/a	25	3	n/a	20.0	n/a	826
Chicken strips, Boston barbecue	1/4	115	n/a	8	0	n/a	4.0	n/a	367

RUBY TUESDAY continued

Item	Serving Size	Calories	Protein	Carb	Fiber	Sugar	Total Fat	Sat Fat	Sodium
Chicken strips, buffalo	1/4	114	n/a	4	1	n/a	6.0	n/a	375
Chicken strips, Thai phoon	1/4	179	n/a	4	0	n/a	13.0	n/a	297
Chicken strips, traditional	1/4	94	n/a	3	0	n/a	4.0	n/a	222
Club house salad	as served	926	n/a	21	9	n/a	59.0	n/a	2203
Dip trio	1/4	467	n/a	27	8	n/a	33.0	n/a	821
Fire wings	1/4	159	n/a	1	1	n/a	9.0	n/a	647
Four-way sampler	1/4	311	n/a	14	2	n/a	17.0	n/a	864
Fresh guacamole dip	1/4	357	n/a	22	10	n/a	24.0	n/a	417
Fried mozzarella	1/4	182	n/a	11	2	n/a	11.0	n/a	484
Jumbo Lump crab cake	1/4	68	n/a	3	1	n/a	4.0	n/a	201
Pimento cheese dip	1/4	284	n/a	16	2	n/a	20.0	n/a	505
Queso dip	1/4	317	n/a	26	3	n/a	20.0	n/a	535
Santa Fe chicken salad	as served	681	n/a	30	8	n/a	35.0	n/a	1099
Southwestern beef salad	as served	1139	n/a	48	10	n/a	81.0	n/a	2345
Southwestern spring rolls	1/4	173	n/a	14	1	n/a	10.0	n/a	324
Spinach artichoke dip	1/4	310	n/a	23	3	n/a	19.0	n/a	470
Thai phoon shrimp	1/4	191	n/a	11	1	n/a	13.0	n/a	502
Wing sampler	1/4	232	n/a	6	1	n/a	12.0	n/a	915

SMART EATING CHOICES

Item	Serving Size	Calories	Protein	Carb	Fiber	Sugar	Total Fat	Sat Fat	Sodium
Baked potato, plain	as served	282	n/a	46	10	n/a	2.0	n/a	113
Brown-rice pilaf	as served	226	n/a	33	2	n/a	7.0	n/a	585
Chicken Bella	as served	417	n/a	9	1	n/a	14.0	n/a	1601
Creamy mashed cauliflower	as served	136	n/a	9	5	n/a	8.0	n/a	714
Creole catch	as served	277	n/a	2	1	n/a	13.0	n/a	303
Fresh steamed broccoli	as served	84	n/a	3	3	n/a	6.0	n/a	222
Grilled chicken salad	as served	547	n/a	9	7	n/a	27.0	n/a	1589

RUBY TUESDAY continued

Item	Serving Size	Calories	Protein	Carb	Fiber	Sugar	Total Fat	Sat Fat	Sodium
Grilled chicken wrap	as served	465	n/a	43	4	n/a	16.0	n/a	1396
Lite ranch dressing	as served	50	n/a	1	0	n/a	5.0	n/a	300
New Orleans seafood	as served	389	n/a	3	1	n/a	22.0	n/a	865
Plain grilled chicken	as served	260	n/a	0	0	n/a	3.0	n/a	150
Plain grilled salmon	as served	167	n/a	0	0	n/a	9.0	n/a	30
Sautéed baby portabella mushrooms	as served	98	n/a	10	0	n/a	4.0	n/a	353
Sugar snap peas	as served	113	n/a	6	3	n/a	6.0	n/a	202
Turkey burger wrap	as served	658	n/a	45	3	n/a	33.0	n/a	2514
White bean chicken chili	as served	233	n/a	21	8	n/a	8.0	n/a	1454
White cheddar mashed potatoes	as served	169	n/a	19	2	n/a	10.0	n/a	520

SONIC DRIVE-IN

Item	Serving Size	Calories	Protein	Carb	Fiber	Sugar	Total Fat	Sat Fat	Sodium
BREAKFASTS									
Breakfast Toaster® with bacon, egg, and cheese	1 order	530	20	40	2	7	32.0	10.0	1440
CroisSONIC® Breakfast sandwich with bacon	1	510	18	29	0	5	36.0	15.0	1400
CroisSONIC® Breakfast sandwich with ham	1	430	21	25	1	4	27.0	12.0	1510
CroisSONIC® breakfast sandwich with sausage	1	600	19	29	0	5	46.0	18.0	1340
French toast sticks	4 sticks	500	7	49	2	9	31.0	5.0	490
Sausage Biscuit Dippers™ with gravy	1 order	690	16	57	0	7	44.0	18.0	1770
Steak and egg breakfast burrito	1	590	28	47	5	3	34.0	12.0	1370
SuperSonic® breakfast burrito	1	570	19	48	3	3	36.0	12.0	1650

SONIC DRIVE-IN continued

Item	Serving Size	Calories	Protein	Carb	Fiber	Sugar	Total Fat	Sat Fat	Sodium
BURGERS & SANDWICHES									
Bacon cheeseburger Toaster® sandwich	1	670	29	52	3	13	39.0	14.0	1440
BLT Toaster® sandwich	1	500	17	45	2	7	29.0	7.0	950
Breaded pork fritter sandwich	1	640	22	66	7	11	33.0	6.0	840
California cheeseburger	1	690	29	57	5	13	39.0	13.0	1060
Chicken club Toaster® sandwich	1	740	29	55	4	7	46.0	11.0	1740
Chili cheeseburger	1	660	31	56	5	11	35.0	14.0	990
Country-fried steak Toaster® sandwich	1	670	14	71	4	6	37.0	10.0	1370
Fish sandwich	1	650	22	71	7	12	31.0	5.0	1160
Green chili cheeseburger	1	630	29	56	5	12	31.0	12.0	1070
Hickory cheeseburger	1	640	28	61	5	17	31.0	12.0	1170
Jalapeño burger	1	550	25	53	5	10	26.0	9.0	880
Sonic® bacon cheeseburger	1	780	33	57	5	12	48.0	16.0	1300
Sonic® burger	1	650	26	55	5	11	37.0	10.0	720
Sonic® cheeseburger	1	720	29	56	5	12	42.0	14.0	1040
Thousand island burger	1	610	26	56	5	13	32.0	10.0	810
SHAKES, MALTS & SLUSHES									
Banana cream pie shake	Regular	640	9	87	1	77	29.0	20.0	330
Banana malt	Regular	510	8	62	1	55	26.0	18.0	290
Banana shake	Regular	500	8	60	1	54	26.0	18.0	280
Barq's® root beer float/blended float	Regular	340	4	51	0	50	14.0	10.0	170
Blue coconut CreamSlush® treat	Regular	350	4	53	0	51	14.0	10.0	170
Butterfinger® Sonic Blast®	Regular	730	11	87	0	75	38.0	26.0	410
Caramel malt	Regular	570	8	75	0	68	27.0	19.0	430

SONIC DRIVE-IN continued

Item	Serving Size	Calories	Protein	Carb	Fiber	Sugar	Total Fat	Sat Fat	Sodium
Cherry CreamSlush® treat	Regular	350	4	54	0	53	14.0	10.0	170
Chocolate cream pie shake	Regular	700	8	101	0	88	29.0	20.0	410
Chocolate malt	Regular	580	8	76	0	66	26.0	18.0	370
Chocolate shake	Regular	560	8	74	0	65	26.0	18.0	360
Coca-Cola® float/ blended float	Regular	330	4	49	0	47	14.0	10.0	160
Coconut cream pie shake	Regular	600	8	78	0	72	29.0	20.0	330
Diet Coke® float/ blended float	Regular	260	4	29	0	27	14.0	10.0	160
Diet Dr Pepper® float/ blended float	Regular	260	4	28	0	27	14.0	10.0	190
Dr Pepper® float/ blended float	Regular	320	4	48	0	46	14.0	10.0	180
Grape CreamSlush® treat	Regular	350	4	53	0	52	14.0	10.0	170
Hot fudge malt	Regular	610	8	72	1	63	31.0	23.0	350
Hot fudge shake	Regular	590	8	70	1	62	31.0	22.0	340
Java chiller, caramel	Regular	500	7	64	0	58	25.0	18.0	360
Java chiller, chocolate	Regular	500	7	64	0	56	24.0	17.0	320
Lemon–berry CreamSlush® treat	Regular	400	5	66	1	58	14.0	10.0	180
Lemon CreamSlush® treat	Regular	350	4	54	0	51	14.0	10.0	170
Lemon real fruit slush with Wacky Pack®	Regular	170	0	46	0	44	0.0	0.0	25
Lime CreamSlush® treat	Regular	350	4	54	0	50	14.0	10.0	170
MandM's® Sonic Blast®	Regular	750	11	86	1	81	40.0	28.0	380
Orange CreamSlush® treat	Regular	350	4	54	0	51	14.0	10.0	170
Oreo® Sonic Blast®	Regular	680	11	78	1	70	37.0	25.0	460
Peanut butter malt	Regular	690	12	63	0	56	45.0	22.0	420
Peanut butter shake	Regular	660	12	60	0	54	44.0	21.0	400
Pineapple malt	Regular	510	8	67	0	58	26.0	18.0	300
Pineapple shake	Regular	520	8	65	0	57	26.0	18.0	290

SONIC DRIVE-IN continued

Item	Serving Size	Calories	Protein	Carb	Fiber	Sugar	Total Fat	Sat Fat	Sodium
Reese's peanut butter Cups® Sonic Blast®	Regular	710	13	88	1	77	35.0	25.0	430
Snickers® Sonic Blast®	Regular	770	11	96	0	88	38.0	25.0	530
Sprite® float/ blended float	Regular	330	4	48	0	47	14.0	10.0	170
Sprite Zero™ float/blended float	Regular	260	4	28	0	27	14.0	10.0	160
Strawberry cream pie shake	Regular	670	9	95	1	83	29.0	20.0	340
Strawberry CreamSlush® treat	Regular	400	5	65	1	58	14.0	10.0	180
Strawberry malt	Regular	540	9	70	1	61	26.0	18.0	300
Strawberry shake	Regular	530	8	68	1	59	26.0	18.0	290
Vanilla malt	Regular	480	8	53	0	50	26.0	18.0	290
Vanilla shake	Regular	460	8	51	0	49	26.0	18.0	280
Watermelon CreamSlush® treat	Regular	350	4	54	0	51	14.0	10.0	170

SIDES

Item	Serving Size	Calories	Protein	Carb	Fiber	Sugar	Total Fat	Sat Fat	Sodium
Apple slices	1 order	35	0	9	2	7	0.0	0.0	0
Apple slices with fat-free caramel dipping sauce	1 order	120	0	27	2	23	0.0	0.0	60
Ched 'R' Bites®	12 pieces	280	13	22	1	0	15.0	6.0	740
Ched 'R' Peppers®	4 pieces	330	8	36	2	2	17.0	6.0	1110
French fries	small	200	2	30	2	0	8.0	1.5	270
French fries with cheese	small	270	5	32	2	1	13.0	5.0	590
French fries with chili and cheese	small	300	8	33	3	1	16.0	6.0	540
Mozzarella sticks	1 order	440	19	40	2	1	22.0	9.0	1050
Pickle-O's®	1 order	310	5	36	2	2	16.0	3.0	1020

STARBUCKS COFFEE

Item	Serving Size	Calories	Protein	Carb	Fiber	Sugar	Total Fat	Sat Fat	Sodium
BREAKFASTS									
Bacon, gouda cheese, & egg frittata on artisan roll	as served	350	17	30	0	n/a	18.0	n/a	n/a
Black Forest ham, parmesan frittata, & cheddar on artisan roll	as served	370	23	32	0	n/a	16.0	n/a	n/a
Brown sugar topping for Starbucks® Perfect Oatmeal	as served	50	0	13	0	n/a	0.0	n/a	n/a
Chicken Santa Fe panini	as served	400	27	47	2	n/a	11.0	n/a	n/a
Chicken & vegetable wrap	as served	290	19	36	4	n/a	9.0	n/a	n/a
Dark cherry yogurt parfait	as served	310	10	61	3	n/a	4.0	n/a	n/a
Dried fruit topping for Starbucks® Perfect Oatmeal	as served	100	<1	24	2	n/a	0.0	n/a	n/a
Egg white, spinach, & feta wrap	as served	280	18	33	6	n/a	10.0	n/a	n/a
Greek yogurt honey parfait	as served	290	8	43	<1	n/a	12.0	n/a	n/a
Huevos rancheros wrap	as served	330	16	35	8	n/a	15.0	n/a	n/a
Nut medley topping for Starbucks® Perfect Oatmeal	as served	100	2	2	<1	n/a	9.0	n/a	n/a
Roasted vegetable panini	as served	350	13	48	4	n/a	12.0	n/a	n/a
Roma tomato & mozzarella sandwich	as served	380	16	40	2	n/a	18.0	n/a	n/a
Sausage, egg, & cheese on English muffin	as served	500	19	41	<1	n/a	28.0	n/a	n/a
Starbucks® Perfect Oatmeal	as served	140	5	25	4	n/a	2.5	n/a	n/a
Strawberry & blueberry yogurt parfait	as served	300	7	60	3	n/a	3.5	n/a	n/a

STARBUCKS COFFEE continued

Item	Serving Size	Calories	Protein	Carb	Fiber	Sugar	Total Fat	Sat Fat	Sodium
Tarragon chicken salad sandwich	as served	480	35	62	3	n/a	11.0	n/a	n/a
Tuna melt panini	as served	390	22	49	3	n/a	12.0	n/a	n/a
Turkey & swiss sandwich	as served	390	34	36	2	n/a	13.0	n/a	n/a

COFFEE DRINKS

Item	Serving Size	Calories	Protein	Carb	Fiber	Sugar	Total Fat	Sat Fat	Sodium
Cappuccino, with nonfat milk	tall	80	8	11	0	10	0.0	0.0	110
Frappuccino, mocha	tall	230	6	44	0	36	3.0	2.0	180
Latte, iced, with nonfat milk	tall	70	7	10	0	9	0.0	0.0	100
Mocha, with nonfat milk	tall	180	12	33	1	28	2.0	0.5	150

SIDES & SNACKS

Item	Serving Size	Calories	Protein	Carb	Fiber	Sugar	Total Fat	Sat Fat	Sodium
8-grain roll	as served	350	10	67	5	n/a	8.0	n/a	n/a
Apple bran muffin	as served	350	6	64	7	n/a	9.0	n/a	n/a
Apple fritter	as served	420	5	59	<1	n/a	20.0	n/a	n/a
Asiago bagel	as served	310	13	54	2	n/a	4.5	n/a	n/a
Banana nut loaf	as served	490	7	75	4	n/a	19.0	n/a	n/a
Birthday cake mini doughnut	as served	130	<1	17	0	n/a	6.0	n/a	n/a
Blueberry oat bar	as served	370	6	47	5	n/a	14.0	n/a	n/a
Blueberry scone	as served	460	7	61	2	n/a	22.0	n/a	n/a
Blueberry streusel muffin	as served	360	7	59	2	n/a	11.0	n/a	n/a
Butter croissant	as served	310	5	32	<1	n/a	18.0	n/a	n/a
Cheese danish	as served	420	7	39	<1	n/a	25.0	n/a	n/a
Chicken on flatbread with hummus artisan snack plate	as served	250	17	27	5	n/a	9.0	n/a	n/a
Chocolate chunk cookie	as served	360	4	50	2	n/a	17.0	n/a	n/a
Chocolate croissant	as served	300	5	34	2	n/a	17.0	n/a	n/a
Chocolate old-fashioned doughnut	as served	420	5	57	2	n/a	21.0	n/a	n/a
Chonga bagel	as served	310	12	52	3	n/a	5.0	n/a	n/a

STARBUCKS COFFEE continued

Item	Serving Size	Calories	Protein	Carb	Fiber	Sugar	Total Fat	Sat Fat	Sodium
Cinnamon chip scone	as served	480	7	70	3	n/a	18.0	n/a	n/a
Cranberry orange scone	as served	490	8	73	2	n/a	18.0	n/a	n/a
Double chocolate brownie	as served	410	6	46	3	n/a	24.0	n/a	n/a
Double fudge mini doughnut	as served	130	<1	16	0	n/a	7.0	n/a	n/a
Double iced cinnamon roll	as served	490	7	70	3	n/a	20.0	n/a	n/a
Fruit, nut, & cheese artisan snack plate	as served	460	19	33	6	n/a	29.0	n/a	n/a
Ginger molasses cookie	as served	360	3	58	<1	n/a	12.0	n/a	n/a
Hawaiian bagel	as served	360	12	60	2	n/a	8.0	n/a	n/a
Iced lemon pound cake	as served	490	5	68	<1	n/a	23.0	n/a	n/a
Lowfat red raspberry muffin	as served	340	7	65	2	n/a	6.0	n/a	n/a
Mallorca sweet bread	as served	420	7	42	<1	n/a	25.0	n/a	n/a
Maple oat pecan scone	as served	440	8	59	3	n/a	18.0	n/a	n/a
Protein artisan snack plate	as served	370	13	36	4	n/a	19.0	n/a	n/a

SUBWAY

Item	Serving Size	Calories	Protein	Carb	Fiber	Sugar	Total Fat	Sat Fat	Sodium
SANDWICHES									
Beef steak and cheese, with white	6"	390	24	48	5	7	14.0	5.0	1210
Breakfast, egg and bacon, deli style	1	320	14	34	3	3	16.0	4.5	520
Breakfast, egg and cheese, deli style	1	320	14	34	3	3	15.0	5.0	550
Chicken breast, with white	6"	320	23	47	5	7	5.0	2.0	1000
Club, with white	6"	320	24	46	4	6	6.0	2.0	1300

SUBWAY continued

Item	Serving Size	Calories	Protein	Carb	Fiber	Sugar	Total Fat	Sat Fat	Sodium
Cold cut trio, with white	6"	440	21	47	4	6	21.0	7.0	1680
Ham, with honey mustard, with white	6"	310	18	52	4	12	5.0	1.5	1260
Italian BMT, with white	6"	480	23	46	4	6	24.0	9.0	1900
Meatball, with white	6"	530	24	53	6	7	26.0	10.0	1360
Roast beef, with white	6"	290	19	45	4	6	5.0	2.0	910
Tuna, with light mayonnaise, with white	6"	450	20	46	4	5	22.0	6.0	1190
Turkey bacon, Southwest, with white	6"	410	21	48	4	7	17.0	4.5	1230
Turkey, with white	6"	280	18	46	4	5	4.5	1.5	1010
Veggie Delite, with white	6"	230	9	44	4	5	3.0	1.0	510

SOUPS

Item	Serving Size	Calories	Protein	Carb	Fiber	Sugar	Total Fat	Sat Fat	Sodium
Black bean	1 cup	180	9	27	15	4	4.5	2.0	1160
Chicken noodle	1 cup	90	7	7	1	1	4.0	1.0	1180
Cream of broccoli	1 cup	130	5	15	2	0	6.0	0.0	860
Cream of potato with bacon	1 cup	210	5	20	4	3	12.0	4.0	970
Minestrone	1 cup	70	3	11	2	2	1.0	0.0	610
Rice with chicken	1 cup	190	6	17	2	3	11.0	4.5	990
Tomato bisque	1 cup	90	1	15	3	7	2.5	0.5	750
Vegetable beef	1 cup	90	5	14	2	4	1.5	0.5	1340

TACO BELL

Item	Serving Size	Calories	Protein	Carb	Fiber	Sugar	Total Fat	Sat Fat	Sodium
TACOS									
Beef	1	170	8	12	3	1	10.0	3.5	330
Chicken, soft	1	190	13	20	1	1	6.0	2.5	660
Chicken supreme, soft	1	230	15	21	1	3	10.0	5.0	570
Double-decker supreme	1	380	15	40	6	4	18.0	8.0	820
Supreme	1	220	9	14	3	2	14.0	7.0	360
BURRITOS									
Bean	1	340	12	56	11	4	8.0	2.5	1290
Beef, fiesta	1	390	14	50	5	4	15.0	5.0	1150
Chicken, fiesta	1	370	18	48	3	4	12.0	3.5	1090
Chicken, supreme	1	340	18	50	8	4	8.0	2.5	1410
Chili cheese	1	390	16	40	3	3	18.0	9.0	1080
Seven-layer	1	530	18	67	10	6	22.0	8.0	1360
Steak, fiesta	1	370	16	48	4	4	13.0	4.0	1080

TGI FRIDAY'S

Item	Serving Size	Calories	Protein	Carb	Fiber	Sugar	Total Fat	Sat Fat	Sodium
APPETIZERS									
Bruschetta chicken pasta	as served	1172	42	191	27	7	29.0	5.6	1260
Buffalo wings	1 box	574	38	6	0	2	38.0	10.0	3542
Chicken quesadilla rolls	1 box	821	26	67	6	3	38.0	12.0	1172
French fries	1 order	140	2	14	0	1	8.0	2.0	370
Honey BBQ wings	3 pieces	190	11	5	0	6	12.0	3.0	630
Mozzarella cheese stick, breaded, fried	1 stick	110	4	7	0	1	6.0	2.0	260
Potato skins with cheddar and bacon	3 pieces	211	8	19	2	1	12.0	4.0	382
Shrimp, medium, breaded, fried	1 shrimp	27	2	1	0	0	1.4	0.3	54
Spinach, cheese, & artichoke dip	1 oz	50	2	2	2	1	3.5	2.0	150

TGI FRIDAY'S continued

Item	Serving Size	Calories	Protein	Carb	Fiber	Sugar	Total Fat	Sat Fat	Sodium
ENTRÉES									
Cedar-seared salmon pasta	as served	500	30	55	9	34	12.0	6.0	400
Complete skillet meals, Cajun-style Alfredo chicken & shrimp	as served	280	21	34	2	4	7.0	3.0	760
Complete skillet meals, chicken & broccoli Alfredo	as served	270	19	28	3	2	9.0	4.0	520
Gourmet mac 'n' five cheese	as served	792	38	76	2	12	35.0	20.5	800
Sirloin beef steak	as served	185	31	0	0	0	7.0	2.8	194
Spicy Cajun chicken pasta	as served	1100	53	144	8	8	32.0	16.0	1760

WENDY'S

Item	Serving Size	Calories	Protein	Carb	Fiber	Sugar	Total Fat	Sat Fat	Sodium
Bacon cheeseburger	junior	380	20	34	2	6	19.0	7.0	890
Baked potato, bacon cheese	1 potato	580	18	79	7	6	22.0	6.0	950
Baked potato with broccoli cheese	1 potato	480	9	81	9	6	14.0	3.0	510
Cheeseburger	single	480	28	38	2	8	24.0	10.0	1230
Chicken club sandwich	1 sandwich	470	30	47	2	6	19.0	4.0	920
Chicken nuggets for kids	4 pieces	334	16	15	1	0	23.2	4.9	679
Chili	small	200	17	21	5	5	6.0	2.5	870
Garden Sensations salad, BLT	1 salad	310	33	10	4	4	16.0	8.0	1100
Garden Sensations, salad with chicken and mandarin oranges	1 salad	150	20	17	3	11	1.5	0.0	650
Garden Sensations, spring mix salad	1 salad	180	11	12	5	5	11.0	6.0	230
Garden Sensations, taco salad supremo, without chips	1 salad	360	27	29	8	8	16.0	9.0	1090

WENDY'S continued

Item	Serving Size	Calories	Protein	Carb	Fiber	Sugar	Total Fat	Sat Fat	Sodium
Hamburger	single	470	26	43	2	10	21.0	8.0	880
Hamburger, Big Bacon	classic	570	34	46	3	11	29.0	12.0	1460

WHITE CASTLE

Item	Serving Size	Calories	Protein	Carb	Fiber	Sugar	Total Fat	Sat Fat	Sodium
BURGERS & SANDWICHES									
Bacon cheeseburger	single	200	10	13	0	2	12.0	5.0	500
Cheeseburger with jalapeños	single	170	8	13	0	2	10.0	5.0	410
Chicken ring sandwich	single	350	8	16	1	1	28	4.5	320
Chicken supreme sandwich	single	230	14	22	0	2	10.0	6.0	750
Fish sandwich	single	310	9	18	12	1	22	3	270
Hamburger, Slyder	single	140	6	13	0	1	7.0	3.0	360
Pulled pork BBQ sandwich	single	170	9	25	1	12	4.5	1	460
Surf and turf sandwich	single	390	20	27	1	3	22.0	9.0	720
White Castle	single	140	7	13	1	1	6	2.5	360
SIDES									
Chicken rings	3 pieces	260	9	6	0	0	24	4	300
Clam strips	regular	210	8	5	0	1	17	2	620
Fish nibblers	14 pieces	280	19	24	5	0	16.0	3.5	870
French fries	saver	350	3	32	3	2	24	4	50
Mozzarella cheese sticks	3 pieces	440	12	22	1	1	33	8	850
Onion chips	kids	510	4	35	6	4	38	6	730
Onion rings	saver	220	1	21	2	3	14	2.5	190